Hot Topics in Acute Care Surgery and Trauma

Endorsed by the World Society for Emergency Surgery (WSES) and the American Association for Trauma Surgery, the series covers the most debated topics in acute care and trauma surgery, from perioperative management to organisational and health policy issues, to the complex management of acute and trauma surgical patients. It is a valuable resource for both trainees and acute surgical professionals.

Etrusca Brogi • Federico Coccolini
Alex Valadka • Eric J. Ley
Editors

Traumatic Spinal Cord Injury

Springer

Editors
Etrusca Brogi
Neuroscience Intensive Care Unit
ASST Grande Ospedale Metropolitano Niguarda
Milan, Italy

Federico Coccolini
General, Emergency and Trauma Surgery Department
Pisa University Hospital
Pisa, Italy

Alex Valadka
Department of Neurological Surgery
University of Texas Southwestern Medical Center
Dallas, TX, USA

Eric J. Ley
R. Adams Cowley Shock Trauma Center
University of Maryland, Baltimore
Baltimore, MD, USA

ISSN 2520-8284 ISSN 2520-8292 (electronic)
Hot Topics in Acute Care Surgery and Trauma
ISBN 978-3-031-99889-8 ISBN 978-3-031-99890-4 (eBook)
https://doi.org/10.1007/978-3-031-99890-4

This Springer imprint is published by the registered company Springer Nature Switzerland AG
The registered company address is: Gewerbestrasse 11, 6330 Cham, Switzerland

Foreword to the Series

Research is fundamentally altering the daily practice of acute care surgery (trauma, surgical critical care, and emergency general surgery) for the betterment of patients around the world. Management for many diseases and conditions is radically different than it was just a few years previously. For this reason, concise up-to-date information is required to inform busy clinicians. Therefore, since 2011 the World Society of Emergency Surgery (WSES), in a partnership with the American Association for the Surgery of Trauma (AAST), endorses the development and publication of the "Hot Topics in Acute Care Surgery and Trauma," realizing the need to provide more educational tools for young in-training surgeons and for general physicians and other surgical specialists. These new forthcoming titles have been selected and prepared with this philosophy in mind. The books will cover the basics of pathophysiology and clinical management, framed with the reference that recent advances in the science of resuscitation, surgery, and critical care medicine have the potential to profoundly alter the epidemiology and subsequent outcomes of severe surgical illnesses and trauma.

General, Emergency and Trauma Surgery Department
Pisa University Hospital
Pisa, Italy
Federico Coccolini

Riverside University Health System Medical Center
Riverside, CA, USA
Raul Coimbra

Department of Surgery and Critical Care Medic
Foothills Medical Centre
Calgary, AB, Canada
Andrew W. Kirkpatrick

Department of Surgery
Madonna Del Soccorso Hospital
San Benedetto del Tronto, Italy
Salomone Di Saverio

Preface

Spinal cord injury remains one of the most complex and life-altering conditions in medicine, requiring coordinated expertise across multiple disciplines. This textbook is designed to provide a comprehensive, evidence-based foundation for clinicians, researchers, and students dedicated to the care and recovery of individuals living with spinal cord injury. Our goal is to equip readers not only with knowledge but also with the clinical insight and compassion essential to improving outcomes and quality of life.

Milan, Italy — Etrusca Brogi
Pisa, Italy — Federico Coccolini
Dallas, TX, USA — Alex Valadka
Baltimore, MD, USA — Eric J. Ley

Contents

Part I

General Considerations and Prehospital Management

Epidemiology and Socioeconomic Impact of Traumatic Spinal Cord Injury

1

Nicoló Marchesini, Andreas K. Demetriades, Filippo Pasqualini, Riccardo Boccaletti, and Edoardo Picetti

1.1 Introduction

Traumatic spinal injury (TSI) encompasses a wide array of conditions, including damage to the osseous structures, and disco-ligamentous components of the spinal column that may or may not be associated with injuries to the neural elements in the spinal canal (spinal cord and cauda equina). Such injuries can result from either blunt or penetrating trauma, involving mechanisms of both high and low energy. Traumatic spinal cord injury (TSCI) constitutes a subset of traumatic spinal injuries, specifically referring to acute traumatic injuries to the spinal cord and/or nerve roots resulting in temporary or permanent sensory deficit, motor deficit, or bladder/bowel dysfunction of different degrees of severity [1–3].

The possible consequences of TSCI for individuals and families are profound and the understanding of its epidemiology and socioeconomic impact is crucial for several reasons. First, insights into the prevalence, incidence, and distribution of TSCI cases are essential for developing effective prevention strategies and allocating resources appropriately. By identifying risk factors and high-risk populations, healthcare systems can implement targeted interventions to reduce the incidence of

N. Marchesini
Department of Neuroscience, Section of Neurosurgery, Azienda Ospedaliera Universitaria Integrata di Verona, Verona, Italy

A. K. Demetriades
Department of Neurosurgery, Royal Infirmary Edinburgh, Scotland, UK

F. Pasqualini
Department of Neuroscience, Biomedicine and Movement, Section of Neurosurgery, University of Verona, Verona, Italy

R. Boccaletti
Department of Neurosurgery, Parma University Hospital, Parma, Italy

E. Picetti (✉)
Department of Anesthesia and Intensive Care, Parma University Hospital, Parma, Italy

E. Brogi et al. (eds.), *Traumatic Spinal Cord Injury*, Hot Topics in Acute Care Surgery and Trauma, https://doi.org/10.1007/978-3-031-99890-4_1

TSCI. Furthermore, by understanding and quantifying the socioeconomic impact of TSCI, policymakers can advocate for improved access to healthcare services, rehabilitation programs, and support services for individuals with TSCI, ultimately enhancing their quality of life and societal inclusion. Additionally, realizing the economic impact of spinal cord injury (SCI) enables the evaluation of the cost-effectiveness of interventions and informs healthcare resource allocation decisions. Finally, a comprehensive knowledge of the epidemiology and socioeconomic impact of TSCI is essential for developing evidence-based strategies to mitigate its burden on individuals, families, and societies as a whole.

This chapter provides an overview of the epidemiological patterns of TSCI and examines its multifaceted socioeconomic implications.

1.2 Epidemiology of Traumatic Spinal Cord Injury

A premise is essential before presenting epidemiological data about TSI and TSCI. Despite the significant efforts and advances in epidemiology research for these conditions, several issues still limit the comparability and interpretation of data, starting with a wide variation within the scientific literature due to heterogeneous data-gathering methods, the populations included, and the definitions employed for TSI and TSCI. For instance, the explanation and process for identifying cases of TSCI are ambiguous in many reports. Some studies exclude cauda equina cases, while others include American Spinal Injury Association (ASIA) grade E patients as TSCIs, leading to plausible heterogeneities. Additionally, some other studies use coding from the International Classification of Diseases (ICD) to report on SCI incidence and prevalence. However, the list of diagnostic codes often includes all conditions considered as SCI, both traumatic and nontraumatic [2]. Differences in reported incidences can also be found within the same population but vary according to the source of data (e.g., rehabilitation program vs hospital discharge data vs population-based datasets). Finally, the inclusion or exclusion of pre-hospital and in-hospital mortality can lead to significant differences in the reported incidence of TSCI cases [3]. For these and other reasons, reported data can differ according to the source of information, hindering their generalization and comparability [1–2, 4–5].

The recently published update of the Global Burden of Diseases, Injuries and Risk Factors Study (GBD) aimed to quantify epidemiological trends of SCIs between 1990 and 2019 on a global scale [2]. Data for SCI were accessible for 93 out of 204 countries (46%) for which GBD provides estimates. Nonetheless, GBD generated predictions for all 204 locations using statistical methods that incorporate predictive covariates and a geographical cascade. This approach allowed areas lacking data to leverage information from neighboring regions. However, it must be noted that, within this study, the SCI data cannot be separated with regard to traumatic and nontraumatic etiology. In 2019, it was estimated that 20.6 million people (95% UI 18.9 to 23.6) were living with SCI, and the global age-standardized incidence of SCI was 900.000 new cases. The study also reported that from 1990 to

2019, there was an estimated increase in the prevalence of SCI by 81.5% and an increase in incidence by 52.7%. However, when data were standardized by age, rates showed only slight increases. On a regional basis, in 2019, high-income North America had the highest age-standardized incidence rate, with 22 cases per 100.000 population (95% UI 17 to 29). This was followed by Australasia, with an incidence rate of 14 per 100.000 (95% UI 11 to 17), and tropical Latin America, which also had a rate of 14 per 100.000 (95% UI 10 to 19). The lowest age-standardized incidence rates were estimated in Andean Latin America and central sub-Saharan Africa (4 per 100.000 each). Age-standardized incidence rates of SCI exhibited considerable variation between countries, ranging from 43 per 100.000 (95% UI 11.8 to 131.7) in Afghanistan and 31.9 per 100.000 (95% UI 24.1 to 42.6) in Greenland to 3 per 100.000 (95% UI 2.4 to 3.8) in North-Korea and 3 per 100.000 (95% UI 2.5 to 3.8) in Kiribati (95% UI 18.9 to 23.6) were living with SCI (Fig. 1.1).

A systematic review by Kumar et al. published in 2018, which included 102 articles representing 32 separate countries and all World Health Organization (WHO) regions, reported that the global incidence of TSI is approximately 10.5 cases per 100.000 individuals (95% CI 8.6 to 12.84), translating to roughly 768.473–790.695 new cases each year. The study indicated that globally, around 37% of TSI patients suffered from TSCI [4]. This translates into an incidence of TSCI ranging from 3.3 to 195.4 cases per million based on subnational studies and from 5.1 to 150.48 based on national studies [1]. The study also revealed a substantial contrast in the percentage of TSI patients with TSCI between high-income (25.27%; standard deviation: 26.8), middle-income (36.6%; standard deviation: 26.9), and low-income countries (70.4%; standard deviation: 6.0) [4]. These significant differences are unlikely to stem solely from differences in causes, as road traffic accidents and falls remain the primary injury mechanisms across all income levels. Nevertheless, the severity of injuries resulting from these incidents might be

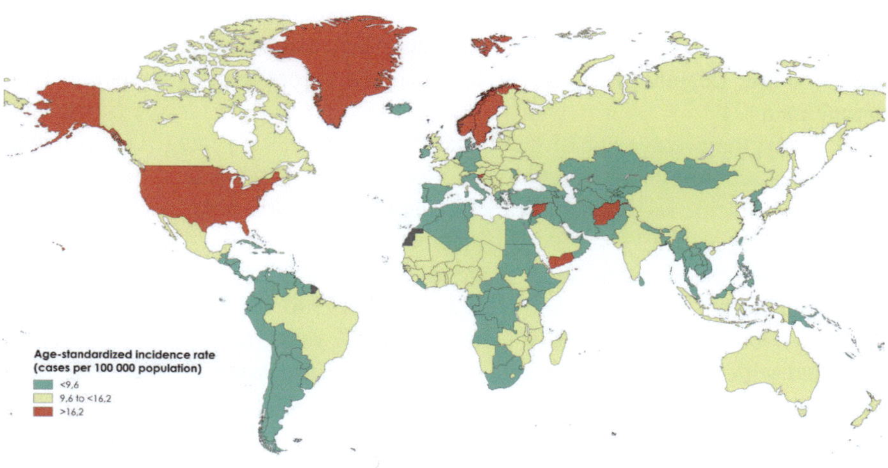

Fig. 1.1 Age-standardized incidence rate of SCI. (Modified from Safdarian et al. [2], licensed under CC-BY 4.0)

more pronounced in low- and middle-income countries (LMICs) due to inadequate safety standards, potentially resulting in a higher SCI prevalence. Another plausible factor could be that individuals in LMICs experiencing TSI without neurological deficits may forego seeking medical attention due to limited access to healthcare and financial barriers. Conversely, those in HICs, reporting only pain following a traumatic incident, might be more inclined to seek medical assistance and consequently receive a diagnosis of TSI. This pattern may contribute to an underestimation of TSI cases in LMICs. Despite these considerations, these findings suggest that preventive and management approaches should consider loco-regional trends. In the same review, the occurrence of TSI varied across WHO regions, ranging from 3.4 per 100.000 in Europe (95% CI 1.8 to 6.6) to 13.7 per 100.000 in the South-East Asia region. When categorized by income classification following the World Bank Country and Lending Groups, TSI incidence was notably higher in LMICs (13.7 per 100.000 individuals; 95% CI 6.4 to 21.0) compared with HICs (8.7 per 100.000 individuals; 95% CI 6.6 to 10.9) [4]. However, despite the apparently higher incidence in LMICs, it is not possible to exclude less accurate data registration in those regions, and further examination of the data on a national scale could enhance comprehension of these variations. Several additional recent systematic reviews with meta-analyses have reported on the incidence of TSCI globally and specifically for LMICs. From these data, the wide variation in incidence from study to study is confirmed, both between regions and within the same nation [1, 6].

Almost invariably across epidemiological studies, TSI and TSCI predominantly impact males, with an average male-to-female (M/F) ratio of 3.37 globally across all geographic and income regions. The highest M/F ratio recorded was 7.35 in a study on cervical spine injuries in Brazil. Conversely, only two reports identified women as more commonly affected than men. In general, the M/F ratio seems greater in LMICs compared to HICs [1–2, 4–5]. Some studies indicate that the proportion of TSCIs between males and females shifts as individuals age past 54 years. This may imply that younger men experience TSCI more frequently than younger women, with the incidence gradually increasing among women in later stages of life. Despite this trend, SCIs still remain more than twice as prevalent among men [7].

Globally, the average age of individuals with TSI is 39.8 years (SD 12.2), with differences according to geographic and income areas. Patients tend to be older in the Western Pacific region and younger in the United States of America (USA) and Canada (46.21 vs 29.33 years). By income classification, low-income countries (LICs) exhibit the youngest average age at the time of injury (36.4 years) [4]. The GBD study found that, in contrast to the scenario in 1990 when a singular incidence peak was observed among individuals aged 20–24 years, in 2019 the occurrence escalated with advancing age and sustained levels surpassing 50,000 cases from approximately age 20 to about age 84. In 2019, two distinct peaks emerged, occurring at ages 30–34 years and 50–54 years, respectively, followed by a subsequent decline. The prevalence shows similar trends. The reported increase in prevalence and incidence and the change in age patterns could be at least partially explained by the increased life expectancy of the ageing population and improvements in global healthcare access and quality. Indeed, mortality for people with SCI has substantially decreased in the last decades [8]. It must also be considered that the incidence of nontraumatic SCI (included in the report) steadily increases with age and could have influenced the reported data.

With respect to the etiology of TSCI, available studies use different definitions of falls, violence, road traffic accidents, and sports. Moreover, some studies refer to specific mechanisms of injury (e.g., motor vehicle accidents can include one or more among driver, passengers, pedestrians, cyclists, or motorcycle drivers). The GBD study reported that on a global scale, falls accounted for the highest number of SCI in 2019, totaling 477.000 cases (95% UI 327 to 683), followed by road injuries, amounting to 230.000 cases (95% UI 122 to 389). The incidence rates standardized by age revealed that in 2019, falls had the highest rate at 6.2 cases per 100.000 population (95% UI 4·2 to 8·8), followed by road injuries at 3 per 100.000 (1.6 to 5). The study by Kumar et al. supports the notion that, regardless of the definitions used, road accidents and falls are the leading causes of TSI, representing 39.5% and 38.8% of cases, respectively. They also reported no differences in the mechanism of injury between studies, including only TSI and those with both TSI and SCI. There seem to be differences across income regions, with road accidents causing TSI being more common in HICs (41.6%) than in middle-income (40.7%) and low-income countries (27.2%). The higher number of motor vehicles per capita in HICs may at least partially explain this difference. Despite the lower number of vehicles per-capita in LMICs, the burden of TSI due to road accidents remains high. Several reasons can explain this observation: inadequate safety legislation and law enforcement in those regions, as well as poor road infrastructure and signaling. Falls represent a frequent cause of TSI in both HICs and LMICs. However, the age distribution of fall-related TSI varies across income areas. In HICs, most TSI due to falls occur in the elderly from self-standing height, while in LMICs, they occur in younger people and are more often related to work environments. Some specific countries report violence as a leading cause of TSI [4]. Additional but less commonly reported causes of TSI and TSCI are sports and other recreational activities [5].

1.3 Risk Factors Associated with Traumatic Spinal Cord Injury and Prevention

Understanding the risk factors associated with TSCI is paramount for developing effective prevention strategies to avoid these injuries. Indeed, the American Trauma Society suggests that the most effective method for managing injuries is through prevention [9]. Actively altering behaviors to enhance safety can reduce the risk of sustaining a TSCI. In other words, by addressing demographic, behavioral, and environmental influences combined with comprehensive prevention measures, policymakers can work towards reducing the incidence and burden of this condition. Prevention measures are also extremely cost-effective. For example, it has been estimated that the USA could save approximately $400 billion by implementing preventive and therapeutic interventions for SCI [10]. For these reasons, the recently published intersectoral WHO global action plan on epilepsy and other neurological disorders (2022–2031) includes, amongst its strategic objectives, the implementation plan for the prevention of TSI and TSCI [11].

Risk factors associated with TSI and TSCI can be divided into modifiable and non-modifiable. Non-modifiable risk factors include age (older adults are at increased risk of TSCI due to age-related changes in bone density and mobility), gender (males have a higher incidence of TSCI compared to females, attributed to differences in risk-taking behavior and occupational exposure), and pre-existing spinal conditions. For example, degenerative spinal disease, such as spinal stenosis or degenerative disc disease, can increase susceptibility to TSCI even after minor traumas [12]. Modifiable risk factors include behavioral and environmental elements such as alcohol and substance abuse, occupational variables, and adherence to safety laws and measures. Substance consumption is a behavior that can serve as both a trigger and a cause of post-injury difficulties for patients with TSCI. Studies reporting combined toxicology tests found that up to 80% of patients admitted for TSCI had a positive screen, with opioids (37.5%) and alcohol (25%) being the most frequently encountered [13]. Overall, between 20% and 47% of people who experience TSCI are documented to have had a heightened blood alcohol content when their injury occurred, suggesting that behavioral misconduct due to impaired judgment and coordination might have led to trauma (road traffic crashes, violence, and falls). However, these data may vary widely according to the setting. Furthermore, some studies suggest an increased risk of complications, prolonged ICU length of stay, and an overall increase in hospital morbidity in this population [14, 15]. Educational campaigns and law-enforcements focused on eradicating the substances' abuse and driving under alcohol and drug influence represent effective primary preventive measures to mitigate the burden of TSCI in such cases. Despite most TSCIs occurring due to falls or motor vehicle accidents, certain occupations have higher rates of TSCI due to exposure to hazardous environments and activities. Studies reveal that between 13% and 18% of TSCI can occur during the course of employment and that within this group, falls and motor vehicle accidents still bear the highest burden [16–17]. Most studies report construction workers as the population with the highest risk of TSCI [17]. However, work-related epidemiology and features can be closely influenced by specific environmental factors, and efforts should be made to collect and analyze data on a locoregional basis. This would translate into preventive measures tailored to specific needs. Many sports and recreational activities can also result in TSCI, with differences in incidence rate according to the examined study. Diving seems to be the sport causing the greatest number of TSCI overall, followed by skiing, rugby, and horseback riding [18]. Defining the increased risk for specific subsets of activities is important to raise awareness, design laws and policies to educate sports professionals and athletes, and implement tailored interventions. General preventive measures include ensuring that team sport players compete against others of similar skill, maturity, and size levels, providing adequate protective gear to athletes and keeping fields and playgrounds well maintained and lit [10]. Primary preventive measures can also be tailored for specific sports and recreational activities. For example, it has been reported that 75% of TSCI resulting from diving headfirst occurred in swimming pools without depth indicators and that 95% of people who sustain a TSCI from a swimming accident dove into water less than 8 feet deep [10]. Hence, the use of clearly marked depths in swimming pools can be used as a simple primary prevention technique. In rugby, new rules were implemented in specific stages of the game when opponents collide with each other and have an increased risk of cervical hyperflexion trauma. This strategy resulted in a 48% reduction of TSCI during this phase of the game in some regions [18].

Primary risk factors to road traffic injuries encompass excessive speed, failure to wear helmets, absence of seat belts and child restraints, poor visibility for pedestrians, driver distractions or fatigue, and insufficient enforcement of traffic regulations. Driving under the influence of drugs or alcohol also plays a crucial role. Accordingly, primary preventive measures focus on reducing these risk factors and include consistently wearing a seat belt, using an airbag, adhering to speed limits, staying attentive, and following traffic rules. For children, essential preventive measures include the use of safety seats and proper restraints [10]. Distracted driving has become a significant issue with the advent of smartphones, and even using a hands-free device is considered unsafe, as drivers while talking on the phone have a slower response time [19]. In fact, studies have shown that drivers who use cell phones while driving are four times more likely to be involved in a motor vehicle accident. Prevention tips include limiting cell phone use while driving and enforcing hands-free laws, along with associated penalties and fines, to deter smartphone usage while driving [20].

Regarding falls, primary preventive measures are particularly relevant for the elderly. Examples of simple strategies that can be implemented to increase safety in living settings include holding onto handrails while climbing stairs, keeping floors free of debris, immediate cleaning of spills, using only non-skid rugs or no rugs at all, keeping electrical cords out of walkways, installing grab bars in bathrooms and showers [10].

Different types of educational and awareness campaigns have been used worldwide, varying by methods, intensity of application, and duration [21–22]. Some include the testimonies and the views of people who suffered a TSCI, while others use virtual reality and audiovisual mediums to enhance adherence and involvement of the audience [23]. In general, such campaigns can be tailored to specific subgroups or to the general population and can use different didactive and learning approaches, empowering individuals to make safer choices.

1.4 Socieconomic Impact of Traumatic Spinal Cord Injury

The socioeconomic consequences and costs of TSCI are significant for healthcare systems, individuals, and caregivers. These injuries often occur in younger people, leading to permanent disability, increased morbidity, and mortality. Direct healthcare costs include initial hospitalization, rehabilitation services, transportation, and personal assistance. Indirect costs can be defined as “the value of potential output that is lost as a result of any reduction or elimination of work or other activity due to SCI” [24]. While direct costs peak during the first year following trauma and gradually decline, indirect costs can have long-term impacts, potentially surpassing health care expenses [25].

A recent systematic review provided data on direct healthcare costs for SCI from countries with varying levels of socioeconomic development and across different phases of care [26]. However, it must be noted that the majority of the 30 included studies were conducted in North America, highlighting a general paucity of data from Europe and LMICs. The study reported relevant variation in direct healthcare costs from one study to another. The average cost of acute care ranged from $290 to $612.590, inpatient rehabilitation costs varied from $19.536 to $44.044, expenses for the first year after the initial injury ranged from $32.238 to $1.156.406, and costs for the subsequent years following the first ranged from $4.392 to $200.810. The highest costs were generally observed in HICs, in patients with cervical injuries, in ASIA A and B patients, in individuals with concomitant injuries, in those who developed complications, in cases of surgical delay greater than 24 hours, in transfer delay to specialized SCI care, in older and female individuals, and in those with higher injury severity scores. Other studies confirmed that the ratios of costs to total health care expenses were higher for inpatient care, followed by outpatient care and pharmacy costs. The most significant factors influencing the cost of care were the presence of pressure ulcers, the cervical level of injury, the specific time period (such as the first year post-injury and end-of-life year), and the severity of the SCI [27]. However, caution is warranted against generalizing these findings to contexts with different economic statuses and healthcare systems. Regarding indirect costs, different methods were used to estimate them according to the study [24]. An estimate from Canada valued their range between $0.7 million and $1.3 million, assuming injury at age 35 years. These costs accounted for 41% of the 2.67 billion total economic burden associated with SCI in the country. Annual indirect costs ranged from $12.726 to $50.470 in older studies [28]. A more recent observational study from the USA quantified the average annual indirect costs at $29.354 and found that lifetime costs for individuals injured at 25 varied by severity of injury, from $0.5 to $2.3 million. For people injured at age 50, lifetime indirect costs ranged from $0.3 to $0.6 million. The same study reported an employment rate decrease from 87% at the time of injury to 35% after injury [24]. A recent survey in 22 countries found an average 38% employment rate after injury, with considerable differences across countries, ranging from 10.3% to 61.4%, and slightly higher among men compared with women [29]. Advancements in several areas are necessary to reduce the burden of indirect costs of SCI, including promoting higher educational attainment, offering job retraining programs, eliminating financial disincentives, and removing both environmental and attitudinal barriers. Employers willing to accommodate modifications (job adjustments, reduced or flexible work hours, and structural changes to the work environment) can facilitate individuals to return to work post-SCI. Earnings gaps also significantly impact indirect costs, especially for those who transition to new employment after trauma. Vocational rehabilitation practices should be promoted to support quality employment throughout a person's career, motivating individuals towards higher earnings, better job positions, and longer work life expectancy. Finally, to improve employment outcomes for individuals with SCI, it is essential to address the disparities between males and females. A model was developed in Canada to forecast changes in demographics and healthcare financial resources between 2012 and 2032. By 2032, the projected median age of individuals with TSCI will be 57, with those aged 61 and older comprising 46% of TSCI cases. Admissions to acute and rehabilitation facilities in 2032 are expected to rise by 31% and 25%, respectively. Due to the demographic shift toward an older population, a 13% increase in total life expectancy for those with TSCI is estimated [30]. Care costs are projected to increase by 54%, and the lifetime cost is expected to rise by 37% in 2032. This progressive shift towards an aging population with an associated increase in direct and indirect costs represents a compelling call for policymakers in planning healthcare delivery after TSCI.

Apart from the economic burden for health systems, individuals suffering from TSCI and those around them undergo profound and enduring changes in their lives with significant psychosocial impact (Fig. 1.2). These psychosocial consequences

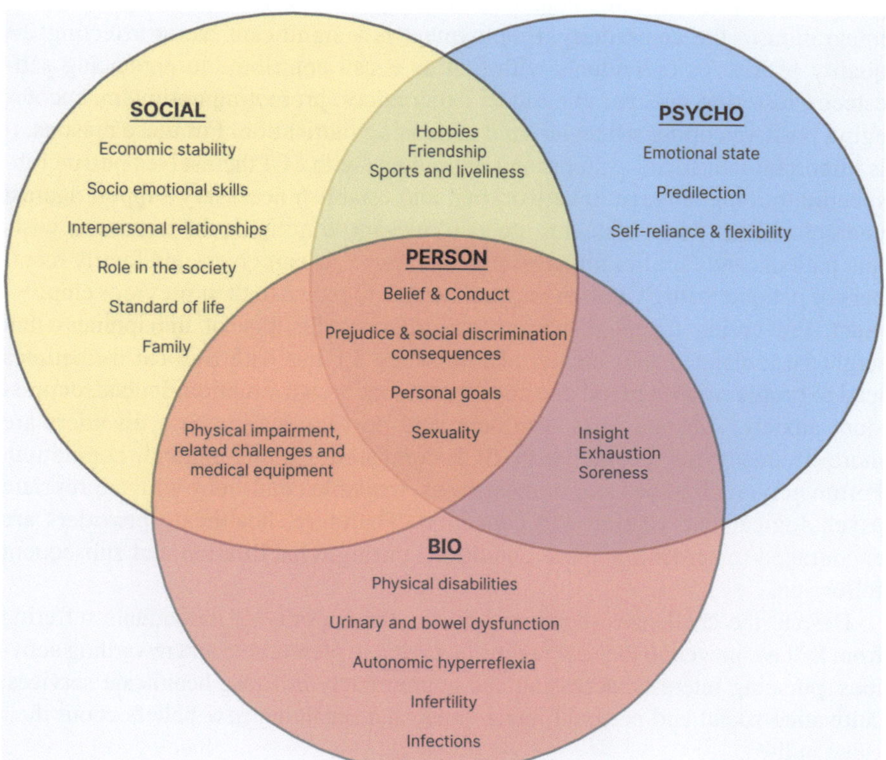

Fig. 1.2 Relevant psychosocial factors in SCI patients. (Modified from ref. [31])

extend well beyond the acute phase of injury, necessitating lifelong, daily adjustments for both the individual with SCI and their caregivers. A detailed description of these topics is outside the scope of this chapter, and the following paragraphs focus only on a part of the psychosocial issues. More specifics can be found in the literature [31–33].

Patients with SCI are frequently compelled to reassess and reconstruct their personal and social goals and identities within their family, professional, and social background. This often results from the shift towards increased dependency, which can initially disrupt usual interactions and traditional expectations among spouses or family members. Accepting the disability, maintaining a solution-focused approach, emphasizing abilities and values, and engaging in socialization and supportive communication can help individuals with SCI and their family members adapt more effectively. While rehabilitation facilities are usually equipped to support the mobility and functioning of people with SCI, the everyday outside world is not. For this reason, some individuals may not be able to return to their previous residence and must be admitted to assisted-living facilities, delaying community reintegration and social participation, with both psychological and economic impacts. Therefore, it is fundamental to boost the role of facilitators (availability of professional services, positive attitudes, social support, self-confidence, and competence of caregivers) while mitigating barriers to integration in the community. Employment is a significant factor affecting the quality of life for individuals with SCI as it can contribute to enhancing self-esteem, fostering positive role model experiences, promoting optimism, encouraging positive coping strategies, and increasing motivation. For these reasons, it is important that social systems and individuals with SCI themselves pursue job-specific training, engage in networking, and establish necessary support against unemployment. Such strategies are also relevant to mitigate the enormous costs that patients and families undergo after discharge, as caregivers and family members of patients with SCI often may not be able to return to their previous employment. Preventing financial burnout can alleviate feelings of unhappiness that might be translated into mental health issues. Living with SCI can sometimes lead to problems with mood and coping with one's own situation. Indeed, depression, anxiety, substance use disorders, and post-traumatic stress disorders are more frequent for people with SCI compared to the general population. Fortunately, such issues are, in most cases, treatable conditions with appropriate psychological intervention and education. Therefore, healthcare providers are encouraged to screen for these conditions during rehabilitation and subsequent follow-up.

Despite the challenges mentioned above, the majority of individuals suffering from SCI adapt well to the new reality, engaging in pleasurable and rewarding activities, pursuing interests, accessing and appropriately utilizing healthcare services, cultivating social and personal interactions, and obtaining new beliefs about their value in life.

To conclude, healthcare professionals within healthcare systems are typically the initial points of contact for individuals who have recently experienced a

SCI. Consequently, there exists a responsibility to thoughtfully prioritize "the individual" in their overall complexity and related psychosocial aspects, beyond the mere medical treatment.

References

1. Jazayeri SB, Maroufi SF, Mohammadi E, et al. Incidence of traumatic spinal cord injury worldwide: a systematic review, data integration, and update. World Neurosurg X. 2023;18:100171. https://doi.org/10.1016/j.wnsx.2023.100171.
2. Safdarian M, Trinka E, Rahimi-Movaghar V, et al. Global, regional, and national burden of spinal cord injury, 1990–2019: a systematic analysis for the Global Burden of Disease Study 2019. Lancet Neurol. 2023;22(11):1026–47. https://doi.org/10.1016/S1474-4422(23)00287-9.
3. Sabre L, Remmer S, Adams A, et al. Impact of fatal cases on the epidemiology of traumatic spinal cord injury in Estonia. Eur J Neurol. 2015;22(5):768–72. https://doi.org/10.1111/ene.12478.
4. Kumar R, Lim J, Mekary RA, et al. Traumatic spinal injury: global epidemiology and worldwide volume. World Neurosurg. 2018;113:e345–63. https://doi.org/10.1016/j.wneu.2018.02.033.
5. Singh A, Tetreault L, Kalsi-Ryan S, Nouri A, Fehlings MG. Global prevalence and incidence of traumatic spinal cord injury. Clin Epidemiol. 2014;6:309–31. https://doi.org/10.2147/CLEP.S68889.
6. Golestani A, Shobeiri P, Sadeghi-Naini M, et al. Epidemiology of traumatic spinal cord injury in developing countries from 2009 to 2020: a systematic review and meta-analysis. Neuroepidemiology. 2022;56(4):219–39. https://doi.org/10.1159/000524867.
7. Ferro S, Cecconi L, Bonavita J, Pagliacci MC, Biggeri A, Franceschini M. Incidence of traumatic spinal cord injury in Italy during 2013-2014: a population-based study. Spinal Cord. 2017;55(12):1103–7. https://doi.org/10.1038/sc.2017.88.
8. Strauss DJ, Devivo MJ, Paculdo DR, Shavelle RM. Trends in life expectancy after spinal cord injury. Arch Phys Med Rehabil. 2006;87(8):1079–85. https://doi.org/10.1016/j.apmr.2006.04.022.
9. American Trauma Society. https://www.amtrauma.org/. Accessed 21 May 2024.
10. Bellon K, Kolakowsky-Hayner S, Chen D, McDowell S, Bitterman B, Klaas S. Evidence-based practice in primary prevention of spinal cord injury. Top Spinal Cord Injury Rehabil. 2013;19(1):25–30. https://doi.org/10.1310/sci1901-25.
11. Organization WH. Intersectoral global action plan on epilepsy and other neurological disorders 2022–2031. World Health Organization; 2023. https://iris.who.int/handle/10665/371495. Accessed 29 April 2024.
12. Yoo DS, Lee SB, Huh PW, Kang SG, Cho KS. Spinal cord injury in cervical spinal stenosis by minor trauma. World Neurosurg. 2010;73(1):50–2; discussion e4. https://doi.org/10.1016/j.surneu.2009.05.021.
13. Eldridge LA, Piatt JA, Agley J, Gerke S. Relationship between substance use and the onset of spinal cord injuries: a medical chart review. Top Spinal Cord Inj Rehabil. 2019;25(4):316–21. https://doi.org/10.1310/sci2504-316.
14. Levy DT, Mallonee S, Miller TR, et al. Alcohol involvement in burn, submersion, spinal cord, and brain injuries. Med Sci Monit. 2004;10(1):CR17–24.
15. Crutcher CL, Ugiliweneza B, Hodes JE, Kong M, Boakye M. Alcohol intoxication and its effects on traumatic spinal cord injury outcomes. J Neurotrauma. 2014;31(9):798–802. https://doi.org/10.1089/neu.2014.3329.
16. Rosenberg NL, Gerhart K, Whiteneck G. Occupational spinal cord injury. Neurology. 1993;43(7):1385. https://doi.org/10.1212/WNL.43.7.1385.

17. Bae SW, Shin HI, Bang MS, Lee MY. Epidemiology of work-related traumatic spinal cord injury. J Occup Environ Med. 2023;65(7):e453–7. https://doi.org/10.1097/JOM.0000000000002852.
18. Chan CW, Eng JJ, Tator CH, Krassioukov A, Team the SCIRE. Epidemiology of sport-related spinal cord injuries: a systematic review. J Spinal Cord Med. 2016;39(3):255. https://doi.org/10.1080/10790268.2016.1138601.
19. Bellinger DB, Budde BM, Machida M, Richardson GB, Berg WP. The effect of cellular telephone conversation and music listening on response time in braking. Transport Res F. 2009;12(6):441–51. https://doi.org/10.1016/j.trf.2009.08.007.
20. Ending Distracted Driving is Everyone's Responsibility - National Safety Council. https://www.nsc.org/road/safety-topics/distracted-driving/distracted-driving-home. Accessed 21 May 2024.
21. Saving Lives on Country Roads Initiative | Towards Zero. https://towardszero.nsw.gov.au/saving-lives-on-country-roads. Accessed 21 May 2024.
22. Campaigns—THINK! https://www.think.gov.uk/campaigns/. Accessed 21 May 2024.
23. Cogollos-Paja M, García-Reneses JA, Herruzo R. Assessment of increased knowledge about traffic accidents prevention, one month after a presentation included in the program "it can happen to you" of AESLEME. Spinal Cord. 2023;61(7):368–73. https://doi.org/10.1038/s41393-023-00887-1.
24. Cao Y, Krause JS. Estimation of indirect costs based on employment and earnings changes after spinal cord injury: an observational study. Spinal Cord. 2020;58(8):908–13. https://doi.org/10.1038/s41393-020-0447-1.
25. Soendergaard PL, Norup A, Kruse M, Biering-Sørensen F. Socioeconomic consequences of traumatic and non-traumatic spinal cord injuries: a Danish nationwide register-based study. Spinal Cord. 2022;60(7):647–54. https://doi.org/10.1038/s41393-021-00724-3.
26. Malekzadeh H, Golpayegani M, Ghodsi Z, et al. Direct cost of illness for spinal cord injury: a systematic review. Global Spine J. 2022;12(6):1267–81. https://doi.org/10.1177/21925682211031190.
27. Furlan JC, Gulasingam S, Craven BC. The health economics of the spinal cord injury or disease among veterans of war: a systematic review. J Spinal Cord Med. 2017;40(6):649–64. https://doi.org/10.1080/10790268.2017.1368267.
28. Krueger H, Noonan VK, Trenaman LM, Joshi P, Rivers CS. The economic burden of traumatic spinal cord injury in Canada. Chronic Dis Inj Can. 2013;33(3):113–22.
29. Post MW, Reinhardt JD, Avellanet M, et al. Employment among people with spinal cord injury in 22 countries across the world: results from the international spinal cord injury community survey. Arch Phys Med Rehabil. 2020;101(12):2157–66. https://doi.org/10.1016/j.apmr.2020.05.027.
30. Ahn H, Lewis R, Santos A, et al. Forecasting financial resources for future traumatic spinal cord injury care using simulation modeling. J Neurotrauma. 2017;34(20):2917–23. https://doi.org/10.1089/neu.2016.4936.
31. Budd MA, Gater DR, Channell I. Psychosocial consequences of spinal cord injury: a narrative review. J Pers Med. 2022;12(7):1178. https://doi.org/10.3390/jpm12071178.
32. Cieza A, Kirchberger I, Biering-Sørensen F, et al. ICF Core sets for individuals with spinal cord injury in the long-term context. Spinal Cord. 2010;48(4):305–12. https://doi.org/10.1038/sc.2009.183.
33. Jenkins HT, Cosco TD. Spinal cord injury and aging: an exploration of the interrelatedness between key psychosocial factors contributing to the process of resilience. Health Psychol Behav Med. 2021;9(1):315–21.

Mechanism and Pathophysiology of Spinal Cord Injury

2

Ted Chung and Felix Yong

2.1 Introduction

Spinal cord injury (SCI) is a devastating medical condition resulting from trauma or damage to the spinal cord, often leading to permanent neurological deficits and impairments [1]. The spinal cord, a crucial component of the central nervous system (CNS), serves as a pathway for transmitting sensory information (i.e., proprioception, temperature, vibration), conveying motor commands, and facilitating autonomic nervous system function. Any disruption to the integrity of the spinal cord can result in profound sensory, motor, and autonomic dysfunction below the level of injury [5].

SCI can occur because of various traumatic events, such as motor vehicle accidents, falls, sports injuries, other recreational activities, and acts of violence. The severity and extent of neurological deficits depend on several factors such as the level of injury, the extent of spinal cord damage (complete or incomplete), and the presence of secondary complications. The pathophysiology of SCI involves both primary and secondary injury mechanisms [2]. The primary injury results from the initial mechanical trauma to the spinal cord, leading to immediate disruption of neuronal tissues and blood flow [8]. Secondary injury mechanisms, which include ischemia, inflammation, excitotoxicity, oxidative stress, and apoptosis, exacerbate tissue damage and contribute to progressive neurological deficits [6].

SCI has profound implications for the affected individuals, impacting various aspects of their physical, functional, psychological, and social well-being. Management of SCI requires a multidisciplinary approach, involving acute medical stabilization, rehabilitation interventions, management of secondary complications, psychosocial support, and long-term care [7].

T. Chung · F. Yong (✉)
Division of General Surgery, Department of Surgery, John A. Burns School of Medicine, University of Hawai'i, Honolulu, HI, USA

E. Brogi et al. (eds.), *Traumatic Spinal Cord Injury*, Hot Topics in Acute Care Surgery and Trauma, https://doi.org/10.1007/978-3-031-99890-4_2

Despite advances in medical treatment and rehabilitation strategies, SCI remains a challenging condition with significant morbidity and long-term consequences. Ongoing research efforts seek to improve our understanding of SCI pathophysiology, develop innovative therapeutic approaches, and enhance outcomes for individuals living with this debilitating condition.

In this context, understanding the complexities of SCI, its mechanisms, management, and impact on individuals' lives is essential for healthcare professionals, researchers, policymakers, and the broader community to address the needs of those affected by this condition effectively.

2.2 Mechanism of Primary Spinal Cord Injury

Primary SCI occurs as a result of mechanical trauma, which can be classified into two main categories: penetrating injuries and non-penetrating injuries [9]. Penetrating injuries are often the result of gunshot wounds, stab wounds, or other sharp objects that penetrate the spinal column and directly damage the neural tissue. Penetrating injuries cause immediate disruption of the spinal cord's structure and function at the site of penetration, leading to neurological deficits corresponding to the affected spinal cord segment. Non-penetrating injuries encompass a variety of mechanisms that do not involve direct penetration of the spinal cord but still result in direct axonal damage. These mechanisms include compression, contusion, and distraction forces [9].

Compression of the spinal cord occurs when external forces exert pressure on the spinal column, leading to compression of neural tissues. Vertebral fractures, intervertebral disc herniation, spinal stenosis, or tumors can cause compression of the spinal cord, resulting in mechanical disruption of neuronal pathways and impairment of neurological function [3].

Contusion injuries occur due to direct blunt trauma to the spinal cord [4]. The force of impact can cause the spinal cord to be compressed against bony structures within the vertebral column. This can, in turn, cause regional injury that ruptures capillaries and forms contusions.

Distraction injuries involve the stretching or elongation of the spinal cord beyond its normal limits. These injuries commonly occur during accidents where the spine is subjected to excessive traction forces, such as in motor vehicle accidents, falls from heights, or sporting injuries. Distraction forces can lead to mechanical disruption of neuronal structures, stretching of axons, and damage to blood vessels within the spinal cord [10].

2.3 Mechanism of Secondary Spinal Cord Injury

The secondary mechanism of injury in SCI refers to the cascade of pathological processes that occur following the initial insult. While the primary injury causes immediate damage to the spinal cord tissues, the secondary injury exacerbates tissue damage, leading to further neurological deficits. Understanding these secondary processes is crucial for developing therapeutic strategies to mitigate damage and promote recovery. The secondary mechanisms of SCI include ischemia, hypoxia, inflammation, excitotoxicity, oxidative stress, and apoptosis and necrosis [11].

After the primary injury causes mechanical axonal injury and disruption of blood flow to the spinal cord, there is subsequent ischemia and hypoxia to the affected segment of spinal cord tissue. Disruption of blood flow to the spinal cord can occur through a variety of different mechanisms. One is direct vascular damage leading to bleeding and clot formation. A second is swelling, which increases pressure around the spinal cord tissue and, in turn, compresses blood vessels. The ensuing ischemia and hypoxia exacerbate neuronal injury and cell death by depriving cells of oxygen and nutrients.

As spinal cord injury progresses, there is an acute inflammatory response characterized by the activation of resident immune cells in the central nervous system, known as microglia. Microglia, such as astrocytes, become activated and release pro-inflammatory cytokines and chemokines in response to the injury. In addition to the activation of microglia, there is infiltration of peripheral immune cells (i.e., macrophages, lymphocytes, neutrophils, monocytes) to the site of injury. These cells play various roles in the inflammatory response, including phagocytosis of cellular debris, release of pro-inflammatory mediators, and modulation of the immune response. Inflammatory mediators, including cytokines (i.e., IL-1a, IL-1b, IL-6, TNF-α) and reactive oxygen species (ROS), contribute to tissue damage and neuronal death [12, 13].

Excitotoxicity occurs due to the excessive release of excitatory neurotransmitters, particularly glutamate, in the injured spinal cord, leading to the accumulation of glutamate in the extracellular space. Glutamate binds to N-methyl-D-aspartate (NMDA) receptors and other glutamate receptors, causing an influx of calcium ions into the cells. The excessive calcium levels then trigger various toxic cascades within the cell, causing mitochondrial dysfunction and ultimately leading to neuronal death. Cell death resulting from excitotoxicity releases damage-associated molecular patterns (DAMPs) that further activate pro-inflammatory mediators.

SCI induces oxidative stress, which is described as an imbalance between ROS production and antioxidant defenses. ROS, including superoxide radicals and hydrogen peroxide, cause oxidative damage to the cell membrane, proteins, and DNA. This causes exacerbation of neuronal injury, slows regeneration of nerve tissue, and leads to cell death.

Programmed cell death pathways, including apoptosis and necrosis, are activated following SCI [14]. Apoptosis involves controlled cell death characterized by DNA fragmentation and cellular shrinkage, whereas necrosis is a form of uncontrolled cell death associated with cellular swelling and membrane rupture.

The disruption of the blood-spinal cord barrier (BSCB) following SCI leads to increased permeability and leakage of blood components into the spinal cord parenchyma [15]. The BSCB is a specialized barrier system that regulates the exchange of substances between the bloodstream and the spinal cord tissue. Similar to the blood brain barrier (BBB), the BSCB helps maintain the homeostasis of the spinal cord by selectively allowing certain molecules to pass while restricting others. During SCI, the disruption of the BSCB can lead to the influx of immune cells, inflammatory mediators, and toxins into the spinal cord.

Progressive axonal degeneration occurs following SCI, resulting from both primary mechanical damage and secondary pathological processes. Progressive axonal degeneration refers to the gradual breakdown and deterioration of axons, not only at the site of initial trauma but also in surrounding areas over time. This progressive axonal degeneration contributes to the extension of functional deficits and neurological impairments observed.

Reactive gliosis, characterized by the proliferation and activation of astrocytes, leads to the formation of a glial scar at the injury site [16]. Reactive gliosis is a process in which glial cells, particularly astrocytes and microglia, become activated in response to injury or damage to the CNS. Reactive gliosis occurs as a protective mechanism to limit the spread of damage, regulate inflammation, and promote tissue repair. Astrocytes undergo morphological and functional changes during reactive gliosis, forming a glial scar around the site of injury. While the glial scar may prevent the spread of inflammatory cells and toxins, it can also create a physical biochemical barrier that hinders axonal regeneration and functional recovery in the spinal cord. Microglia, the resident immune cells of the CNS, become activated during reactive gliosis and participate in the inflammatory response. While microglia normally play a role in clearing cellular debris and releasing inflammatory factors, their prolonged activation can lead to secondary tissue damage and neuroinflammation.

2.4 Acute Phase of Spinal Cord Injury

The acute phase of SCI refers to the initial period immediately following the traumatic event, typically lasting from minutes to days [5]. During this phase, a series of pathological processes unfold rapidly, contributing to further tissue damage and neurological dysfunction. Understanding the events that occur during the acute phase is crucial for providing timely medical interventions and optimizing patient outcomes. The acute phase of SCI is characterized by the following key events:

The acute phase begins with the primary injury, which involves the initial mechanical trauma to the spinal cord. This injury can result from various mechanisms, such as compression, contusion, distraction, or penetrating trauma. The primary injury disrupts the integrity of the spinal cord tissues, leading to immediate neurological deficits corresponding to the level and severity of injury.

The primary injury often causes damage to blood vessels within the spinal cord, leading to hemorrhage and disruption of blood flow. Vascular disruption results in spinal ischemia and hypoxia in the injured tissues, exacerbating tissue damage and compromising cellular viability.

Following SCI, there are cytotoxic, ionic, and vasogenic edemas. There is an acute inflammatory response characterized by the infiltration of immune cells and the release of inflammatory mediators. Increased vascular permeability and the influx of fluid into the spinal cord parenchyma lead to the formation of edema. Edema exacerbates tissue compression, impairs blood flow, and further compromises neurological function. Water molecules influx through aquaporin water channels, and disturbances in the balance between solute and water cause cell swelling and loss of cytoskeletal integrity, promoting cell death [17]. Ionic edema occurs due to increased permeability of the blood–spinal cord barrier (BSCB). An increase in trans-endothelial ion transport leads to increased permeability and leakage of blood components into the spinal cord parenchyma [18]. Disruption of the BSCB exacerbates inflammation, edema formation, and neuronal injury, further compromising tissue integrity. Endothelial injury and inflammation increase pore size and allow large plasma molecules to pass through the cell membrane, resulting in vasogenic edema.

The primary injury triggers the release of excitatory neurotransmitters, particularly glutamate, into the extracellular space. Glutamate is an excitatory neurotransmitter that is released in the CNS and interacts with N-methyl-D-aspartate (NMDA) and α-amino-3-hydroxy-5-methyl-4-isoxazolepropionic acid (AMPA) receptors [18]. Excessive glutamate binding to NMDA receptors and other glutamate receptors causes calcium influx and neuronal hyperexcitability, a phenomenon known as excitotoxicity [18]. Neuronal excitotoxicity leads to apoptosis and necrosis, failure of Na^+/K^+ ATPase in the axonal membrane, and lipid peroxidation [19]. Rising Ca^{2+} concentration inhibits mitochondrial respiration, causing energy depletion. Alteration of Na^+/K^+ ATPase function increases axonal membrane depolarization. This ionic dysregulation produces axonal acidosis, activation of phospholipases, increased ROS generation, and mitochondrial dysfunction [17, 18].

The acute phase of SCI is characterized by a spectrum of clinical manifestations, including motor deficits, sensory deficits, autonomic dysfunction, and spinal shock. The severity and extent of neurological deficits depend on the level, severity, and type of injury. Spinal shock, characterized by temporary loss of reflexes and flaccid paralysis below the level of injury, is a common feature of the acute phase.

In summary, the acute phase of SCI is marked by a complex interplay of pathological processes. Timely medical interventions aimed at stabilizing the spinal cord, minimizing secondary damage, and optimizing neurological outcomes are critical during this phase.

2.5 Subacute Phase of Spinal Cord Injury

The subacute phase of SCI extends from days to weeks post-injury and is characterized by mitochondrial phosphorylation, increased production of ROS, and ongoing neuroinflammation [5]. During this phase, the pathological processes initiated in the acute phase continue to evolve, and additional mechanisms come into play, influencing the progression of tissue damage and the potential for neurological recovery. Understanding the events that occur during the subacute phase is essential for guiding therapeutic interventions and optimizing patient outcomes. The subacute phase of SCI is characterized by the following key events:

CNS cells contain a large number of mitochondrial complex 1 and generate ROS. Coenzyme Q and cytochrome regulate electron transport in the electron transport chain (ETC) [5]. The ability to control electrons reduces the production of ROS. In SCI, elevated cytosolic Ca^{2+} levels activate mitochondrial complex 1, increase ATP generation, and promote ROS production. The accumulation of high cytosolic Ca^{2+} leads to increased mitochondrial permeability transition pores (mPTPs) [20]. The opening of mPTPs inactivates ATP production, increases water influx, and leads to cell swelling and death [20, 21]. Calcium overload upregulates protein kinases and phospholipases, which lead to calpain-associated protein degradation and oxidative damage [22, 23]. High ROS and reactive nitrogen species (RNS) generation induce lipid peroxidation. ROS reacts with the membrane's polyunsaturated fatty acids and generates reactive lipid species [23].

Neuroinflammation is associated with SCI and involves numerous cell types such as neutrophils, microglia, macrophages, astrocytes, dendritic cells, T-lymphocytes, and B-lymphocytes. They also involve molecular components such as cytokines and prostanoids [23, 24]. The inflammatory responses following SCI produce neurotoxic or neuroprotective effects depending on the duration of the responses. Early inflammatory cells and mediators, such as macrophages, may have beneficial functions by assisting in inflammation, repair, and recovery [24]. However, during SCI, the abnormal activation of autophagosomes and lysosomes triggers rapid cell death [25].

Despite ongoing tissue damage, some individuals may begin to show signs of clinical recovery during the subacute phase. In summary, the subacute phase of SCI is characterized by mitochondrial phosphorylation, increased production of ROS, and ongoing neuroinflammation. Despite the persistence of pathological processes, this phase also represents a critical period for potential clinical recovery and interventions aimed at maximizing functional outcomes.

2.6 Chronic Phase of Spinal Cord Injury

The chronic phase of SCI encompasses the period extending from weeks to months post-injury and is characterized by acute axonal degeneration (AAD), axonal remodeling and demyelination, Wallerian degeneration, and glial scar formation (gliosis or astrogliosis) [5]. During this phase, the acute and subacute pathological processes gradually resolve, giving rise to a new equilibrium characterized by persistent neurological deficits, ongoing neuroplasticity, and potential secondary complications. Understanding the events that occur during the chronic phase is crucial for managing long-term sequelae and optimizing the quality of life for individuals living with SCI. The chronic phase of SCI is characterized by the following key features:

AAD is initiated by a high Ca^{2+} influx into axons. A high Ca^{2+} deposition increases AAD risk in axons [26]. AAD induces other effectors, such as cysteine protease calpain and promotes axonal degeneration [26]. The later phase of AAD is called Wallerian degeneration and typically occurs between 24 and 48 hours after injury [27]. The Wallerian degeneration is propagated by retraction bulbs, which are a microtubule network that inhibits axonal regeneration [27]. Anterograde degeneration is known as Wallerian degeneration, while retrograde degeneration is known as axonal dieback [28, 29].

Oligodendrocytes that promote the myelination of axons in CNS [30] are sensitive to glutamate excitotoxicity caused by hyperactivation of AMPA and NMDA receptors [17]. During SCI, high glutamate levels increase Ca^{2+} influx that provokes oligodendrocytes apoptosis and necrosis [17]. Damage to oligodendrocytes is caused by ROS and RNS production, glutathione reduction, and an increase in peroxisome hyperactivation [31]. ROS production by neutrophils and microglia leads to the release of pro-inflammatory cytokines (i.e., TNFα, IL-2, IFN-γ, proteases) and propagates oligodendrocyte apoptosis [31]. The apoptosis of oligodendrocytes leads to demyelination of axons and increases expression of Fas-receptors that release caspases 3 and 8, which mediate apoptosis [31, 32, 38, 39].

Glial scar formation (gliosis) is a reactive mechanism mediated by astrocytes. The scarring of astrocytes (astrogliosis) is a process that starts the healing process following SCI [33]. The other major components of scar tissue are pericytes and connective tissue. At baseline, the number of astrocytes is ten times higher than pericytes in the spinal cord parenchyma. Approximately 2 weeks after SCI, pericytes outnumber astrocytes two to one [34]. Pericytes secrete markers that promote fibroblasts to express extracellular matrix (ECM) such as fibronectin. This serves as the main component of scar tissue [35].

The continuous formation of cysts is the hallmark feature of SCI. The formation of cysts indicates ongoing apoptotic responses. Astrocytes undergo apoptosis through TLR4/MyD88 signalling [36]. Additionally, cyst formation may lead to syringomyelia in some patients with SCI. Syringomyelia is a condition in which a cyst develops in the spinal cord and over time damages the spinal cord. The damage to the spinal cord may lead to sensation loss, paralysis, weakness, and stiffness [37].

Neurological deficits stabilize during the chronic phase, with the severity and extent of impairment reaching a plateau. While some spontaneous recovery may occur in the initial months post-injury, further improvement in neurological function is typically limited beyond the chronic phase.

Individuals with SCI are at risk of developing secondary complications, which can significantly impact their quality of life and long-term outcomes. Common secondary complications include neuropathic pain, muscle spasticity, urinary and bowel dysfunction, pressure ulcers, osteoporosis, and respiratory complications. Management of these complications is essential for minimizing morbidity and optimizing functional independence.

SCI has profound psychosocial implications, affecting various aspects of an individual's life, including mental health, social relationships, sexual health, and vocational status. Depression, anxiety, social isolation, and decreased quality of life are common psychosocial issues experienced by individuals with SCI. Psychosocial support services, counseling, and peer support groups play an integral role in promoting emotional well-being.

Rehabilitation interventions continue to be important in the chronic phase of SCI, focusing on maximizing functional independence, enhancing quality of life, and preventing secondary complications. Multidisciplinary rehabilitation teams, including physiatrists, physical therapists, occupational therapists, speech therapists, psychologists, and social workers, collaborate to provide comprehensive care tailored to the individual's needs.

Technological advancements in assistive devices, mobility aids, and adaptive equipment have greatly improved the quality of life for individuals with SCI. Wheelchairs, orthotic devices, electronic aids for activities of daily living, and functional electrical stimulation systems are examples of assistive technologies that enhance independence and mobility.

Ongoing research efforts seek to develop novel therapeutic approaches for SCI, including stem cell therapies, neuroprotective agents, tissue engineering strategies, and neurorehabilitation interventions. Advances in regenerative medicine, neuroimaging, and neurorehabilitation hold promise for improving outcomes and enhancing recovery in individuals with SCI.

In summary, the chronic phase of SCI is characterized by neurological stabilization, ongoing neuroplasticity, management of secondary complications, psychosocial adaptation, long-term rehabilitation and care, technological advancements, and research innovation. Comprehensive management strategies addressing physical, functional, psychological, and social aspects are essential for optimizing outcomes and improving the quality of life for individuals living with SCI.

2.7 Conclusion

Spinal cord injury represents a complex and multifaceted pathological process involving both primary and secondary injury mechanisms. Understanding the intricate interplay between mechanical trauma, neuroinflammation, and neurodegenerative processes is essential for developing targeted therapeutic interventions aimed at minimizing tissue damage and promoting functional recovery in individuals with SCI.

References

1. Kabu S, Gao Y, Kwon BK, Labhasetwar V. Drug delivery, cell-based therapies, and tissue engineering approaches for spinal cord injury. J Control Release. 2015;219:141–54. https://doi.org/10.1016/j.jconrel.2015.08.060. Epub 2015 Sep 4
2. Zhang Y, Al Mamun A, Yuan Y, Lu Q, Xiong J, Yang S, Wu C, Wu Y, Wang J. Acute spinal cord injury: pathophysiology and pharmacological intervention (Review). Mol Med Rep. 2021;23(6):417. https://doi.org/10.3892/mmr.2021.12056. Epub 2021 Apr 13
3. Yisheng W, Fuying Z, Limin W, Junwei L, Guofu P, Weidong W. First aid and treatment for cervical spinal cord injury with fracture and dislocation. Indian J Orthop. 2007;41(4):300–4. https://doi.org/10.4103/0019-5413.36991.

4. van Den Hauwe L, Sundgren PC, Flanders AE. Spinal Trauma and Spinal Cord Injury (SCI). In: Hodler J, Kubik-Huch RA, von Schulthess GK, editors. Diseases of the brain, head and neck, spine 2020–2023: diagnostic imaging [Internet]. Cham (CH): Springer; 2020. Chapter 19.
5. Anjum A, Yazid MD, Fauzi Daud M, Idris J, Ng AMH, Selvi Naicker A, Ismail OHR, Athi Kumar RK, Lokanathan Y. Spinal Cord Injury: pathophysiology, multimolecular interactions, and underlying recovery mechanisms. Int J Mol Sci. 2020;21(20):7533. https://doi.org/10.3390/ijms21207533.
6. Hellenbrand DJ, Quinn CM, Piper ZJ, Morehouse CN, Fixel JA, Hanna AS. Inflammation after spinal cord injury: a review of the critical timeline of signaling cues and cellular infiltration. J Neuroinflammation. 2021;18(1):284. https://doi.org/10.1186/s12974-021-02337-2.
7. Tian T, Zhang S, Yang M. Recent progress and challenges in the treatment of spinal cord injury. Protein Cell. 2023;14(9):635–52. https://doi.org/10.1093/procel/pwad003.
8. Li S, Dinh HTP, Matsuyama Y, Sato K, Yamagishi S. Molecular mechanisms in the vascular and nervous systems following traumatic Spinal Cord Injury. Life (Basel). 2022;13(1):9. https://doi.org/10.3390/life13010009.
9. Roach MJ, Chen Y, Kelly ML. Comparing blunt and penetrating trauma in Spinal Cord Injury: analysis of long-term functional and neurological outcomes. Top Spinal Cord Inj Rehabil. 2018;24(2):121–32. https://doi.org/10.1310/sci2402-121.
10. Han B, Liang W, Hai Y, Liu Y, Chen Y, Ding H, Yang J, Yin P. Elucidating the potential mechanisms underlying distraction Spinal Cord injury-associated neuroinflammation and apoptosis. Front Cell Dev Biol. 2022;10:839313. https://doi.org/10.3389/fcell.2022.839313.
11. He Z, Zhang C, Liang JX, Zheng FF, Qi XY, Gao F. Targeting mitochondrial oxidative stress: potential neuroprotective therapy for Spinal Cord Injury. J Integr Neurosci. 2023;22(6):153. https://doi.org/10.31083/j.jin2206153.
12. Li C, Xiong W, Wan B, Kong G, Wang S, Wang Y, Fan J. Role of peripheral immune cells in spinal cord injury. Cell Mol Life Sci. 2022;80(1):2. https://doi.org/10.1007/s00018-022-4644-0.
13. Gu C, Kong F, Zeng J, Geng X, Sun Y, Chen X. Remote ischemic preconditioning protects against spinal cord ischemia-reperfusion injury in mice by activating NMDAR/AMPK/PGC-1α/SIRT3 signaling. Cell Biosci. 2023;13(1):57. https://doi.org/10.1186/s13578-023-00999-4.
14. Xiao S, Zhang Y, Liu Z, Li A, Tong W, Xiong X, Nie J, Zhong N, Zhu G, Liu J, Liu Z. Alpinetin inhibits neuroinflammation and neuronal apoptosis via targeting the JAK2/STAT3 signaling pathway in spinal cord injury. CNS Neurosci Ther. 2023;29(4):1094–108. https://doi.org/10.1111/cns.14085. Epub 2023 Jan 10
15. Jiang T, Qin T, Gao P, Tao Z, Wang X, Wu M, Gu J, Chu B, Zheng Z, Yi J, Xu T, Huang Y, Liu H, Zhao S, Ren Y, Chen J, Yin G. SIRT1 attenuates blood-spinal cord barrier disruption after spinal cord injury by deacetylating p66Shc. Redox Biol. 2023;60:102615. https://doi.org/10.1016/j.redox.2023.102615. Epub 2023 Jan 24
16. Kwiecien JM, Dabrowski W, Dąbrowska-Bouta B, Sulkowski G, Oakden W, Kwiecien-Delaney CJ, Yaron JR, Zhang L, Schutz L, Marzec-Kotarska B, Stanisz GJ, Karis JP, Struzynska L, Lucas AR. Prolonged inflammation leads to ongoing damage after spinal cord injury. PLoS One. 2020;15(3):e0226584. https://doi.org/10.1371/journal.pone.0226584.
17. Jha RM, Kochanek PM, Simard JM. Pathophysiology and treatment of cerebral edema in traumatic brain injury. Neuropharmacology. 2019;145:230–46.
18. Vanzulli I, Butt AM. mGluR5 protect astrocytes from ischemic damage in postnatal CNS white matter. Cell Calcium. 2015;58:423–30.
19. O'Shea TM, Burda JE, Sofroniew MV. Cell biology of spinal cord injury and repair. J Clin Invest. 2017;127:3259–70.
20. Cao Y, Lv G, Wang YS, Fan ZK, Bi YL, Zhao L, Guo ZP. Mitochondrial fusion and fission after spinal sacord injury in rats. Brain Res. 2013;1522:59–66.
21. Pivovarova NB, Andrews SB. Calcium-dependent mitochondrial function and dysfunction in neurons. FEBS J. 2010;277:3622–36.
22. Alizadeh A, Dyck SM, Karimi-Abdolrezaee S. Traumatic spinal cord injury: an overview of pathophysiology, models and acute injury mechanisms. Front Neurol. 2019;10:282.
23. Hall ED. Antioxidant therapies for acute spinal cord injury. Neurotherapeutics. 2011;8:152–67.

24. Miron VE, Franklin RJ. Macrophages and CNS remyelination. J Neurochem. 2014;130:165–71.
25. Yu WR, Fehlings MG. Fas/FasL-mediated apoptosis and inflammation are key features of acute human spinal cord injury: implications for translational, clinical application. Acta Neuropathol. 2011;122:747–61.
26. Ginet V, Spiehlmann A, Rummel C, Rudinskiy N, Grishchuk Y, Luthi-Carter R, Clarke PG, Truttmann AC, Puyal J. Involvement of autophagy in hypoxic-excitotoxic neuronal death. Autophagy. 2014;10:846–60.
27. Williams PR, Marincu BN, Sorbara CD, Mahler CF, Schumacher AM, Griesbeck O, Kerschensteiner M, Misgeld T. A recoverable state of axon injury persists for hours after spinal cord contusion in vivo. Nat Commun. 2014;5:1–11.
28. Wang JT, Medress ZA, Barres BA. Axon degeneration: molecular mechanisms of a self-destruction pathway. J Cell Biol. 2012;196:7–18.
29. Couillard-Despres S, Bieler L, Vogl M. Pathophysiology of traumatic spinal cord injury. Neurological aspects of Spinal Cord Injury. Cham: Springer; 2017. p. 503–28.
30. Cohen-Adad J, El Mendili MM, Lehéricy S, Pradat PF, Blancho S, Rossignol S, Benali H. Demyelination and degeneration in the injured human spinal cord detected with diffusion and magnetization transfer MRI. NeuroImage. 2011;55:1024–33.
31. Domingues HS, Portugal CC, Socodato R, Relvas JB. Oligodendrocyte, astrocyte, and microglia crosstalk in myelin development, damage, and repair. Front Cell Dev Biol. 2016;4:71.
32. Almad A, Sahinkaya FR, McTigue DM. Oligodendrocyte fate after spinal cord injury. Neurotherapeutics. 2011;8:262–73.
33. Mekhail M, Almazan G, Tabrizian M. Oligodendrocyte-protection and remyelination post-spinal cord injuries: a review. Prog Neurobiol. 2012;96:322–39.
34. Yuan YM, He C. The glial scar in spinal cord injury and repair. Neurosci Bull. 2013;29:421–35.
35. Billakanti R, Karimi-Abdolrezaee S. Reactive astrogliosis after spinal cord injury-beneficial and detrimental effects. Mol Neurobiol. 2012;46:251–64.
36. Göritz C, Dias DO, Tomilin N, Barbacid M, Shupliakov O, Frisén J. A pericyte origin of spinal cord scar tissue. Science. 2011;333:238–42.
37. Fan H, Zhang K, Shan L, Kuang F, Chen K, Zhu K, Ma H, Ju G, Wang YZ. Reactive astrocytes undergo M1 microglia/macrohpages-induced necroptosis in spinal cord injury. Mol Neurodegener. 2016;11:14.
38. Liu S, Li Y, Choi HMC, Sarkar C, Koh EY, Wu J, Lipinski MM. Lysosomal damage after spinal cord injury causes accumulation of RIPK1 and RIPK3 proteins and potentiation of necroptosis. Cell Death Dis. 2018;9:476.
39. Sobrido-Cameán D, Barreiro-Iglesias A. Role of caspase-8 and Fas in cell death after spinal cord injury. Front Mol Neurosci. 2018;11:101.

Prehospital Evaluation and Management, Part I: Clinical Presentation, Spine Stabilization, Airway Management

3

Adham M. Khalafallah, Seth Stravers Tigchelaar, and Kristine O'Phelan

3.1 Background/Epidemiology

Traumatic spinal cord injury (tSCI) is a devastating condition resulting in lifelong disability, affecting approximately 54 cases per million people in the United States, resulting in about 18,000 new tSCI cases each year [1–4]. The National Spinal Cord Injury Statistical Center (NSCISC) estimates that there are around 305,000 individuals living with tSCI in the United States [1, 5]. As of June 2024, the NSCISC maintains the world's largest and longest-running research database on tSCI, which includes information on 53,494 patients who have sustained tSCI [1]. The average age at injury has increased from 29 years during the 1970s to 43 years since 2015 [1], with males constituting about 79% of new tSCI cases [6]. In terms of race and ethnicity, the data indicated that approximately 25% of tSCI cases have occurred among non-Hispanic Blacks, which is notably higher than their representation in the general population at 13%. These statistics underscore the demographic trends and disparities within the tSCI population in the United States [1, 2]. According to the NSCISC's 2023 report on the causes of tSCI, vehicular accidents accounted for the highest proportion at 38%, followed by falls at 31%. Gunshot wounds (13%) and sports and recreational activities (8%) were also notable contributors [5]. Hospital stays in acute care units have decreased from an average of 30 days in the 1970s to 19 days. Similarly, the average length of rehabilitation stays decreased from 110 days in the 1970s to 37 days [1].

A. M. Khalafallah · S. S. Tigchelaar
Department of Neurosurgery, University of Miami, Miller School of Medicine, Miami, FL, USA

K. O'Phelan (✉)
Department of Neurology, Division of Neurocritical Care, University of Miami, Miller School of Medicine, Miami, FL, USA
e-mail: KOPhelan@med.miami.edu

E. Brogi et al. (eds.), *Traumatic Spinal Cord Injury*, Hot Topics in Acute Care Surgery and Trauma, https://doi.org/10.1007/978-3-031-99890-4_3

Effective management of tSCI begins with immediate and precise prehospital evaluation and management to prevent or minimize secondary injury and optimize patient outcomes [7–10]. Extensive literature on this topic focuses on key areas we will discuss: clinical presentation, immobilization, spine stabilization during transport, and airway management.

3.2 Clinical Presentation

Patients with tSCI may present with a variety of symptoms depending on the level and severity of the injury [11]. The clinical presentation can include pain, paralysis, paresthesia, loss of sensation, and loss of autonomic function below the level of injury. The International Standards for Neurological Classification of SCI (ISNCSCI) scale is commonly used to assess and classify the severity of SCI [12]. A detailed neurological examination, including motor and sensory testing, is essential for determining the level of injury and guiding further management [13]. The pathophysiology of tSCI involves primary and secondary injury mechanisms. The primary injury occurs at the moment of impact, causing immediate damage to the spinal cord tissues, including neuronal and glial cells, blood vessels, and supporting structures. This is followed by secondary injury processes that involve a cascade of biochemical and cellular events, leading to further neuronal damage, inflammation, and edema [14, 15]. Early intervention in the pre-hospital phase aims to mitigate these secondary injury mechanisms.

3.3 Clinical Symptoms and Signs

3.3.1 Pain and Sensory Changes

Patients with tSCI often experience acute pain at the injury site. This pain can be due to direct trauma to the spine, concomitant injuries (such as fractures or dislocations), or inflammatory processes. The pain may radiate along the dermatomal distribution of the affected spinal nerves. Sensory deficits, such as numbness, tingling (paresthesias), and loss of sensation, are common and can be indicative of the spinal level and extent of the spinal cord injury [16, 17].

3.3.2 Motor Deficits

Motor deficits are a hallmark of tSCI. The severity and distribution of motor impairment depend on the level of injury. Injuries to the cervical spine can result in tetraplegia (quadriplegia), where there is paralysis of all four limbs. Thoracic and lumbar injuries typically result in paraplegia, affecting the lower limbs. The presence of muscle weakness or complete paralysis below the level of injury is a critical finding. Muscle strength is assessed using the Medical Research Council (MRC) scale, which grades muscle power on a scale from 0 to 5 where a score of 0 indicates no voluntary movement and a score of 5 represents normal strength [18].

3.3.3 Autonomic Dysfunction

Autonomic dysfunction is a significant concern in tSCI, particularly in injuries above the T6 level. This can lead to neurogenic shock, characterized by hypotension and bradycardia due to the loss of sympathetic tone. Patients may also experience autonomic dysreflexia, a potentially life-threatening condition triggered by noxious stimuli below the level of injury, leading to severe hypertension, bradycardia, and other autonomic responses [19].

3.3.4 Spinal Shock

Spinal shock is an immediate and temporary physiological response to acute tSCI, characterized by a complete loss of motor, sensory, and autonomic functions below the level of the lesion [20]. This state of areflexia and flaccid paralysis can last from days to weeks, and its resolution marks the return of reflex activity. During spinal shock, the absence of all reflexes, including deep tendon reflexes, makes it difficult to assess the full extent of the spinal cord injury. Clinically, patients present with flaccid paralysis, loss of sensation, and absent reflexes below the injury level. Autonomic functions are also affected, leading to issues such as urinary retention and bowel dysfunction. The return of reflexes, such as the bulbocavernosus reflex, signals the end of spinal shock. The period of spinal shock is critical for managing the patient to prevent secondary complications such as pressure ulcers, deep vein thrombosis, and respiratory issues. Supportive care, including fluid management, maintaining adequate perfusion, and preventing infections, is essential during this phase. Understanding spinal shock is crucial for clinicians as it impacts the initial assessment and long-term prognosis of patients with tSCI.

3.3.5 Neurogenic Shock

Neurogenic shock is a severe and life-threatening condition that arises from the disruption of the autonomic pathways within the spinal cord, often occurring in the context of high spinal cord injuries (typically above the T6 level) [21]. This disruption results in a loss of sympathetic tone, leading to a predominance of parasympathetic activity. Clinically, neurogenic shock is characterized by hypotension, bradycardia, and peripheral vasodilation. The hallmark of neurogenic shock is the combination of low blood pressure and a slow heart rate, which is counterintuitive as shock states usually present with tachycardia. The vasodilation and pooling of blood in the periphery reduce venous return to the heart, exacerbating hypotension. The management of neurogenic shock requires immediate medical intervention to stabilize the patient. Fluid resuscitation is the first line of treatment to address hypotension, but vasopressors are often required to maintain adequate perfusion pressures. Atropine may be administered to counteract symptomatic bradycardia. Identifying and managing neurogenic shock promptly is crucial to prevent organ dysfunction, preserve spinal perfusion, and improve outcomes. Continuous monitoring and supportive care, including respiratory support if necessary, are essential components of the management strategy.

3.3.6 Neurogenic Shock Versus Spinal Shock

Neurogenic shock and spinal shock are two distinct phenomena that can occur following tSCI, each with different pathophysiological mechanisms and clinical implications. Neurogenic shock is primarily characterized by a disruption of the sympathetic nervous system pathways, leading to a loss of sympathetic tone. This results in severe hypotension and bradycardia due to unopposed parasympathetic activity, often occurring in injuries above the T6 level where sympathetic outflow is significantly impaired. Neurogenic shock is a life-threatening condition that requires prompt recognition and management to prevent further complications such as organ ischemia and failure. Treatment typically involves fluid resuscitation and the administration of vasopressors to maintain adequate blood pressure and perfusion.

In contrast, spinal shock refers to a transient physiological response to acute tSCI, marked by a complete loss of motor, sensory, and autonomic function below the level of the lesion. This state of areflexia and flaccid paralysis occurs immediately after the injury and can last from days to weeks. During spinal shock, the absence of reflexes makes it challenging to assess the true extent of the injury. As spinal shock resolves, reflexes return, and the extent of permanent injury can be more accurately determined. The management of spinal shock focuses on supportive care, close monitoring, and preventing secondary complications. Differentiating between neurogenic and spinal shock is crucial for clinicians as it guides specific therapeutic interventions and has significant prognostic implications.

3.4 Immobilization and Transport

Studies have highlighted the critical role of prehospital providers in preventing further trauma to the spinal cord. Research suggests that between 3% and 25% of all spinal cord injuries occur after the initial traumatic event, either during transportation or early in the treatment process [22–26]. Considering the mechanism of injury is pivotal during the on-field assessment, as significant spinal injury may not immediately manifest with focal neurological signs or symptoms. Therefore, assessing the spine initially in such cases can be challenging. While still in the field, the prevention of further insult to the spinal cord is the single most important objective. Although there is expert consensus supporting immobilization of the spine after acute injury, data to determine standards for immobilization during emergency transport remain sparse and inconclusive [7, 8, 13, 22, 27–30].

Biomechanical studies recommend the combination of a rigid cervical collar with supportive blocks on a hard backboard with straps. Abdominal straps fastened to the backboard reduce lateral thoracolumbar spinal motion, and excess slack between the patient and backboard should be eliminated to reduce further injury. However, tissue necrosis may occur from the pressure of the rigid backboard during prolonged transport, and/or short periods of rigid immobilization. A padded board may reduce the risk of pressure necrosis by relieving the excess pressure between the board surface and the occiput and/or sacrum. Although cervical stabilization protocols are implemented in many health care systems, there is limited data to suggest true benefit. Generally, immobilization protocols are ubiquitous across health care institutions, are relatively easy to standardize and implement, and are unlikely to have negative effects—provided they do not interfere with rapid patient transport to a trauma center, and do not produce pressure ulcers.

3.5 Spine Stabilization

Prehospital spine stabilization is a critical step in the management of patients with suspected SCI [8, 22]. The goal is to immobilize the spine to prevent further injury. This is typically achieved through rigid cervical collars, spinal boards, and securing straps. The literature emphasizes the importance of maintaining spinal alignment during extrication and transport. Log-rolling techniques and scoop stretchers may be used to minimize movement of the spine during patient handling. In the case of blunt trauma, immobilization is typically indicated in the following situations: Low GCS or evidence of intoxication, midline tenderness in the cervical spine, obvious spinal deformity, or the presence of other distracting injuries.

3.5.1 Spinal Immobilization in the Prehospital Setting Involves Several Key Components

3.5.1.1 Rigid Cervical Collars

Cervical collars are applied to maintain alignment of the cervical spine and prevent further injury. It is crucial to ensure that the collar fits properly and is applied correctly to avoid causing additional harm (Table 3.1).

3.5.1.2 Spinal Boards and Scoop Stretchers

Spinal boards provide a rigid support surface for patients suspected of having spinal injuries. Scoop stretchers can be used to lift and transport patients onto the spinal board with minimal movement.

Table 3.1 Spine immobilization strategies

Spinal stabilization strategy	Recommendation	Risks
Rigid cervical collar	The American Association of Neurological Surgeons recommends the rigid cervical collar as a method for stabilizing the cervical spine in pre-hospital scenarios [8]	Low-quality evidence supports its positive influence on the neurological outcome of cervical spine injury, with potential negative effects including a significant rise of intracranial pressure and dysphagia [31]
Spinal boards, padded board/ mattresses, and securing straps	The original spinal longboard is used in conjunction with the hard collar, blocks, and straps to achieve immobilization of the spine. There may be benefit of use of the vacuum mattress versus the spine board alone in preventing motion at an unstable, subaxial cervical spine injury [32]	There is currently evidence of increased risk for pressure sores over the sacrum when placed on spinal boards for extended periods of time [33]
Log rolling technique	Particularly imperative in the patient found prone, in which case the patient should be log rolled directly onto the spine board using a push technique.	Studies suggest the log roll produces more motion than placing a patient on a spine board, removing a spine board, performing continuous lateral therapy, and positioning a patient prone for surgery.

3.5.1.3 Securing Straps

Securing straps are used to immobilize the patient on the spinal board. These straps should be applied snugly to prevent any movement during transport, but should not be so tight as to cause discomfort or impede circulation.

3.5.1.4 Log-Rolling Technique

The log-rolling technique is employed to move patients with suspected spinal injuries. This technique involves rolling the patient onto their side in a coordinated manner, maintaining spinal alignment throughout the process.

3.5.1.5 Padded Boards

Padded boards or mattresses can be used to reduce the risk of pressure injury during prolonged transport. These devices help distribute pressure more evenly and provide additional comfort to the patient. Alternatively, spinal motion restriction (SMR) with use of a cervical collar and cot to maintain neutral alignment of the spine during transport of a patient with concern for spinal injury has been shown to be noninferior to traditional spinal immobilization and to confer lower risks of pressure ulcers and pain [34, 35].

3.6 Fluid Resuscitation and Perfusion

Maintaining adequate perfusion to the injured spinal cord is crucial to prevent secondary injury. Hypotension can exacerbate spinal cord ischemia and worsen neurological outcomes [36–38]. Prehospital providers should aim to maintain a systolic blood pressure of at least 90 mmHg in patients with tSCI.

3.6.1 Key Aspects of Fluid Resuscitation Include

3.6.1.1 Intravenous Access

Establishing intravenous (IV) access is a priority. Large-bore IV catheters should be used to facilitate rapid fluid administration.

3.6.1.2 Fluid Administration

Crystalloids such as normal saline or Lactated Ringer's solution are typically used for initial fluid resuscitation. The goal is to maintain adequate blood pressure and tissue perfusion.

3.6.1.3 Avoiding Hypotension

Hypotension should be avoided at all costs. Vasopressors may be administered if fluid resuscitation alone is insufficient to maintain blood pressure.

3.6.1.4 Monitoring for Fluid Overload

Care should be taken to avoid fluid overload, which can lead to complications such as pulmonary edema. Monitoring urine output and signs of fluid overload is important.

3.7 Pain Management

Pain management is an important aspect of prehospital care for patients with tSCI. Effective pain control can prevent additional stress and discomfort, which may exacerbate secondary injury processes.

3.7.1 Key Considerations in Pain Management Include

3.7.1.1 Assessment of Pain

Pain should be assessed using appropriate pain scales. Patients should be asked to describe the location, intensity, and quality of their pain.

3.7.1.2 Administration of Analgesics

Analgesics such as opioids may be administered to control pain. Care should be taken to avoid respiratory depression, especially in patients with high cervical injuries.

3.7.1.3 Non-pharmacological Interventions

Non-pharmacological interventions such as immobilization and positioning can also help alleviate pain. Patients should be positioned comfortably and immobilized to prevent further injury.

3.8 Communication About Transport

Effective communication between EMS providers and receiving facilities is crucial for optimizing patient outcomes. Key aspects include:

3.8.1 Pre-arrival Notification

Providing timely and accurate pre-arrival notifications to the receiving hospital ensures that the trauma team is prepared for the patient's arrival. Information should include the mechanism of injury, vital signs, neurological status, and any interventions performed.

3.8.2 Transport Considerations

Rapid and safe transport to a specialized spinal injury center is essential. Helicopter transport may be considered for patients in remote or inaccessible areas to minimize transport time.

3.9 Challenges and Considerations

3.9.1 The Prehospital Management of tSCI Presents Several Challenges

3.9.1.1 Environmental Factors

Managing tSCI in adverse environmental conditions, such as remote locations, extreme weather, or hazardous terrains, can complicate the assessment and transport of patients.

3.9.1.2 Resource Limitations

Limited resources, such as insufficient immobilization equipment, lack of advanced airway management tools, or inadequate training of first responders, can impact the quality of care provided.

3.9.1.3 Patient Factors

Factors such as obesity, concomitant injuries, and patient cooperation can influence the ease of assessment and management. Tailoring interventions to individual patient needs is essential.

3.9.1.4 Protocols and Guidelines

Variability in pre-hospital protocols and adherence to evidence-based guidelines can affect the consistency and quality of care provided [39–42]. Standardized protocols and continuous education for EMS providers are necessary to ensure optimal outcomes.

3.9.2 Airway Management in Patients with Acute Cervical SCI

Patients with cervical spine injury comprise approximately 2.5% of patients treated for spinal fractures and only 0.8% sustain acute cervical SCI [43]. However, this subset of patients is uniquely at risk for respiratory complications and airway compromise. Additionally, up to 40% of cervical spine fractures are deemed to be unstable, which makes manipulation of the head and neck during airway management particularly problematic. Assessment and proper management of the airway are essential because preservation of oxygenation and ventilation is paramount to avoid worsening secondary cord injury. Patients should be evaluated for inability to protect the airway, failure to oxygenate, and failure to ventilate. Emergent or urgent airways may be needed if there is acute distress or rapidly progressing respiratory compromise.

When tracheal intubation is needed in patients with acute cervical SCI, there are techniques commonly used to minimize associated cervical spine movement. The risk of cervical movement is highest with facemask ventilation, and tracheal intubation is likely to be beneficial. Rapid sequence intubation (RSI) should be performed with manual-in-line stabilization with the anterior portion of the cervical collar removed to allow mouth opening [44].

Most airway maneuvers are associated with some movement of the cervical spine; the goal is to minimize movement and maximize oxygenation and ventilation. The jaw thrust maneuver moves the tongue anteriorly with the mandible and decreases upper airway obstruction without extending the neck.

Sniffing position is used in patients without cervical spine injury to best visualize the larynx during intubation. It involves flexion of the lower cervical spine and extension of the atlanto-axial joint. Clearly, this is not an option in patients with acute or suspected cervical spine injury, so intubation must be performed using maneuvers that avoid cervical spine motion and provide the best visualization of the larynx for intubation. For stable, cooperative patients, awake intubation using a flexible bronchoscope has traditionally been used. However, if a more urgent airway is required, RSI should be performed as described above. Manual- in-line stabilization of the head and neck has been shown to limit the view of the larynx during direct laryngoscopy, and use of a bougie is recommended to improve the rate of successful tracheal intubation. Use of videolaryngoscopy improves the rate of first-attempt intubation with minimal cervical movement, and its use is recommended when available. Table 3.2 lists various intubation techniques and the associated risks and benefits. The incidence of neurologic worsening related to tracheal intubation is low; however, the neurologic exam should be documented before airway stabilization if possible.

During RSI, induction agents are used to provide amnesia and to blunt the sympathetic response. In patients with cervical spinal cord injury and neurogenic shock, sympathetic tone is already diminished; therefore, hemodynamic complications may be magnified. Medications used for sedation and RSI induction should be chosen carefully to avoid excessive hypotension. The addition of a sedative to neuromuscular blockade improves intubating conditions by improving laryngoscopic view of the airway. Frequently used medications for RSI induction in these patients include etomidate and ketamine.

Etomidate 0.3 mg/kg IV has an onset of 15–45 seconds, a duration of 3–12 minutes, and is hemodynamically neutral. Etomidate does not provide analgesia, so the addition of an analgesic or topical anesthetic is recommended.

Ketamine is a dissociative anesthetic agent that provides analgesia along with amnesia and sedation. The usual dose is 1–2 mg/kg with a time to effect of 45–60 seconds and a duration of 10–20 minutes. Ketamine does not blunt the respiratory drive, so it can be used with a topical anesthetic for "awake" intubations when neuromuscular blockade is not used due to concerns for a difficult airway. Ketamine may cause hypotension in patients with blunted sympathetic drive or depleted catecholamines [45].

Neuromuscular blockade for RSI is generally provided with succinylcholine but should be used with caution in patients with spinal cord injury unless injury is within less than 24 hours due to the risk of extra-junctional receptors and hyperkalemic complications, including cardiac arrest [46, 47].

Table 3.2 Airway management options

Device	Benefits	Risks
Awake fiberoptic intubation	Allows for neuro exam before and after	Requires time to perform, not for anxious or uncooperative patients, provider expertise needed
Video laryngoscopy	Excellent laryngeal visualization, less mouth opening spine movement	Not available in the field
Direct laryngoscopy	Available, most rapid approach	Poor views with MILS, more spinal movement
Laryngeal mask airway	Essential adjunct to difficult airway	Not a definitive airway for the cervical SCI patient

3.10 Conclusion

Traumatic spinal cord injury affects many people in the United States each year. Attention to the clinical presentation aids early identification of these patients and allows for rapid management to prevent secondary injury. Protocols for spine stabilization and clear communication between EMS and hospital teams are critical to optimizing the early care of patients with tSCI. Rapid correction of hemodynamic instability and airway compromise can avoid secondary injury and improve functional recovery after tSCI.

References

1. Birmingham AU of A at B. National Spinal Cord Injury Statistical Center, traumatic spinal cord injury facts and figures at a glance. Published online 2024. Accessed July 21, 2024. https://www.nscisc.uab.edu/public/Facts%20and%20Figures%202024%20-%20Final.pdf
2. University of Alabama at Birmingham: Birmingham Alabama. National Spinal Cord Injury Statistical Center. 2023 Annual Statistical Report for the Spinal Cord Injury Model Systems. Accessed July 21, 2024. University of Alabama at Birmingham: Birmingham, Alabama.
3. Lasfargues JE, Custis D, Morrone F, Cars Well J, Nguyen T. A model for estimating spinal cord injury prevalence in the United States. Spinal Cord. 1995;33(2):62–8. https://doi.org/10.1038/sc.1995.16.
4. Cripps RA, Lee BB, Wing P, Weerts E, Mackay J, Brown D. A global map for traumatic spinal cord injury epidemiology: towards a living data repository for injury prevention. Spinal Cord. 2011;49(4):493–501. https://doi.org/10.1038/sc.2010.146.
5. Birmingham AU of A at B. National Spinal Cord Injury Statistical Center, Recent trends in causes of traumatic spinal cord injury. Published online 2024. Accessed July 21, 2024. https://www.nscisc.uab.edu/Public/Recent%20Trends%20in%20Causes%20of%20SCI%20-%202023.pdf
6. Furlan JC, Fehlings MG. The impact of age on mortality, impairment, and disability among adults with acute traumatic spinal cord injury. J Neurotrauma. 2009;26(10):1707–17. https://doi.org/10.1089/neu.2009.0888.
7. Ahn H, Singh J, Nathens A, et al. Pre-hospital care management of a potential spinal cord injured patient: a systematic review of the literature and evidence-based guidelines. J Neurotrauma. 2011;28(8):1341–61. https://doi.org/10.1089/neu.2009.1168.
8. Theodore N, Hadley MN, Aarabi B, et al. Prehospital cervical spinal immobilization after trauma. Neurosurgery. 2013;72(suppl 2):22–34. https://doi.org/10.1227/NEU.0b013e318276edb1.
9. Hadley MN, Walters BC. The case for the future role of evidence-based medicine in the management of cervical spine injuries, with or without fractures. J Neurosurg Spine. 2019;31(4):457–63. https://doi.org/10.3171/2019.6.SPINE19652.
10. ATLS Subcommittee, American College of Surgeons' Committee on Trauma, International ATLS Working Group. Advanced trauma life support (ATLS®). J Trauma Acute Care Surg. 2013;74(5):1363–6. https://doi.org/10.1097/TA.0b013e31828b82f5.
11. Silva NA, Sousa N, Reis RL, Salgado AJ. From basics to clinical: a comprehensive review on spinal cord injury. Prog Neurobiol. 2014;114:25–57. https://doi.org/10.1016/j.pneurobio.2013.11.002.
12. Rupp R, Biering-Sørensen F, Burns SP, et al. International standards for neurological classification of spinal cord injury. Top Spinal Cord Inj Rehabil. 2021;27(2):1–22. https://doi.org/10.46292/sci2702-1.

13. Hachem LD, Ahuja CS, Fehlings MG. Assessment and management of acute spinal cord injury: from point of injury to rehabilitation. J Spinal Cord Med. 2017;40(6):665–75. https://doi.org/10.1080/10790268.2017.1329076.
14. Hachem LD, Fehlings MG. Pathophysiology of spinal cord injury. Neurosurg Clin N Am. 2021;32(3):305–13. https://doi.org/10.1016/j.nec.2021.03.002.
15. Kwon B, et al. Pathophysiology and pharmacologic treatment of acute spinal cord injury. Spine J. 2004;4(4):451–64. https://doi.org/10.1016/j.spinee.2003.07.007.
16. Yue JK, Winkler EA, Rick JW, et al. Update on critical care for acute spinal cord injury in the setting of polytrauma. Neurosurg Focus. 2017;43(5):E19. https://doi.org/10.3171/2017.7.FOCUS17396.
17. Jain NB, Ayers GD, Peterson EN, et al. Traumatic spinal cord injury in the United States, 1993–2012. JAMA. 2015;313(22):2236. https://doi.org/10.1001/jama.2015.6250.
18. Compston A. Aids to the Investigation of Peripheral Nerve Injuries. Medical Research Council: Nerve Injuries Research Committee. His Majesty's Stationery Office: 1942; pp. 48 (iii) and 74 figures and 7 diagrams; with Aids to the Examination of the Peripheral Nervous System. By Michael O'Brien for the Guarantors of Brain. Saunders Elsevier: 2010; pp. [8] 64 and 94 Figures. Brain. 2010;133(10):2838–44. https://doi.org/10.1093/brain/awq270.
19. Eldahan KC, Rabchevsky AG. Autonomic dysreflexia after spinal cord injury: systemic pathophysiology and methods of management. Auton Neurosci. 2018;209:59–70. https://doi.org/10.1016/j.autneu.2017.05.002.
20. Ditunno JF, Little JW, Tessler A, Burns AS. Spinal shock revisited: a four-phase model. Spinal Cord. 2004;42(7):383–95. https://doi.org/10.1038/sj.sc.3101603.
21. Ruiz IA, Squair JW, Phillips AA, et al. Incidence and natural progression of neurogenic shock after traumatic spinal cord injury. J Neurotrauma. 2018;35(3):461–6. https://doi.org/10.1089/neu.2016.4947.
22. Podolsky S, Baraff LJ, Simon RR, Hoffman JR, Larmon B, Ablon W. Efficacy of cervical spine immobilization methods. J Trauma. 1983;23(6):461–5. https://doi.org/10.1097/00005373-198306000-00003.
23. Streijger F, Lee JHT, Manouchehri N, et al. Responses of the acutely injured spinal cord to vibration that simulates transport in helicopters or mine-resistant ambush-protected vehicles. J Neurotrauma. 2016;33(24):2217–26. https://doi.org/10.1089/neu.2016.4456.
24. Dvorak MF, Noonan VK, Fallah N, et al. The influence of time from injury to surgery on motor recovery and length of hospital stay in acute traumatic spinal cord injury: an observational Canadian cohort study. J Neurotrauma. 2015;32(9):645–54. https://doi.org/10.1089/neu.2014.3632.
25. Dvorak MF, Fisher CG, Hoekema J, et al. Factors predicting motor recovery and functional outcome after traumatic central cord syndrome. Spine (Phila Pa 1976). 2005;30(20):2303–11. https://doi.org/10.1097/01.brs.0000182304.35949.11.
26. Fehlings MG, Rabin D, Sears W, Cadotte DW, Aarabi B. Current practice in the timing of surgical intervention in spinal cord injury. Spine (Phila Pa 1976). 2010;35(Suppl):S166–73. https://doi.org/10.1097/BRS.0b013e3181f386f6.
27. Fehlings MG, Tetreault LA, Wilson JR, et al. A clinical practice guideline for the management of acute spinal cord injury: introduction, rationale, and scope. Gllobal Spine J. 2017;7(3_suppl):84S–94S. https://doi.org/10.1177/2192568217703387.
28. Ahuja CS, Martin AR, Fehlings MG. Recent advances in managing a spinal cord injury secondary to trauma. F1000Res. 2016;5:1017. https://doi.org/10.12688/f1000research.7586.1.
29. Walters BC, Hadley MN, Hurlbert RJ, et al. Guidelines for the management of acute cervical spine and spinal cord injuries. Neurosurgery. 2013;60(Supplement 1):82–91. https://doi.org/10.1227/01.neu.0000430319.32247.7f.
30. Lewis NE, Tabarestani TQ, Cellini BR, et al. Effect of acute physical interventions on pathophysiology and recovery after spinal cord injury: a comprehensive review of the literature. Neurospine. 2022;19(3):671–86. https://doi.org/10.14245/ns.2244476.238.

31. Hood N, Considine J. Spinal immobilisaton in pre-hospital and emergency care: a systematic review of the literature. Australas Emerg Nurs J. 2015;18(3):118–37. https://doi.org/10.1016/j.aenj.2015.03.003.
32. Prasarn ML, Hyldmo PK, Zdziarski LA, et al. Comparison of the vacuum mattress versus the spine board alone for immobilization of the cervical spine injured patient. Spine (Phila Pa 1976). 2017;42(24):E1398–402. https://doi.org/10.1097/BRS.0000000000002260.
33. Main PW, Lovell ME. A review of seven support surfaces with emphasis on their protection of the spinally injured. Emerg Med J. 1996;13(1):34–7. https://doi.org/10.1136/emj.13.1.34.
34. Castro-Marin F, Gaither JB, Rice AD, Blust RN, Chikani V, Vossbrink A, Bobrow BJ. Prehospital protocols reducing long spinal board use are not associated with a change in incidence of spinal cord injury. Prehosp Emerg Care. 2020;24(3):401–10.
35. White CC, Domeier RM, Millin MG, Standards and Clinical Practice Committee, National Association of EMS Physicians. EMS spinal precautions and the use of the long backboard – resource document to the position statement of the National Association of EMS Physicians and the American College of Surgeons Committee on Trauma. Prehosp Emerg Care. 2014;18(2):306–14.
36. Squair JW, Bélanger LM, Tsang A, et al. Spinal cord perfusion pressure predicts neurologic recovery in acute spinal cord injury. Neurology. 2017;89(16):1660–7. https://doi.org/10.1212/WNL.0000000000004519.
37. Williams AM, Manouchehri N, Erskine E, et al. Cardio-centric hemodynamic management improves spinal cord oxygenation and mitigates hemorrhage in acute spinal cord injury. Nat Commun. 2020;11(1):5209. https://doi.org/10.1038/s41467-020-18905-8.
38. Ryken TC, Hurlbert RJ, Hadley MN, et al. The acute cardiopulmonary management of patients with cervical spinal cord injuries. Neurosurgery. 2013;72(suppl 2):84–92. https://doi.org/10.1227/NEU.0b013e318276ee16.
39. Heary RF, Vaccaro AR, Vaccaro AR, et al. Steroids and gunshot wounds to the spine. Neurosurgery. 1997;41(3):576–84. https://doi.org/10.1097/00006123-199709000-00013.
40. Bracken MB. Steroids for acute spinal cord injury. Cochrane Database Syst Rev. 2012;2018(9) https://doi.org/10.1002/14651858.CD001046.pub2.
41. Guest JD, Kelly-Hedrick M, Williamson T, et al. Development of a systems medicine approach to spinal cord injury. J Neurotrauma. 2023;40(17–18):1849–77. https://doi.org/10.1089/neu.2023.0024.
42. Parent S, Barchi S, LeBreton M, Casha S, Fehlings MG. The impact of specialized centers of care for spinal cord injury on length of stay, complications, and mortality: a systematic review of the literature. J Neurotrauma. 2011;28(8):1363–70. https://doi.org/10.1089/neu.2009.1151.
43. Hasler RM, Exadaktylos AK, Bouamra O, et al. Epidemiology and predictors of cervical spine injury in adult major trauma patients. J Trauma Acute Care Surg. 2012;72(4):975–81. https://doi.org/10.1097/TA.0b013e31823f5e8e.
44. Higgs A, McGrath BA, Goddard C, et al. Guidelines for the management of tracheal intubation in critically ill adults. Br J Anaesth. 2018;120(2):323–52. https://doi.org/10.1016/j.bja.2017.10.021.
45. April MD, Arana A, Schauer SG, et al. Ketamine versus etomidate and peri-intubation hypotension: a national emergency airway registry study. Acad Emerg Med. 2020;27(11):1106–15. https://doi.org/10.1111/acem.14063.
46. Wiles MD. Airway management in patients with suspected or confirmed traumatic spinal cord injury: a narrative review of current evidence. Anaesthesia. 2022;77(10):1120–8. https://doi.org/10.1111/anae.15807.
47. Austin N, Krishnamoorthy V, Dagal A. Airway management in cervical spine injury. Int J Crit Illn Inj Sci. 2014;4(1):50. https://doi.org/10.4103/2229-5151.128013.

Pre-hospital Evaluation and Management, Part II: Fluid and Blood Pressure Management, Assessment of Hemostasis and Correction of Coagulopathy

4

Davide Corbella and Andrea Fanti

4.1 Introduction

The pathophysiologic model of traumatic spinal cord injury (tSCI) is directly derived from the one of traumatic brain injury (TBI). An initial mechanical insult creates primary damage, which is the area where the mechanical insult disrupts the organ's structure, leading to tissue death. The secondary spread of this initial insult to the surrounding areas, the secondary damage, leads to a temporary and, eventually, permanent loss of function in the adjacent areas. Primary damage is amenable only to preventive measures that reduce the mechanical impact. Secondary damage is an appealing possible target for therapeutic intervention. Several mechanisms play a role that can be synergic in the spread of the damage. So far, the scientific research has focused on hemodynamic, immunologic, and excitotoxic mechanisms. Figure 4.1 briefly shows their general mechanism of action; a chapter in this book addresses the pathophysiology basis of tSCI damages.

In 2013, the American Association of Neurological Surgeons, jointly with the Congress of Neurological Surgeons (AANS/CNS), rolled out the first guideline for hemodynamic management of tSCI [1]. Since then, several papers have challenged specific recommendations made by those guidelines. A decade after those guidelines, the World Society of Emergency Surgeons (WSES) surveyed many physicians treating tSCI with representatives from many countries, both from high and low-middle income [2]. This survey showed widespread knowledge of the current

D. Corbella (✉)
NeuroTrauma Intensive Care Unit, Department of Anesthesia, Emergency and Critical Care, Azienda Socio-Sanitaria Territoriale Papa Giovanni XXIII, Bergamo, Italy
e-mail: dcorbella@asst-pg23.it

A. Fanti
Neurosurgery Unit, Department of Neurosciences, Azienda Socio-Sanitaria Territoriale Papa Giovanni XXIII, Bergamo, Italy
e-mail: afanti@asst-pg23.it

E. Brogi et al. (eds.), *Traumatic Spinal Cord Injury*, Hot Topics in Acute Care Surgery and Trauma, https://doi.org/10.1007/978-3-031-99890-4_4

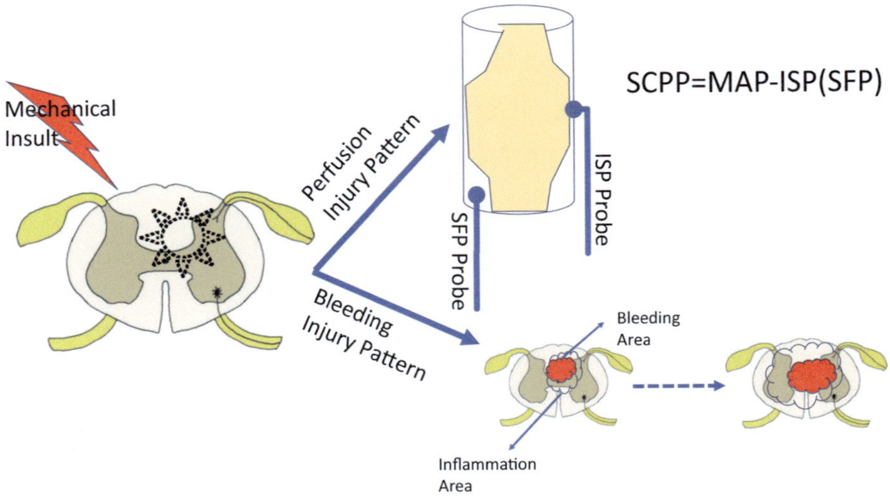

Fig. 4.1 This image illustrates the two injury mechanisms—the perfusion injury pattern and the bleeding injury pattern—that can be effectively managed in a pre-hospital setting through hemodynamic optimization and early coagulation support. The abbreviations are as follows: SCPP (Spinal Cord Perfusion Pressure), ISP (Intraspinal Pressure), SFP (Spinal Fluid Pressure), and MAP (Mean Arterial Pressure) (adapted from [https://commons.wikimedia.org/wiki/Commons:SMART-Servier_Medical_Art/Nervous_system#/media/File:Nervous_system_-_Spinal_cord_section_2_--_Smart-Servier.png], licensed under CC-BY 4.0)

guidelines and a general adherence to them. At the same time, some of the therapeutic goals were felt to be unfeasible in daily practice, and the recommendations were considered partly outdated.

Urged by this and other reports in 2024, the WSES and a multidisciplinary guideline development group under the auspices of the AO Spine and the Praxis Spinal Cord Institute produced two different guidelines [3, 4] addressing tSCI treatment options in the early phase of trauma. Those guidelines provided recommendations on several aspects, including hemodynamic treatment, use of steroids, immobilizations, multidisciplinary approach, spinal cord evaluation, and early surgery.

Pre-hospital management of tSCI is an active research area with very little established evidence and even less effective therapeutic intervention. This chapter will focus on pre-hospital hemodynamic treatment and early coagulation support.

4.2 Optimization of Spinal Cord Perfusion

Treatment options to improve neurologic function in SCI patients are limited, primarily involving urgent surgical decompression and hemodynamic management. The ultimate goal of both treatments is to enhance vascular perfusion and oxygen delivery to the injured spinal cord, thereby minimizing secondary ischemic damage to vulnerable neural tissue and improving neurologic recovery. Hemodynamic management aims to deliver enough blood flow to the spinal cord to prevent further tissue ischemia. Pivotal to hemodynamic management is the concept of "optimal blood pressure," which is influenced by two main factors: the peculiar anatomy of the spinal cord blood supply and the intraspinal parenchymal pressure (ISP) that leads to a spinal compartment syndrome similar to the concept of intracranial hypertension in TBI patients.

4.2.1 Spinal Cord Blood Supply

Spinal cord circulation has been documented in several classic anatomic studies [5–7], which many surgeons still reference. The most influential among these papers is from Albert W. Adamkiewicz (1850–1921). His description and detailed drawings suggested that the most critical input into the anterior spinal artery (ASA) is a single dominant branch of a segmental artery (SA) in the lower thoracic or upper lumbar region, characterized by a characteristic hairpin turn, the artery of Adamkiewicz [8].

Since then, further steps have been taken to understand the spinal cord's vascularization. Many studies stem from the need to preserve the spinal cord's vascularization during surgeries for the repair of thoracoabdominal aortic aneurysms. Etz et al. [9] undertook a series of anatomic explorations in pigs due to their physiologic responses similar to humans.

These anatomic studies establish the presence of an extensive collateral network that supports spinal cord perfusion. The collateral system involves a widespread axial arterial network in the spinal canal, the paravertebral tissues, and the paraspinous muscles, in which vessels anastomose with one another and the nutrient arteries of the spinal cord. The configuration of the arterial network includes inputs from the segmental vessels (intercostal and lumbar arteries) and the subclavian and hypogastric arteries. This extensive network implies a considerable reserve to ensure spinal cord perfusion when some inputs are compromised, but it also presents opportunities for vascular steal [10].

The thoracic and lumbar Segmental Arteries give rise to three major vessel groups, which anastomose within each group and with one another [9]. A schematic representation is presented in Fig. 4.2. The main feeding vessels of the network are:

- Intrathecal vessels: the ASA (anterior spinal artery) and a longitudinal chain of epidural arcades between the spinal cord and the vertebral bodies;
- Interconnecting vessels that sit outside the spinal canal along the dorsal processes of the vertebral bodies;
- Interconnecting vessels supply the paraspinous muscles, including the iliopsoas anteriorly and the erector spinae posteriorly.

The existence of this vast vascular system, rich in collaterals, must be supported by adequate perfusion pressures. Research has been conducted in the clinical setting of thoracic aorta aneurysm repair. Mean arterial pressure (MAP) augmentation and spinal fluid drain (SFD) are the most effective interventions. Both of them define

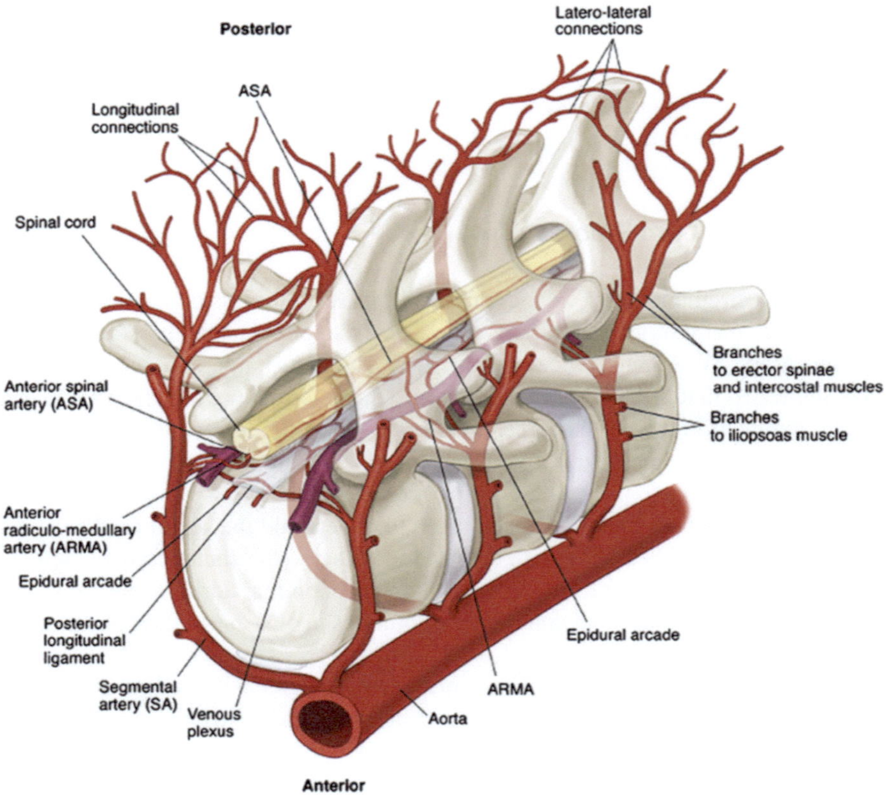

Fig. 4.2 A schematic diagram of the blood supply to the spinal cord demonstrates the relationships, relative sizes, and interconnections among the segmental arteries (SAs), the anterior radiculomedullary arteries (ARMAs), the epidural arcades, and the anterior spinal artery (ASA). The longitudinal anastomoses along the dorsal processes of the spine as well as dorsal communications (interstitial connections) between the right and the left branches of segmental arteries, are also shown. (Reprinted with permission from Etz et al. [9])

spinal cord perfusion pressure (SCPP) as the difference between MAP and spinal fluid pressure (SFP) as a proxy of the parenchymal intra spinal pressure (ISP). This model of spinal cord preservation is simple: the SCPP decreases due to segmental artery sacrifice, but the SCCP is restored by increasing the MAP or decreasing the SFP. These interventions aim to increase flow through collateral in the acute phase. The same collaterals will eventually become permanently "recruited" and give a new balance to the spinal circulation even at the return to baseline MAP and SFP [11]. However, it is unknown whether such redundancy of vascularization is present at the distal level within the spinal cord. This site is the most affected following acute post-traumatic spinal cord injury. Spinal cord swelling and extradural compressions (fragments of bone from vertebrae, intervertebral discs, and hematomas) reduce or interrupt microvascularization at this level through direct compression.

4.2.2 Spinal Cord Compartment Syndrome

The model of SCPP, defined as the difference between MAP and SFP, aligns with the physiology of a spinal cord experiencing a vascular ischemic insult. However, it does not necessarily reflect the ongoing ischemia in a traumatized spinal cord. In TBI, intracranial pressure is assumed to be the same regardless of whether it is measured with a probe inserted in the brain parenchyma or the ventricular system. Even though this is not true for every TBI patient, it can be considered a good approximation of reality. In 2015, Phang [12] demonstrated that the spinal cord swollen against the dura creates three non-communicating compartments with different SFP when directly measured, advancing a catheter in the subdural space. Data from a subset of patients from the ISCoPE study [13] confirmed this finding, showing no correlation between ISP and SFP. These findings indicate the lack of correlation between SFP and ISP when the space between the spinal cord and dura is obliterated. Furthermore, the space between the spinal cord and the dura is limited, permitting only a small amount of edema to accumulate before the cord is compressed against the dura. In the wake of spinal cord injury, the relationship between spinal cord edema and SCPP has been interpreted through the model of vascular pressure reactivity, akin to the brain autoregulation curve [14]. The spinal cord reactivity index (sPRX) ranges from −1 to +1 (sPRx≤0 indicates intact vascular reactivity, whereas sPRx >0 indicates impaired reactivity) and, when plotted against SCPP, shows a classical U-shaped curve, which defines the optimum SCPP (SCPPopt) as the SCPP that minimizes sPRx [15]. Figure 4.2 shows sPRX plotted against SCPP and the potential mechanism of damage. In the case of TBI patients, there is evidence of a better outcome if the therapy keeps the patient as long as possible and as close as possible to the optimal cerebral perfusion pressure. Unfortunately, few studies evaluated this relationship for tSCI patients [16] even though the pathophysiology at its basis is sound.

4.3 MAP Augmentation

Based on the anatomic and pathophysiologic model, increasing MAP and decreasing ISP are the two possible actions to enhance SCPP and improve spinal cord vitality. As observed in several studies, SCPP optimization is probably the fundamental determinant of spinal cord perfusion and vitality [17, 18]. However, in the prehospital setting, directly addressing the SCPP is impossible due to the need to measure ISP invasively or, at least, SFP. MAP is considered a proxy of spinal cord perfusion.

Several older studies [19, 20] and the first clinical practice guidelines [1] on tSCI have recommended that the mean arterial pressure (MAP) be augmented in patients with acute traumatic SCI to facilitate spinal cord perfusion, which often improves spinal cord neurophysiological function.

The 2013 AANS/CNS guideline for hemodynamic management of SCI [1] stated:

- Correction of hypotension in SCI (systolic blood pressure <90 mmHg) when possible and as soon as possible is recommended.
- Maintenance of MAP between 85 and 90 mmHg for the first 7 days following an acute SCI is recommended.

Systemic hypotension, defined as a systolic blood pressure of less than 90 mmHg, can harm the spinal cord and the patient and should, therefore, be avoided or corrected. There is extensive evidence that a low MAP, or systolic blood pressure, is detrimental, with several papers highlighting the close relationship between hypotension and neurological deterioration or long-term lack of improvement. Park et al. [21] evaluated 73 patients with cervical SCI who underwent decompression and stabilization to identify prognostic factors that influenced the outcome. This study determined that patients who arrived at the hospital with a MAP <75 mmHg did worse neurologically than those with a MAP >85 mmHg on admission. However, patients with an average MAP >85 mmHg, between 75 and 85 mmHg, or <75 mmHg for 1 week did not differ in neurologic recovery. These results indicate that while arriving at the hospital with a MAP <75 mmHg is unfavorable, the average MAP over the first week of hospitalization may not influence recovery. The effect of hypotension and the ASIA Grade at arrival at the Emergency Department was relevant not only in the perioperative period but was independently and significantly associated with a lack of neurological improvement at 3 months.

Catapano et al. [22] focused on a threshold of 85 mmHg and reported that patients with AIS A, B, and C injuries who did not improve neurologically had significantly more recordings below 85 mmHg. Hawryluk et al. [23] demonstrated that a higher average MAP correlated with outcome in the first 3 days after injury. The lowest MAP at which patients with no improvement were distinguished from those with 1 AIS grade of improvement was 70–75 mm Hg, suggesting that this may be the lowest blood pressure threshold associated with neurological benefit.

Even though the majority of studies report an apparent effect of hypotension on motor scores or ASIA Grade, five studies failed to demonstrate an association between MAP and neurologic recovery [16, 17, 21, 24, 25]. According to their findings, the variations in motor scores were similar between patients who needed vasopressors and those who did not, as well as between patients who were "relatively hypotensive" and those who kept their MAP within specified targets.

Despite the contrasting results of some studies and the low level of evidence (all the studies are observational, and the majority are retrospective), all the published guidelines agree on avoiding hypotension in the pre-hospital phase and recommend a MAP cut-off; see Table 4.1 for details. In their guidelines and systematic literature review, Kwon et al. [4] recommended a lower MAP limit of 75–80 mmHg. This limit is lower than the ones reported in other papers based on the reviewed studies that suggested worse neurologic outcomes with a MAP below 70, 75, or 80 mmHg or failed to demonstrate an association between neurologic recovery and MAP levels. Moreover, the variability of results across studies was large, and targeting an exact MAP goal can be challenging from a practical standpoint.

Table 4.1 Published guidelines with recommendations for hemodynamic management

	MAP lower limit	MAP upper limit	Duration of treatment after SCI	Strength of recommendation
T C. Ryken et al. [1]	MAP 85–90 mmHg		First 7 days	Weak
B K. Kwon et al. [4]	MAP 75–80 mmHg	MAP 90–95 mmHg	First 3–7 days	Weak
E. Picetti et al. [3]	MAP >85 mmHg		First 7 days	Strong

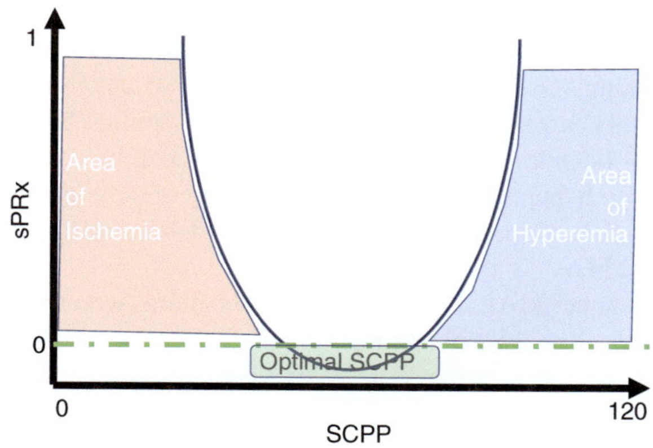

Fig. 4.3 The image illustrates the relationship between Spinal Cord Perfusion Pressure (SCPP) and the Spinal Pressure Reactivity Index (sPRx). The optimal SCPP range, where sPRx is less than or equal to 0, is highlighted in light green. The areas indicating ischemic damage and hyperemia damage are highlighted in light red and purple, respectively

The manipulation of SCPP can be detrimental to spinal cord vitality by two mechanisms, according to the concept of vascular reactivity index, see Fig. 4.3. Whereas a low SCPP exposes the spinal cord to an ischemic insult, an SCPP higher than the optimal SCPP leads to a hyperemic spinal cord. Hyperemia can lead to further damage by cord swelling, cord hemorrhage, and the local steal phenomenon [26].

A recent literature review [4] found three studies that discussed the upper limit of the MAP target range, beyond which there was no further improvement in neurologic recovery. A study by Ehsanian et al. [27] included 25 acute SCI patients and examined the impact of intraoperative MAP, measured at 5 mmHg increments, on neurologic recovery improvement in motor score was not evident in patients whose MAPs were ≥95 mmHg, but occurred when MAP was maintained between 70 and 94 mmHg. Similar results were published by Hawryluk et al. [23] and Hogg et al. [28]. Both studies showed no further neurologic improvement when MAP was ≥95 mmHg, suggesting this as a potential upper limit. Interestingly, one of the main arguments of this last study was that neurologic recovery is more closely associated with SCPP than with MAP, and there is not necessarily a linear relation between these two parameters.

Increasing the MAP beyond a certain level is not only clinically useless but also harmful, not only for the spinal cord but also because it exposes the patients to possible adverse events related to MAP augmentation strategies. Three studies from UCSF [29–31] reported high rates of adverse events (74.0–94.0%) when vasopressors or inotropes were used to maintain a MAP of at least 85 mmHg. Complications associated with the use of vasopressors or inotropes were often cardiogenic. They included bradycardia, atrial fibrillation or flutter, ventricular tachycardia, and elevated troponin or ST changes, almost all of them not life-threatening. Other authors [32] found that although maintaining MAP above 85 mmHg was not associated with an increase in severe adverse events, the use of vasopressors was, pointing out that this is a pharmacologic effect and not a "higher MAP" effect. The neurologic benefit of increasing MAP above an upper limit of 90–95 mmHg is questionable. It can be helpful only in patients with a relatively high optimal SCPP. For others, it exposes them to the side effects of vasopressors and can be detrimental to spinal cord vitality due to hyperemia. With the impossibility of defining an individualized SCPP before hospital admission, an upper limit of 90–95 mmHg can be considered effective and safe [4].

However, this upper MAP limit applies only to patients who require active MAP augmentation (e.g., through volume resuscitation and vasopressors and inotropes) and not to patients who achieve a MAP above 95 mmHg without medical intervention.

Maintaining adequate spinal perfusion pressure seems particularly important during the first week. Within that week, the first few hours (24–48 hours) appear to be the most critical [23, 33]. Considering this data, during the pre-hospital phase, it seems to be mandatory to maintain an adequate MAP range: it is imperative to avoid episodes of hypotension, which are often associated with irreversible spinal cord ischemia.

4.4 How to Achieve MAP Augmentation

Hypovolemia, spinal shock, and obstructive heart failure are the three main mechanisms responsible for hypotension in tSCI. Once obstructive heart failure, particularly pneumothorax, is excluded, distinguishing between hypovolemia and spinal shock in the pre-hospital setting holds limited importance, as the treatment approach—vasopressors and volume resuscitation—remains the same. No trial compared head-to-head in the pre-hospital setting or the acute phase of tSCI, different strategies of MAP augmentation like different types of pressors or fluids, or strategies preferring fluid resuscitation over vasopressors. Some data can be derived from retrospective observational or physiologic studies, but they are of limited generalizability. In 2014, Werndle et al. [34] published the initial findings of the Injured Spinal Cord Pressure Evaluation Study (ISCoPE). In this study, patients affected by severe tSCI underwent laminectomy and bony realignment. During surgery, a catheter was placed subdurally at the site of maximum cord swelling according to a pre-procedural MRI scan. The probe was kept in place for 7 days to monitor the continuous ISP. The authors tested the ability of different interventions to decrease ISP or increase SCPP. Inotropes resulted in an increase in MAP and ISP with a net increase in SCPP. Other interventions routinely used in TBI patients to decrease ICP (i.e., hyperventilation, mannitol boluses, deepening of sedation) did not affect ISP and SCPP. They did not test the administration of hypertonic saline, which has the theoretical potential to increase MAP through its osmotic power and to decrease ISP acting on tissue edema. There is no evidence on the best choice of inotropes to achieve MAP augmentation. Inoue et al. [31] and Readdy et al. [29, 30] found a slightly higher incidence of complications in their retrospective studies when they used dopamine instead of phenylephrine for MAP augmentation. Altaf et al. [35] compared in a cross-over study, the infusion of dopamine vs. norepinephrine increased MAP and SCPP. Despite a similar MAP, SCPP was higher when they used norepinephrine instead of dopamine because the dopamine infusion correlated with an SFP increase. The authors found a 2 mmHg difference in SCPP that, even though significant, was impossible to define as clinically relevant. Furthermore, the study utilized SFP instead of ISP, increasing the risk of an unreliable SCPP read in patients with a swollen spinal cord against the dura.

Volume resuscitation in the pre-hospital setting is challenging. Targeting a normal or supranormal MAP using only crystalloids exposes the patient to the risk of hypothermia, dilutional coagulopathy, and metabolic acidosis, mainly if normal saline is used for volume resuscitation. Several studies referenced in recent guidelines [36] highlight the need to decrease crystalloids in the early phase of trauma and use blood products (i.e., fresh frozen plasma, fibrinogen) and packed red blood cells to restore coagulation and oxygen delivery. A reasonable approach could be an early transfusion of blood products and initiating vasopressors. Hypertonic saline is appealing because it can increase circulating volume and decrease edema. However, as previously mentioned, there are no data on tSCI patients or studies comparing different strategies of fluid resuscitation (for ex., crystalloids vs. blood products).

4.5 Coagulation Support

The mechanical hit in tSCI leads to disruption of blood vessels and breakdown of the blood-spinal cord barrier. The intraparenchymal hemorrhage brings further damage to the spinal cord through two main mechanisms. The first is related to the compression the hematoma exerts on the adjacent structures, impairing the blood flow in those areas, resulting in an enlargement of the ischemic lesions. The second is mediated by generating an inflammatory response associated with vasogenic and cytotoxic edema. A thorough evaluation of these mechanisms is beyond the scope of this chapter. Nevertheless, it is important to remember two key pieces of data, even in the pre-hospital setting. The location of the intraparenchymal bleeding corresponds to the neurological level of the injury [37], its extension correlates with the severity of the final injury [38], and eventually, its evolution into large cystic cavitations predicts poor neurological recovery. Bleeding within the spinal cord indicates not only the site of the most significant energy impact and tissue disruption but also the area where a harmful cycle of bleeding, toxic heme products, free radical production, and leukocyte infiltration occurs. Even with this discouraging perspective, bleeding remains an active process that can be managed. Several papers showed in animal models that bleeding inside the spinal cord is an evolving process, and in the first hours after the mechanical insult, the hemorrhagic area tends to enlarge [39, 40]. Serial MRI studies in humans confirmed the tendency of active bleeding in the first period after the hit [41]. These studies suggest the existence of a time frame early after the hit in which active bleeding is susceptible to control. Fan et al. [42] showed in a rat model of spinal cord injury that early administration of procoagulants reduced the area of hemorrhage and tissue necrosis, resulting in less local inflammation and better functional recovery. In 2019, Yoshizaki et al. [43] evaluated the effect of tranexamic acid (TXA) on spinal cord bleeding in a murine model of contusion tSCI. In their experiment, the administration of TXA reduced the area of intraspinal bleeding compared to mice treated with normal saline or heparin. Bleeding inside the spinal cord was associated with local inflammation and tissue destruction, mainly driven by the presence of heme. In their model of bleeding (direct intraspinal injection of autologous packed red blood cells vs. free heme from lysed autologous red cells), the amount of free heme correlated with the area of demyelination on the spinal cord and with the activation of inflammatory cells. TXA administration significantly reduced inflammation and demyelination, probably by reducing the bleeding and the spread of free-heme products. It eventually led to a better functional recovery of the mice. Although TXA in animal models is usually administered at a dose several times the one used for humans, these results are comforting, suggesting a possible positive role of ultra-early administration of TXA for tSCI patients. To date, no study has defined the effect of pre-hospital administration of any anticoagulants in tSCI. The spinal cord shares several characteristics and mechanisms of injury and repair with the brain. Some advice can be derived from the data of the CRASH-3. The CRASH-3 [44] study showed a reduction in mortality and suggested a trend toward a better functional outcome in mild-moderate TBI patients treated with TXA. Data from pre-clinical studies and data derived from TBI patients suggest the possible positive role of TXA and early coagulation support in patients affected by tSCI. Aggressive early coagulation and reversal of anticoagulation are supported in the WSES guidelines [3] as they reduce bleeding from other sites, decreasing hemodynamic instability and reducing exposure to hypotensive episodes. Moreover, it may reduce intraspinal bleeding, which acts directly on one of the major mechanisms of spinal injury. The Sixth edition of the European guideline on the management of major bleeding and coagulopathy following trauma [36] does not specifically address the treatment of tSCI apart from the indication of keeping a higher MAP than the one pursued in the bleeding patient without TBI or tSCI. The literature on this topic is rather scanty. However, it is probably reasonable to adopt the recommendations used in TBI patients: keeping a higher MAP, early aggressive coagulation support, continuous monitoring of coagulation status by viscoelastic assays or traditional ones, reversal of anticoagulation, platelet transfusion, and possibly reversal of antiplatelet drugs. In the pre-hospital setting, TXA, plasma administration, and local hemostatic agents are the main interventions studied to address traumatic coagulopathy. In tSCI, TXA is probably effective according to pre-clinical data, and in parallel to results in TBI, plasma administration has a strong rationale for reducing bleeding and, hence, increasing hemodynamic stability. However, definitive data are lacking.

4.6 Conclusions

The primary goal in managing a patient with a spinal cord injury (SCI) is to maintain spinal cord perfusion pressure (SCPP) to prevent secondary ischemic damage. SCPP would be the ideal parameter to monitor to assess the adequacy of spinal cord perfusion, but measuring this data is not feasible in a prehospital setting. Scientific literature suggests the use of MAP as a surrogate indicator. Although there are some uncertainties regarding the reliability of MAP for this purpose, there are currently no valid alternatives. Therefore, MAP remains the only option available in the prehospital setting. Early aggressive coagulation support has a strong rationale and is supported by literature from TBI patients and pre-clinical research. Despite the paucity of data in tSCI patients, TXA probably has a role as the reversal of blood thinner medications. However, strong evidence from human trials is lacking.

References

1. Ryken TC, Hurlbert RJ, Hadley MN, et al. The acute cardiopulmonary management of patients with cervical spinal cord injuries. Neurosurgery. 2013;72(Suppl 2):84–92. https://doi.org/10.1227/NEU.0b013e318276ee16.
2. Picetti E, Iaccarino C, Coimbra R, et al. The acute phase management of spinal cord injury affecting polytrauma patients: the ASAP study. World J Emerg Surg. 2022;17:20. https://doi.org/10.1186/s13017-022-00422-2.
3. Picetti E, Demetriades AK, Catena F, et al. Early management of adult traumatic spinal cord injury in patients with polytrauma: a consensus and clinical recommendations jointly developed by the World Society of Emergency Surgery (WSES) & the European Association of Neurosurgical Societies (EANS). World J Emerg Surg. 2024;19:4. https://doi.org/10.1186/s13017-023-00525-4.
4. Kwon BK, Tetreault LA, Martin AR, et al. A clinical practice guideline for the management of patients with acute spinal cord injury: recommendations on hemodynamic management. Global Spine J. 2024;14:187S–211S. https://doi.org/10.1177/21925682231202348.
5. Lazorthes G, Gouaze A, Zadeh JO, et al. Arterial vascularization of the spinal cord. Recent studies of the anastomotic substitution pathways. J Neurosurg. 1971;35:253–62. https://doi.org/10.3171/jns.1971.35.3.0253.
6. Lazorthes G, Poulhes J, Bastide G, et al. Research on the arterial vascularization of the medulla; applications to medullary pathology. Bull Acad Natl Med. 1957;141:464–77.
7. Lazorthes G, Poulhes J, Bastide G, et al. Arterial vascularization of the spine; anatomic research and applications in pathology of the spinal cord and aorta. Neurochirurgie. 1958;4:3–19.
8. Adamkiewicz A. Die Blutgefäße des menschlichen Rückenmarks. Sitzungsberichte der königl. Akademie d Wissenschaften, Wien Math Naturw Classe. 1881;84:496.
9. Etz CD, Kari FA, Mueller CS, et al. The collateral network concept: a reassessment of the anatomy of spinal cord perfusion. J Thorac Cardiovasc Surg. 2011;141:1020–8. https://doi.org/10.1016/j.jtcvs.2010.06.023.

10. Griepp EB, Di Luozzo G, Schray D, et al. The anatomy of the spinal cord collateral circulation. Ann Cardiothorac Surg. 2012;1:350–7. https://doi.org/10.3978/j.issn.2225-319X.2012.09.03.
11. Wynn MM, Acher CW. A modern theory of spinal cord ischemia/injury in thoracoabdominal aortic surgery and its implications for prevention of paralysis. J Cardiothorac Vasc Anesth. 2014;28:1088–99. https://doi.org/10.1053/j.jvca.2013.12.015.
12. Phang I, Papadopoulos MC. Intraspinal pressure monitoring in a patient with spinal cord injury reveals different Intradural compartments: injured spinal cord pressure evaluation (ISCoPE) study. Neurocrit Care. 2015;23:414–8. https://doi.org/10.1007/s12028-015-0153-6.
13. Hogg FRA, Gallagher MJ, Kearney S, et al. Acute spinal cord injury: monitoring lumbar cerebrospinal fluid provides limited information about the injury site. J Neurotrauma. 2020;37:1156–64. https://doi.org/10.1089/neu.2019.6789.
14. Zeiler FA, Donnelly J, Calviello L, et al. Pressure autoregulation measurement techniques in adult traumatic brain injury, part II: a scoping review of continuous methods. J Neurotrauma. 2017;34:3224–37. https://doi.org/10.1089/neu.2017.5086.
15. Saadoun S, Papadopoulos MC. Targeted perfusion therapy in spinal cord trauma. Neurotherapeutics. 2020;17:511–21. https://doi.org/10.1007/s13311-019-00820-6.
16. Chen S, Smielewski P, Czosnyka M, et al. Continuous monitoring and visualization of optimum spinal cord perfusion pressure in patients with acute cord injury. J Neurotrauma. 2017;34:2941–9. https://doi.org/10.1089/neu.2017.4982.
17. Saadoun S, Chen S, Papadopoulos MC. Intraspinal pressure and spinal cord perfusion pressure predict neurological outcome after traumatic spinal cord injury. J Neurol Neurosurg Psychiatry. 2017;88:452–3. https://doi.org/10.1136/jnnp-2016-314600.
18. Squair JW, Bélanger LM, Tsang A, et al. Spinal cord perfusion pressure predicts neurologic recovery in acute spinal cord injury. Neurology. 2017;89:1660–7. https://doi.org/10.1212/WNL.0000000000004519.
19. Levi L, Wolf A, Belzberg H. Hemodynamic parameters in patients with acute cervical cord trauma: description, intervention, and prediction of outcome. Neurosurgery. 1993;33:1007–16; discussion 1016–1017
20. Vale FL, Burns J, Jackson AB, Hadley MN. Combined medical and surgical treatment after acute spinal cord injury: results of a prospective pilot study to assess the merits of aggressive medical resuscitation and blood pressure management. J Neurosurg. 1997;87:239–46. https://doi.org/10.3171/jns.1997.87.2.0239.
21. Park JH, Kim JH, Roh SW, et al. Prognostic factor analysis after surgical decompression and stabilization for cervical spinal-cord injury. Br J Neurosurg. 2017;31:194–8. https://doi.org/10.1080/02688697.2016.1247781.
22. Catapano JS, John Hawryluk GW, Whetstone W, et al. Higher mean arterial pressure values correlate with neurologic improvement in patients with initially complete spinal cord injuries. World Neurosurg. 2016;96:72–9. https://doi.org/10.1016/j.wneu.2016.08.053.
23. Hawryluk G, Whetstone W, Saigal R, et al. Mean arterial blood pressure correlates with neurological recovery after human spinal cord injury: analysis of high frequency physiologic data. J Neurotrauma. 2015;32:1958–67. https://doi.org/10.1089/neu.2014.3778.
24. Martin ND, Kepler C, Zubair M, et al. Increased mean arterial pressure goals after spinal cord injury and functional outcome. J Emerg Trauma Shock. 2015;8:94–8. https://doi.org/10.4103/0974-2700.155507.
25. Sewell MD, Vachhani K, Hockings J, et al. A hemodynamic safety checklist can improve blood pressure monitoring in patients with acute spinal cord injury. World Neurosurg. 2019;128:e225–30. https://doi.org/10.1016/j.wneu.2019.04.106.
26. Gallagher MJ, Hogg FRA, Zoumprouli A, et al. Spinal cord blood flow in patients with acute spinal cord injuries. J Neurotrauma. 2019;36:919–29. https://doi.org/10.1089/neu.2018.5961.
27. Ehsanian R, Haefeli J, Quach N, et al. Exploration of surgical blood pressure management and expected motor recovery in individuals with traumatic spinal cord injury. Spinal Cord. 2020;58:377–86. https://doi.org/10.1038/s41393-019-0370-5.

28. Hogg FRA, Kearney S, Zoumprouli A, et al. Acute spinal cord injury: correlations and causal relations between intraspinal pressure, spinal cord perfusion pressure, lactate-to-pyruvate ratio, and limb power. Neurocrit Care. 2021;34:121–9. https://doi.org/10.1007/s12028-020-00988-2.
29. Readdy WJ, Saigal R, Whetstone WD, et al. Failure of mean arterial pressure goals to improve outcomes following penetrating spinal cord injury. Neurosurgery. 2016;79:708–14. https://doi.org/10.1227/NEU.0000000000001249.
30. Readdy WJ, Whetstone WD, Ferguson AR, et al. Complications and outcomes of vasopressor usage in acute traumatic central cord syndrome. J Neurosurg Spine. 2015;23:574–80. https://doi.org/10.3171/2015.2.SPINE14746.
31. Inoue T, Manley GT, Patel N, Whetstone WD. Medical and surgical management after spinal cord injury: vasopressor usage, early surgerys, and complications. J Neurotrauma. 2014;31:284–91. https://doi.org/10.1089/neu.2013.3061.
32. Weinberg JA, Farber SH, Kalamchi LD, et al. Mean arterial pressure maintenance following spinal cord injury: does meeting the target matter? J Trauma Acute Care Surg. 2021;90:97–106. https://doi.org/10.1097/TA.0000000000002953.
33. Haldrup M, Dyrskog S, Thygesen MM, et al. Initial blood pressure is important for long-term outcome after traumatic spinal cord injury. J Neurosurg Spine. 2020;33:256–60. https://doi.org/10.3171/2020.1.SPINE191005.
34. Werndle MC, Saadoun S, Phang I, et al. Monitoring of spinal cord perfusion pressure in acute spinal cord injury: initial findings of the injured spinal cord pressure evaluation study. Crit Care Med. 2014;42:646–55. https://doi.org/10.1097/CCM.0000000000000028.
35. Altaf F, Griesdale DE, Belanger L, et al. The differential effects of norepinephrine and dopamine on cerebrospinal fluid pressure and spinal cord perfusion pressure after acute human spinal cord injury. Spinal Cord. 2017;55:33–8. https://doi.org/10.1038/sc.2016.79.
36. Rossaint R, Afshari A, Bouillon B, et al. The European guideline on management of major bleeding and coagulopathy following trauma: sixth edition. Crit Care. 2023;27:80. https://doi.org/10.1186/s13054-023-04327-7.
37. Silberstein M, Tress BM, Hennessy O. Prediction of neurologic outcome in acute spinal cord injury: the role of CT and MR. AJNR Am J Neuroradiol. 1992;13:1597–608.
38. Aarabi B, Sansur CA, Ibrahimi DM, et al. Intramedullary lesion length on postoperative magnetic resonance imaging is a strong predictor of ASIA impairment scale grade conversion following decompressive surgery in cervical spinal cord injury. Neurosurgery. 2017;80:610–20. https://doi.org/10.1093/neuros/nyw053.
39. Choo AM-T, Liu J, Liu Z, et al. Modeling spinal cord contusion, dislocation, and distraction: characterization of vertebral clamps, injury severities, and node of Ranvier deformations. J Neurosci Methods. 2009;181:6–17. https://doi.org/10.1016/j.jneumeth.2009.04.007.
40. Malomo T, Allard Brown A, Bale K, et al. Quantifying intraparenchymal hemorrhage after traumatic spinal cord injury: a review of methodology. J Neurotrauma. 2022;39:1603–35. https://doi.org/10.1089/neu.2021.0317.
41. Rutges JPHJ, Kwon BK, Heran M, et al. A prospective serial MRI study following acute traumatic cervical spinal cord injury. Eur Spine J. 2017;26:2324–32. https://doi.org/10.1007/s00586-017-5097-4.
42. Fan H, Chen K, Duan L, et al. Beneficial effects of early hemostasis on spinal cord injury in the rat. Spinal Cord. 2016;54:924–32. https://doi.org/10.1038/sc.2016.58.
43. Yoshizaki S, Kijima K, Hara M, et al. Tranexamic acid reduces heme cytotoxicity via the TLR4/TNF axis and ameliorates functional recovery after spinal cord injury. J Neuroinflammation. 2019;16:160. https://doi.org/10.1186/s12974-019-1536-y.
44. CRASH-3 trial collaborators. Effects of tranexamic acid on death, disability, vascular occlusive events and other morbidities in patients with acute traumatic brain injury (CRASH-3): a randomised, placebo-controlled trial. Lancet. 2019;394 https://doi.org/10.1016/S0140-6736(19)32233-0.

Role of Trauma Networks and Neurocritical Care Specialization in the Treatment of Spinal Cord Injury

5

Umar F. Bhatti and Ara Ko

5.1 Spinal Cord Injury

About 90% of SCIs are traumatic and result from falls, road accidents, sports-related injuries, or violence [7]. The age distribution is bimodal, with the first peak involving young adults and the second peak involving adults over 60 years [8]. Patients with SCI may present with or without neurological deficits. The injury mechanism and neurological symptoms can provide important clues about the nature and location of spinal injury. The four spine sections are the cervical, thoracic, lumbar, and sacral spine, with each section protecting a different group of nerves. About 50% of spinal injuries occur in the cervical region, 35% in the thoracic region, and 11% in the lumbar region [9] (Fig. 5.1).

A sudden traumatic impact on the spinal column can result in fracture or dislocation of the vertebrae. The damaged vertebrae may then deliver the mechanical force to the spinal cord, resulting in primary injury [10]. The mechanical force of impact may damage the ascending and descending spinal tracts, causing spinal shock, systemic hypotension, vasospasm, and progressive ischemia to the spinal cord [11, 12]. The secondary injury follows the primary insult within minutes of impact and may continue for weeks to months, causing progressive damage to the spinal column [13]. Secondary spinal injury refers to cellular biochemical responses to primary insults, such as neuroinflammation, glial activation, oxidative stress, and lipid peroxidation, and may result in delayed neurological deterioration [14].

U. F. Bhatti · A. Ko (✉)
Cedars-Sinai Medical Center, Los Angeles, CA, USA
e-mail: Ara.Ko@cshs.org

E. Brogi et al. (eds.), *Traumatic Spinal Cord Injury*, Hot Topics in Acute Care Surgery and Trauma, https://doi.org/10.1007/978-3-031-99890-4_5

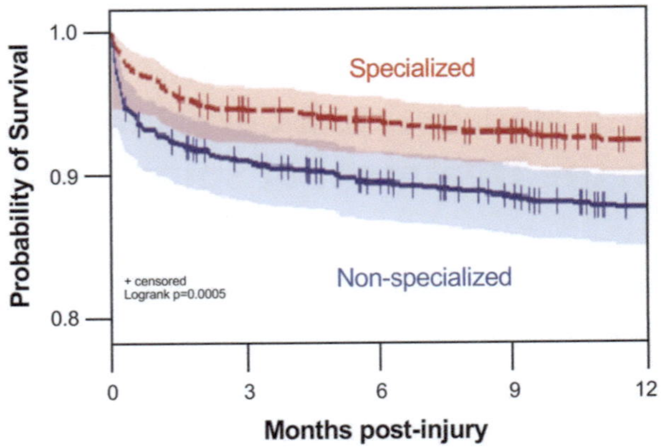

Fig. 5.1 Kaplan–Meier plot or survival among 1920 patients with acute traumatic spinal cord injuries (tSCI) admitted to specialized ($n = 960$) or non-specialized care ($n = 960$) in the province of British Columbia from 2001 to 2017 with number of subjects at risk and 95% Hall–Wellner Bands [1]

5.2 Management of SCI

Despite recent advances in the understanding of the pathophysiology of SCI, it remains a devastating event carrying a high degree of morbidity and mortality [15]. In an alert patient who is not intoxicated, an SCI can be safely excluded when there are no neurological deficits, pain, or tenderness along the spine. However, evaluation can be challenging in comatose patients and those with depressed levels of consciousness. The evaluation of SCI begins in the pre-hospital setting, where any patient suspected of having SCI, regardless of the level of consciousness, should be placed in spinal precautions on a backboard with the head rigidly stabilized with tape and the neck placed in a cervical collar [16].

Spinal injuries rarely occur in isolation and are often associated with polytrauma [17]. Upon arrival in the emergency department, a rapid assessment of injuries should be performed according to the Advanced Trauma Life Support (ATLS) guidelines [18]. Depending on the injury, SCI patients may experience a wide array of symptoms, from simple neurological deficits to paraplegia or quadriplegia, severe neurogenic shock, and even death. About 5% of these patients may experience the onset of neurological symptoms upon arrival to the hospital, usually due to worsening spinal ischemia and progression of cord edema. Excessive spinal movement may exacerbate the injury. Therefore, spinal stabilization is of critical importance in the early management of SCI. Once the spine is stabilized, further evaluation of spinal cord injury can be deferred until other life-threatening conditions, such as respiratory insufficiency and hypotension, are addressed. Ideally, a mean arterial pressure (MAP) goal of 85–90 mmHg is to be maintained for adequate spinal perfusion. However, other life-threatening injuries, such as a significant vascular injury, may require a reduction in blood pressure to control hemorrhage. In such patients, an augmentation of blood pressure may result in worsening hemorrhagic shock, and therefore, spinal perfusion blood pressure goals should be deferred until it's safe to initiate [15]. Once hemodynamically stable, the patient should initially be assessed with computed tomography (CT) imaging to characterize the spinal injury. If a fracture of the cervical column is diagnosed, CT angiography of the head and neck should be performed, given the high likelihood of cerebrovascular injuries with high spinal fractures. In cases where no apparent spinal injury is detected on the CT scan, magnetic resonance imaging (MRI) can demonstrate ligamentous injury and spinal cord injury [15].

Once an SCI is diagnosed, the on-call spine surgeon should be consulted for further management and recommendations. Early management of acute traumatic SCI may include surgical decompression and medical management in an intensive care setting [15]. Since not all hospitals have an on-call spine surgery team and critical care expertise, the emergency physician or trauma surgeon should quickly assess whether the patient will require transfer to a higher level of care. If it is determined that the current hospital is not equipped to care for spine injuries, it is safest to stabilize the patient and transfer to an appropriate center with SCI expertise after consultation with the accepting trauma surgeon.

5.3 Determining the Need to Transfer SCI Patients

Trauma patients who require prompt transfer to a higher level of care in the trauma system can be identified based on physiologic parameters, including significant hypotension as a result of severe injury and depressed neurological function, as determined by the Glasgow Coma Scale (GCS). However, the need to transfer patients for serious injuries that do not result in significant hemodynamic derangements may be less obvious. Therefore, healthcare providers in community hospitals and Level III trauma centers must be diligent in recognizing such injuries and initiating the transfer process in a timely fashion.

Any patient with significant injuries should be triaged for transfer to an appropriate higher-level center. Any signs of paralysis or paresthesia during the primary survey indicate a possible injury to the spine, and such patients should be placed in spinal precautions. Once the injury has been identified, the clinician should quickly assess whether the center can provide appropriate care. Patients with SCIs with concomitant life-threatening injuries should receive care for such injuries and be stabilized before being transferred. All such life-saving procedures should be done expeditiously. The clinician should use their best judgment to determine whether such interventions are critical before transfer, avoiding unnecessary delays as patient outcomes are directly related to the time elapsed after injury and delivery of proper care [19]. If the local center lacks the expertise or appropriate resources, the clinician should promptly communicate with the transfer center to initiate transport to an appropriate higher-level center in the trauma network. Protective measures such as backboards and semi-rigid cervical collars should be used in preparation for transfer. Patients with injuries above the sixth cervical vertebra (C6) carry a significant risk of respiratory collapse due to diaphragmatic dysfunction from interrupted innervation from spinal levels C3–5. In such patients, if there are concerns for adequate respiratory function, endotracheal intubation should be strongly considered before transfer. Any unnecessary delays should be avoided as these patients have a propensity to deteriorate quickly in the absence of proper care.

5.4 Importance of Levels I and II Trauma Centers in Treatment of SCI

SCIs can be fatal, but more commonly, they result in varying degrees of paralysis, subsequent morbidity, need for long-term care, healthcare expenditures, and loss of productivity. In the United States, about 300,000 individuals live with SCI-induced paralysis, adding $9.8 billion to annual healthcare costs [20]. Paralysis from SCI can be reduced by prompt diagnosis, surgical decompression, medical management, and monitoring in the intensive care unit (ICU) [21]. Unfortunately, not all trauma centers have the expertise to care for SCIs. (Figure 5.1) An early transfer to an appropriate center with SCI expertise should be arranged to reduce the risk of death (1). Trauma systems regionalize care for traumatic injuries to allow for an organized approach to injury management (2,3) such that the mortality risk is significantly lower when care is provided at a Level I trauma center compared to a non-trauma center (4). The complex nature of SCIs may warrant advanced care delivered at hospitals with specialized SCI expertise (5). A trauma network comprised of hospitals designated at different levels based on their capability will provide specialized care for acute injuries. Trauma centers are categorized into five levels in the United States based on the resources available to care for acute injuries and the number of patients treated annually [6, 22]. On one end, a Level I trauma center is a tertiary care center capable of providing rapid and total care for every aspect of traumatic injury. On the other end, a Level V trauma center provides initial evaluation, stabilization, and diagnostic capabilities to transport the patient to higher care. In a trauma network, Levels I and II have promptly available neurosurgical expertise and critical care units to provide comprehensive care to SCI patients [23]. While patients with SCI should receive advanced care for their spinal injury at Levels I and II centers, it is to be acknowledged that these patients may be hundreds of miles away from these centers at the time of the traumatic event and may require early stabilization at a nearby lower tier trauma center before being transferred to a Level I or II trauma center. According to a systematic review of the literature by Parent et al., an early transfer to specialized centers is associated with decreased length of stay and overall mortality in SCI patients [24].

5.5 Neurocritical Care and SCI

Patients with life-threatening SCIs may require treatment in a neurocritical care setting. SCI patients have improved morbidity and mortality with aggressive monitoring and management in a critical care setting [25]. Treatment of SCI in a critical care setting focuses on preventing the propagation of secondary SCI [26]. Factors such as hypotension, ischemia, edema, inflammation and free radical production, hemorrhage, impaired autoregulation of micro-circulation, electrolyte disturbances, neurotransmitter accumulation, and excitotoxicity may result from the primary insult to the spinal column, and contribute to the propagation of secondary injury [27]. Worsening secondary injury may result in delayed neurological deterioration, with a reported incidence ranging from 1.8% to 10% [28]. Intensive monitoring and rapid correction of post-traumatic derangements in a critical care setting are, therefore, integral to preventing continued spinal damage after trauma.

Intensive care units specialized to treat spinal cord injured patients address the multifaceted sequelae of spinal cord injury. As mentioned previously, patients with high cervical spine injuries often suffer respiratory failure requiring intubation and mechanical ventilation, with some requiring long-term support with a tracheostomy. Due to compromised respiratory mechanics, these patients often require aggressive pulmonary toilet and respiratory treatments to avoid pneumonia and other complications. Those who have suffered an injury at T6 and above can encounter disruptions to their sympathetic tone, resulting in hemodynamic effects and ultimately autonomic dysfunction [29]. Neurogenic shock from spinal cord injury necessitates judicious volume resuscitation in addition to vasopressor support delivered and titrated in the intensive care unit, especially if required to target an augmented MAP goal of >85 mmHg for spinal perfusion in the first 5–7 days [30]. Other ICU adjuncts in managing the spinal cord injured patient include intensive nursing support, optimization of fluid balance and nutrition, aggressive bowel regimens to combat gastrointestinal dysmotility, intermittent catheterization for urinary retention, frequent turning to avoid pressure injuries, early engagement of physical medicine and rehabilitation, as well as social and psychological support. Level I and II trauma centers can offer these resources with a multidisciplinary approach and can ultimately help coordinate transfer to specialized spinal cord rehabilitation centers for continued optimal therapy.

5.6 Summary

SCIs are a severe healthcare problem resulting in significant morbidity and mortality. Patients with serious SCIs usually have other life-threatening injuries and those presenting to non-specialized centers should be stabilized and treated for concomitant life-threatening injuries expeditiously. Utilizing the resources of trauma networks, an early transfer to an appropriate center with SCI expertise and neurocritical care should be arranged as the treatment of SCI patients at specialized centers is associated with improved overall outcomes.

References

1. Dvorak MF, et al. Impact of specialized versus non-specialized acute hospital care on survival among patients with acute incomplete traumatic spinal cord injuries: a population-based observational study from British Columbia, Canada. J Neurotrauma. 2023;40(23–24):2638–47.
2. MacKenzie EJ, et al. National inventory of hospital trauma centers. JAMA. 2003;289(12):1515–22.
3. American College of Surgeons, Committee on Trauma. Resources for optimal care of the injured patient. American College of Surgeons, Committee on Trauma; 1990.
4. MacKenzie EJ, et al. A national evaluation of the effect of trauma-center care on mortality. N Engl J Med. 2006;354(4):366–78.
5. Chamberlain JD, et al. Mortality and longevity after a spinal cord injury: systematic review and meta-analysis. Neuroepidemiology. 2015;44(3):182–98.

6. Soto JM, et al. An overview of the American trauma system. Chin J Traumatol. 2018;21(2):77–9.
7. World Health Organization. Spinal cord injury. World Health Organization; 2024.
8. Stein DM, et al. Emergency neurological life support: traumatic spine injury. Neurocrit Care. 2015;23:155–64.
9. Alizadeh A, Dyck SM, Karimi-Abdolrezaee S. Traumatic spinal cord injury: an overview of pathophysiology, models and acute injury mechanisms. Front Neurol. 2019;10:282.
10. Oyinbo C. Secondary injury mechanisms in traumatic spinal cord injury: a nugget of this multiply cascade. Acta Neurobiol Exp. 2011;71(2):281–99.
11. Rowland JW, et al. Current status of acute spinal cord injury pathophysiology and emerging therapies: promise on the horizon. Neurosurg Focus. 2008;25(5):E2.
12. Fehlings MG, Sekhon L. Restoration of spinal cord function. Fardon DF. Garfin SR. OKU Spine. 2002;2:483–8.
13. Allen AR. Surgery of experimental lesion of spinal cord equivalent to crush injury of fracture dislocation of spinal column: a preliminary report. JAMA J Am Med Assoc. 1911;57(11):878–80.
14. Fehlings MG, Vaccaro AR, Boakye M. Essentials of spinal cord injury: basic research to clinical practice. Georg Thieme Verlag; 2012.
15. Wang TY, et al. Management of acute traumatic spinal cord injury: a review of the literature. Front Surg. 2021;8:698736.
16. White CC IV, et al. EMS spinal precautions and the use of the long backboard–resource document to the position statement of the National Association of EMS Physicians and the American College of Surgeons Committee on Trauma. Prehosp Emerg Care. 2014;18(2):306–14.
17. Burney RE, et al. Incidence, characteristics, and outcome of spinal cord injury at trauma centers in North America. Arch Surg. 1993;128(5):596–9.
18. Paydar S, Farhadi P, Ghaffarpasand F. Advanced trauma life support (ATLS) tips to be kept in mind. Bull Emerg Trauma. 2013;1(1):49–51.
19. Harmsen AMK, et al. The influence of prehospital time on trauma patients outcome: a systematic review. Injury. 2015;46(4):602–9.
20. National Spinal Cord Injury Statistical Center. Annual report for the model spinal cord injury care systems. Birmingham, AL: National Spinal Cord Injury Statistical Center; 2005.
21. Amar AP, Levy ML. Pathogenesis and pharmacological strategies for mitigating secondary damage in acute spinal cord injury. Neurosurgery. 1999;44(5):1027–39.
22. American Trauma Society. Trauma Center Levels Explained. Saving Lives. Improving Care. Empowering Survivors.
23. Southern AP, Celik DH. EMS, trauma center designation. In: StatPearls. StatPearls Publishing; 2024. Copyright © 2024, StatPearls Publishing LLC.: Treasure Island (FL) ineligible companies. Disclosure: Daniel Celik declares no relevant financial relationships with ineligible companies.
24. Parent S, et al. The impact of specialized centers of care for spinal cord injury on length of stay, complications, and mortality: a systematic review of the literature. J Neurotrauma. 2011;28(8):1363–70.
25. Hadley MN. Management of acute spinal cord injuries in an intensive care unit or other monitored setting. Neurosurgery. 2002;50(3):S51–7.
26. Evans LT, Lollis SS, Ball PA. Management of acute spinal cord injury in the neurocritical care unit. Neurosurg Clin N Am. 2013;24(3):339–47.
27. Hadley MN, Walters BC, Grabb PA, Oyesiku NM, Przybylski GJ, Resnick DK, Ryken TC. Pharmacological therapy after acute cervical spinal cord injury. Neurosurgery. 2002;50(3):S63–72.
28. Harrop JS, et al. The cause of neurologic deterioration after acute cervical spinal cord injury. Spine (Phila Pa 1976). 2001;26(4):340–6.
29. Alwashmi AH. Spinal cord injury and autonomic dysreflexia: a case report on an overlooked complication of spinal cord injury. Cureus. 2022;14(10):e30259.
30. Menacho ST, Floyd C. Current practices and goals for mean arterial pressure and spinal cord perfusion pressure in acute traumatic spinal cord injury: defining the gaps in knowledge. J Spinal Cord Med. 2021;44(3):350–6.

Part II

In Hospital Admission—Diagnosis and Neuromonitoring

6 Spinal Cord Injuries: General Information, Classification, Etiology, Clinical Presentation, and Evaluations

Sean O'Leary, Takara Newsome-Cuby, Usama AlDallal, Mina Guirguis, Umaru Barrie, Mazin Al Tamimi, Carlos A. Bagley, and Salah Aoun

6.1 Introduction

The estimated annual prevalence of acute spinal cord injury (SCI) in the United States is about 40 per million people, or approximately 18,000 cases each year [1]. The age distribution of SCI is bimodal, with a first peak in young adults (around 50% of new injuries) and a second peak in adults over 60 years old [2]. The average age of patients presenting with SCI has risen from 28.7 years in 1979 to approximately 42 years in 2010 [3]. Older adults are more prone to spinal cord injuries because of age-related changes in the spine, like cervical spondylosis and stenosis, the effects of medications, and reduced sensory perception [4]. Clinical outcomes, including motor, sensory, pain, and functional recovery, are generally worse in patients over 60 compared to younger patients [1, 5].

S. O'Leary
Department of Neurosurgery, University of Texas Medical Branch, Galveston, TX, USA

T. Newsome-Cuby
Kansas City University School of Osteopathic Medicine, Kansas City, MO, USA

U. AlDallal
Addenbrooke's Hospital, Cambridge University Hospitals NHS Foundation Trust, Cambridge, UK

M. Guirguis · M. Al Tamimi · S. Aoun (✉)
Department of Neurosurgery, University of Texas Southwestern Medical Center, Dallas, TX, USA
e-mail: salah.aoun@utsouthwestern.edu

U. Barrie
Department of Neurosurgery, New York University Langone Health, New York City, NY, USA

C. A. Bagley
Department of Neurosurgery, St. Lukes Health, Kansas City, MO, USA

E. Brogi et al. (eds.), *Traumatic Spinal Cord Injury*, Hot Topics in Acute Care Surgery and Trauma, https://doi.org/10.1007/978-3-031-99890-4_6

SCIs occur when the spinal cord is damaged, leading to different levels of motor and sensory deficits based on which part of the spinal cord is affected. These injuries can be caused by traumatic events, representing approximately 83% of all SCIs, such as automobile crashes (31.5%), falls (25.3%), gunshot wounds (10.4%), motorcycle crashes (6.8%), diving injuries (4.7%), and iatrogenic injuries (4.3%) [6]. Non-traumatic causes, representing 17% of all SCI, include demyelinating disease (19.1%), neoplasm (34.54%), degenerative disease (10.02%), vascular disease (12.72%), and infectious disease (17.27%) [7, 8]. Additionally, SCI can also result from spinal cord neoplasms and infections, including spinal epidural abscesses and neurosyphilis [7].

The spinal cord can be injured through several mechanisms, including compression, contusion, laceration, or vascular damage. The severity of a spinal cord injury depends on the initial impact and the spinal cord's pre-existing condition. Mechanical failure of the spinal column's osseo-ligamentous structure can lead to SCI through abrupt deformation (contusion) or direct laceration/compression by bone fragments. Gunshot wounds may directly lacerate the cord or indirectly injure it through bone or disc fragments, and the kinetic energy from projectiles can cause injury through blast cavitation. Knife wounds can result in direct, partial, or complete lacerations of the spinal cord.

SCI has a wide distribution of locations along the spinal column, with about 50% of injuries being cervical, 35% thoracic or thoracolumbar, and 11% lumbar, with the remaining 4% being unknown or unreported. The C5 level is the most commonly affected [9]. The most frequently reported post-SCI neurological condition is incomplete tetraplegia (30.1%), followed by complete paraplegia (25.6%), complete tetraplegia (25.6%), and incomplete paraplegia (18.5%) [10]. Additionally, at least 20% of SCI patients have other significant injuries, such as cerebral contusions or flail chest and blunt cerebrovascular injury [11].

6.2 Spinal Cord Tracts and Pathways

Anatomically, the spinal cord can be divided into four axonal tracts when considering injury: the posterior columns, lateral corticospinal tracts, anterior horn, and anterolateral pathways, as visualized in Fig. 6.1a. Specific types of injury are summarized in Table 6.1.

6.2.1 Posterior Column

The posterior column, or dorsal column, is responsible for proprioception and position sense (fine touch, two-point discrimination, and vibratory sensation) below the head. This pathway involves three orders of neurons [12, 13]. First-order neurons, located in the dorsal root ganglia, are pseudounipolar and have peripheral processes that receive sensory inputs from the skin and proprioceptive receptors and central processes that relay these signals to the spinal cord. Tactile mechanoreceptors

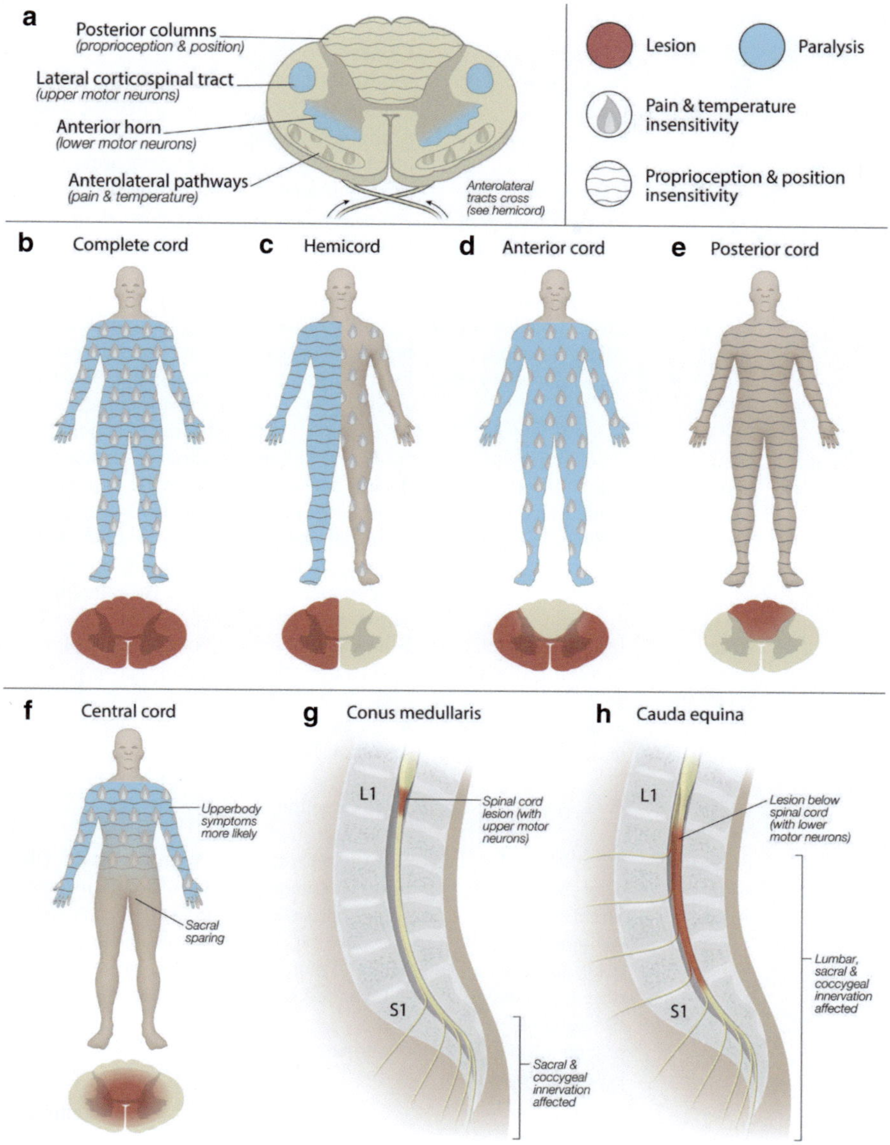

Fig. 6.1 Anatomy of the spinal cord (**a**), with complete cord (**b**), hemicord (**c**), anterior cord (**d**), posterior cord (**e**), central cord (**f**), and terminal lesions including conus medullaris (**g**), and cauda equina syndrome (**h**)

include Meissner corpuscles (fine touch and two-point discrimination), free nerve endings (fine touch), and Pacinian corpuscles (pressure and vibration). Proprioception is mediated by muscle spindles and Golgi tendon organs, which sense muscle length and contraction. The central axons of the dorsal root ganglia enter the spinal cord, primarily forming the fasciculus gracilis (lower extremities) and fasciculus

Table 6.1 Complete, incomplete, and terminal spinal cord injuries (SCI)

Type of injury	Specific injury	Description	Clinical presentation	Prognosis
Complete spinal cord injury	Atlanto-occipital dislocation	Complete or near-complete disruption of ligamentous structures between the occiput and upper cervical spine	Catastrophic neurological injury, often leading to sudden death or severe deficits, including quadriplegia	Poor prognosis with high mortality. Survivors usually have significant neurological impairment
	Complete cord injuries	Complete and irreversible loss of all neural functions below the injury level	No voluntary motor or sensory function below the injury level. No sacral sparing	Poor prognosis for regaining motor function. Minimal recovery if the injury remains complete beyond 72 hours
Incomplete spinal cord injury	Hemicord injury (Brown Sequard syndrome)	Partial injury to one side of the spinal cord, affecting different nerve tracts	Ipsilateral motor deficits and proprioception loss, with contralateral loss of pain and temperature sensation	Variable recovery potential. Patients may recover significant function depending on the severity of the injury
	Anterior cord syndrome	Injury to the anterior two-thirds of the spinal cord, often due to infarction of the anterior spinal artery	Bilateral motor dysfunction and loss of pain and temperature sensation below the injury. Proprioception is preserved	Poor prognosis for motor recovery. Sensory deficits typically persist, with varying degrees of motor recovery
	Posterior cord syndrome	Selective dysfunction of proprioception, vibration sense, two-point discrimination, and deep touch due to ischemia or compression of the posterior spinal cord	Sensory ataxia, positive Romberg sign, Lhermitte's sign, and hypotonia. Minimal motor deficits, prominent sensory disturbances	Prognosis varies, but sensory deficits are typically persistent. Motor function is usually preserved

(continued)

Table 6.1 (continued)

Type of injury	Specific injury	Description	Clinical presentation	Prognosis
	Central cord syndrome	Injury primarily affecting the white matter of the lateral corticospinal tracts, often sparing the central gray matter	Greater motor impairment in the upper extremities compared to the lower extremities. Bladder dysfunction is common	Prognosis is generally favorable, especially in younger patients. Recovery is variable, with lower extremity function typically improving more than upper extremity function
Terminal spinal cord lesions	Conus medullaris syndrome	Injury to the conus medullaris, the tapered end of the spinal cord, leading to a mix of upper and lower motor neuron signs	Motor and sensory deficits in the saddle region and lower extremities, bladder and bowel dysfunction, sexual dysfunction	Prognosis depends on the extent of the injury. Early intervention can improve outcomes, but deficits in bladder, bowel, and sexual function may persist
	Cauda equina syndrome	Injury to the cauda equina, the bundle of lumbar and sacral nerve roots, often due to compression by a herniated disc or other mass	Severe back pain, sciatica, saddle anesthesia, bladder and bowel dysfunction, and varying degrees of lower extremity motor weakness	Prognosis depends on the severity and timing of intervention. Early decompression can lead to significant recovery, but some deficits may persist

cuneatus (upper extremities). These tracts terminate at the nucleus gracilis and nucleus cuneatus in the caudal medulla, respectively. Internal arcuate fibers from these nuclei cross the midline in the medulla, forming the medial lemniscus, which maintains a somatotopic organization as it travels to the ventral posterolateral (VPL) nucleus of the thalamus. From there, third-order neurons project to the primary somatosensory cortex, preserving the somatotopic arrangement.

6.2.2 Lateral Corticospinal Tract and Anterior Horn

Motor impulses are transmitted by the lateral corticospinal tract, containing the upper motor neurons, and the anterior horn, which relays to the lower motor neurons [13–15]. The lateral corticospinal tract, which contains over 90% of the fibers in the corticospinal tract, runs the spinal cord's length and controls the voluntary movement of contralateral limbs. Originating in the primary motor cortex in the precentral gyrus, the upper motor neurons send impulses through the tract, traveling ipsilaterally through the corona radiata, posterior limb of the internal capsule, cerebral peduncle, and basis pontis, decussating at the caudal medulla (pyramidal decussation), and then descending contralaterally into the spinal cord to the anterior horn.

Next, the impulses are transmitted via lower motor neurons in the anterior horn to muscle fibers. Motor fibers exit the spinal cord, passing through the spinal nerve root, plexus, peripheral nerve, and finally reaching the neuromuscular junction to cause muscle contraction. The decussation at the caudal medulla determines whether deficits are ipsilateral or contralateral. For example, a lesion in the left precentral gyrus causes upper motor neuron signs on the right side, while spinal cord damage on the left side (below the pyramidal decussation) results in left-sided motor deficits. Damage at the anterior horn level presents with lower motor neuron signs and ipsilateral deficits.

6.2.3 Anterolateral Pathways

The anterolateral system conveys nociception (pain) and innocuous stimuli such as temperature and some light touch. This system consists of the spinothalamic, spinoreticular, and spinomesencephalic tracts. First-order neurons enter the spinal cord via the lateral division of the dorsal root entry zone and synapse in the spinal cord gray matter. The second-order fibers decussate in the ventral white commissure within one or two segments of entry and ascend in the anterolateral quadrant of the spinal cord white matter. The spinothalamic tract originates primarily in laminae I, IV, and VI and travels to the thalamus. Collateral branches are given off to the reticular formation in the brainstem. Third-order neurons from the thalamus project to the primary sensory cortex. The spinoreticular tract originates from second-order neurons in laminae VII and VIII, synapses in the medullary and pontine reticular formation, and projects to the intralaminar thalamic nuclei. The spinomesencephalic tract originates in laminae I and V, terminates in midbrain nuclei such as the superior colliculus and periaqueductal gray, and is involved with the motivational-affective component of pain and activation of a descending analgesic system [13, 16].

6.3 Classification of Spinal Cord Injury: A Review of ASIA Impairment Scale

The American Spinal Injury Association (ASIA) Impairment Scale (AIS) is a tool for classifying SCI based on the completeness of the injury and the preservation of sensory and motor function after the resolution of spinal shock [17]. This classification system is integral for making informed treatment decisions and providing accurate prognostic information. The AIS aims to (1) standardize the documentation of SCIs, (2) guide further radiographic assessment and treatment, and (3) determine whether injuries are complete or incomplete, an important and often subtle neurologic distinction with significant prognostic implications. The AIS helps providers answer difficult questions such as "will the patient ever walk again?" and may also help predict recovery of autonomic functions such as bowel, bladder, cardiovascular, respiratory, and reproductive functions; however, this remains a topic for further study [17]. A summary of the ASIA impairment scale is presented in Table 6.2.

The AIS uses a standardized examination that includes a myotome-based motor assessment, a dermatomal-based sensory assessment, and an anorectal assessment. These evaluations assign an injury severity grade and level based on specific criteria [17]. The motor examination grades five muscle groups in the upper and lower extremities using a six-point scale (0–5). The maximum bilateral motor score in a healthy individual is 100. The sensory examination evaluates 28 dermatomes bilaterally for light touch and pinprick sensation. Sensation is graded as 0 (absent), 1 (impaired or altered), or 2 (normal), with a total score of 224 points for a fully normal sensory examination. The anorectal examination assesses voluntary motor contraction and deep anal pressure sensation in the external anal sphincter, as well as the bulbocavernosus reflex. This examination is essential for determining the completeness of the injury and evaluating for spinal shock [17].

Additionally, the AIS also classifies injuries as complete or incomplete. Complete injuries (Grade A) show no motor or sensory function below the injury site, including sacral roots. Incomplete injuries (Grades B–E) retain some motor or sensory function. The degree of motor function is further distinguished in Grades C and D based on the muscle strength below the injury level [17]. Studies show good intra- and interobserver reliability for the AIS motor and sensory assessments, with correlation coefficients generally above 0.90 [18]. The AIS has strong prognostic value, particularly in predicting ambulatory outcomes at 1 year.

Patients classified with an ASIA Grade A injury (complete injury) have a poor prognosis for regaining motor function below the level of injury. In complete spinal

Table 6.2 American Spinal Injury Association (ASIA) Impairment Scale (AIS)

Grade	Description	Key features
A	Complete: No motor or sensory function is preserved in the sacral segments S4-S5	No voluntary control of bowel or bladder, and no sensory function below the level of injury, including the sacral area
B	Incomplete: Sensory but not motor function is preserved below the neurological level and includes the sacral segments S4-S5	Some sensation below the level of injury, including sacral regions, but no motor function below the neurological level
C	Incomplete: Motor function is preserved below the neurological level, and more than half of key muscle functions have a muscle grade less than 3	Some voluntary motor function is preserved below the level of injury, but most key muscles are too weak to be functional
D	Incomplete: Motor function is preserved below the neurological level, and at least half of key muscle functions have a muscle grade of 3 or more	Significant motor function is preserved below the level of injury, with most key muscles strong enough to be functional
E	Normal: Motor and sensory function are normal	Normal motor and sensory function, though the individual may have had an SCI

cord lesions, there is no preservation of motor and/or sensory function more than three segments below the level of the injury. Approximately 3% of patients may develop some recovery within 24 hours, but recovery is essentially zero if the injury remains complete beyond 72 hours [19]. In contrast, those with incomplete injuries (Grades B, C, and D) have varying degrees of potential for recovery, with Grade D injuries having the best prognosis for functional improvement, including the possibility of ambulation [17].

6.4 Complete Spinal Cord Injury

Complete spinal cord injury includes atlanto-occipital dislocation as well as complete loss of all spinal cord function from contusions or other pathologies (Fig. 6.1a).

6.4.1 Atlanto-Occipital Dislocation

6.4.1.1 Etiology

Atlanto-occipital dislocation (AOD) is considered quite rare compared to other SCIs, with an incidence of 1% of patients presenting with cervical trauma [20]. Though rare, AOD has a high mortality, with approximately 20–30% of deaths directly related to cervical spinal cord injuries as a result of bulbar-cervical dissociation [21]. High-speed motor vehicle accidents and striking of pedestrians by motor vehicles represent the most common causes of AOD [22, 23]. Additionally, AOD is three times more common in children than adults due to the pediatric cervical spine's relatively horizontal articular surfaces and greater ligamentous laxity as well as larger head size and higher fulcrum point in these patients [20].

6.4.1.2 Anatomical Mechanism

The stability of the occipitocervical junction is maintained by two groups of ligaments [21, 24–26]. The first group, providing direct articulation stability, includes the articular capsule ligaments, anterior and posterior atlanto-occipital ligaments, and lateral atlanto-occipital ligaments. The anterior atlanto-occipital ligament is a continuation of the anterior longitudinal ligament, limiting extension and anterior displacement by connecting the atlas to the foramen magnum. The posterior atlanto-occipital ligament spans the posterior foramen magnum and the atlas, preventing excessive flexion. The lateral atlanto-occipital ligament stabilizes lateral movements, while the cruciate ligament, crossing behind the odontoid process, enhances atlanto-axial joint stability. The second group, ensuring craniocervical stability, comprises the tectorial membrane, alar ligaments, apical dental ligament, and ligamentum nuchae. The tectorial membrane, a continuation of the posterior longitudinal ligament, extends from the odontoid to the foramen magnum and resists hyperextension. Paired alar ligaments extend from the dens to the occipital condyles and atlas, restricting contralateral axial rotation. The apical dental ligament, connecting the dens to the foramen magnum, offers minimal stability. The ligamentum nuchae, extending from the external occipital protuberance to the cervical spinous processes, stabilizes the head and neck, aiding in flexion and extension control. Together, these ligaments are crucial for maintaining occipitocervical stability and preventing dislocation.

AOD results from complete or near-complete disruption of the ligamentous structures between the occiput and the upper cervical spine [22]. This injury typically results from extreme forces applied during hyperextension, hyperflexion, or lateral flexion, either individually or in combination. Hyperextension is often the predominant force, leading to rupture of the tectorial membrane [27, 28]. When the alar ligaments and tectorial membrane are compromised, the cranium can dislocate anteriorly relative to the upper cervical spine [29]. Studies suggest that hyperflexion forces may also contribute to atlanto-occipital dislocation as posterior elements of C1 and C2 are frequently separated in these cases [21, 22]. The second cervical segment of the spinal cord is particularly susceptible to trauma due to the significant forces endured by the atlantoaxial joint's ligaments and bones.

6.4.1.3 Clinical Presentation

Neurological injury from AOD can be catastrophic, frequently leading to sudden death [30]. Patients with vertebral artery insufficiency at this level may develop Wallenberg syndrome, characterized by ipsilateral cranial nerve deficits (V, IX, X, XI), ipsilateral Horner syndrome, dysphagia, and cerebellar dysfunction [31]. Brainstem compression often necessitates mechanical ventilation, complicating definitive neurological assessment. Without intervention, patients with pulmonary or cardiac arrest will succumb rapidly, but immediate artificial resuscitation can restore cardiac and respiratory function, allowing prolonged maintenance on a respirator.

Survivors of AOD typically experience significant neurological impairment, including lower cranial nerve deficits and unilateral or bilateral sensory and motor deficits, cruciate paralysis, or quadriplegia [30, 32, 33]. A reflex examination should be interpreted cautiously due to the possibility of spinal shock. Concomitant traumatic injuries to the brain, chest, abdomen, and extremities can obscure the clinical examination and associated deficits. Autonomic dysregulation, including neurogenic shock, may also be present and must be managed appropriately to ensure hemodynamic stability [30, 34]. Patients may have signs of brainstem, spinal cord, and cranial nerve injury. About 30% of those who survive present as quadriplegic and ventilator-dependent [19].

Despite the severe nature of the injury, up to 20% of patients with AOD may present with a normal neurological examination, with severe neck pain as the only symptom [35]. This highlights the importance of maintaining a high index of suspicion for AOD in any patient involved in high-energy trauma, regardless of clinical findings. Appropriate precautionary measures should be taken until the diagnosis is definitively ruled out to prevent missing an underlying AOD.

Traynelis et al. classified AOD into three distinct types based on the direction of the occiput's dislocation relative to the cervical spine [22]. Type I involves anterior displacement of the occiput in relation to C1, while Type II is characterized by a longitudinal distraction in which the occiput separates from the atlas. Type III denotes a posterior displacement of the occiput relative to C1. This classification highlights the extreme instability of these injuries, where the position of the head relative to the neck is more influenced by external forces than by any inherent characteristic of the injury. However, this system may fail to detect spontaneously repositioned or rotational injuries, such as unilateral alar ligament disruptions.

In a more recent effort to reflect injury severity and stability, Bellabarba et al. introduced the Harborview classification system [36]. This system categorizes occipitocervical injuries into three stages. Stage I represents stable, minimally displaced, or nondisplaced injuries with sufficient ligamentous integrity to allow for nonoperative treatment. Examples include unilateral alar ligament avulsion or partial ligamentous injuries. Stage II includes partially or completely spontaneously reduced bilateral craniocervical dissociation with minimal displacement, defined by Harris lines within 2 mm of the upper limit of normal. Differentiation from Stage I is achieved through a manual traction test. Stage III comprises highly unstable injuries with significant craniocervical malalignment, indicated by Harris lines exceeding 2 mm beyond normal limits, necessitating internal fixation.

6.4.2 Complete Spinal Cord Lesions

6.4.2.1 Etiology

Complete cord injury is the most severe form of spinal cord injury, resulting in total loss of all neural functions below the level of injury. This condition represents the most catastrophic outcome for individuals suffering from spinal trauma [37, 38]. Approximately 45% of SCI cases are ASIA Class A [38]. The etiology of complete cord injuries predominantly includes motor vehicle accidents, falls from height, acts of violence such as gunshot wounds and stabbings, and sports-related injuries [37, 38].

6.4.2.2 Anatomical Mechanism

The anatomical mechanism and pathophysiology of complete cord injuries involve complete loss of all spinal cord function at the level of injured spinal cord, often due to severe contusions of the cord. This disruption affects all ascending and descending neural pathways, leading to the loss of motor and sensory functions below the level of injury, along with disruption of autonomic nervous system function. Consequently, this damage results in the complete loss of voluntary motor control and sensation below the injury level, loss of bladder and bowel control, and potential immediate respiratory complications if the injury is at or above C5 [39]. Additionally, cardiovascular complications such as hypotension, increased vasovagal reflexes, bradyarrhythmia, supraventricular/ventricular ectopic beats, vasodilation, and venous stasis can occur due to autonomic dysfunction [40]. Complete injuries can occur at any level of the spinal cord, with the cervical and thoracic regions being common sites due to their vulnerability in traumatic incidents [41].

6.4.2.3 Clinical Presentation

The clinical presentation of complete cord injury includes a range of severe symptoms. Patients exhibit no voluntary motor function, no sensory function below the level of injury, and no sacral sparing, meaning there is no sensation or motor function in the S4-S5 segments, which helps distinguish complete from incomplete injury [42]. In the acute setting, reflexes such as the bulbocavernosus reflex are absent. Other symptoms include urinary retention and bladder distention, potential priapism in male patients, and variable sympathetic dysfunction, including hypotension and bradycardia in cases of cervical or high thoracic injuries [42].

6.5 Incomplete Spinal Cord Injury

Incomplete spinal cord lesions include hemisection (Fig. 6.1b), anterior (Fig. 6.1c), posterior (Fig. 6.1d), and central lesions (Fig. 6.1e). Because of the partial nature of the cord injury, these lesions are characterized by variable sensory and motor loss at and/or below the level of the lesion.

6.5.1 Unilateral Cord Injuries

6.5.1.1 Etiology

Brown-Séquard syndrome (BSS) arises from both traumatic and nontraumatic causes, with traumatic causes being more common. Although BSS is rare, with approximately 500 reported cases and an estimated prevalence of 1–4% among traumatic SCIs, its true incidence remains unknown [43, 44]. Traumatic mechanisms include gunshot wounds, stab injuries, motor vehicle accidents, blunt trauma, and vertebral fractures from falls. Nontraumatic causes, while less frequent, include vertebral disc herniation, cysts, cervical spondylosis, tumors, multiple sclerosis, radiation myelopathy, and decompression sickness. Vascular causes, such as spinal cord hemorrhage or ischemia, and infectious agents like tuberculosis, transverse myelitis, herpes zoster, empyema, and meningitis have also been implicated. Additionally, spinal cord compression from an epidural hematoma, large cervical disc herniation, spinal arteriovenous malformations (AVMs), and spinal cord herniation contribute to nontraumatic BSS [45–48].

6.5.1.2 Anatomical Mechanism

Unilateral spinal cord lesions affects various nerve tracts: loss of dorsal column function (gracile and cuneate fasciculi) results in ipsilateral loss of fine touch, vibration, and proprioception; damage to the anterior spinothalamic tracts causes contralateral loss of pain, temperature, and crude touch; complete injury to the spinocerebellar tracts results in ipsilateral loss of proprioception; and damage to the corticospinal tracts leads to ipsilateral hemiplegia below the level of injury.

6.5.1.3 Clinical Presentation

As a result of hemi-injury, which affects the dorsal column, anterior spinothalamic tract, and spinocerebellar tract, patients with BSS exhibit a combination of ipsilateral motor deficits and contralateral sensory deficits, reflecting the complex anatomical pathways disrupted by the injury [45–48]. Although pure BSS, characterized by a complete hemisection of the spinal cord, is rare, a more common variant known as Brown-Séquard plus syndrome (BSPS) has been characterized, which encompasses the involved white matter tracts of pure BSS, with additional neurological findings also present [49].

A prospective multicenter cohort study analyzed the neurological and functional recovery in patients with cervical BSPS compared to those with other forms of incomplete tetraplegia [50]. The analysis showed no significant differences in overall neurological and functional recovery between BSPS and non-BSPS patients when matched for injury severity according to their ASIA classification. However, BSPS patients exhibited better bladder function at 12 months compared to non-BSPS patients, although this difference was not deemed clinically significant. The findings suggest that classifying patients strictly as BSS or BSPS based on current criteria may be clinically irrelevant, as the neurological and functional outcomes are similar when adjusted for injury severity [50].

6.5.2 Anterior Cord Syndrome (Anterior Spinal Artery Syndrome)

6.5.2.1 Etiology

Anterior spinal artery syndrome (ASAS) results from direct or indirect injury to the ventral spinal cord, leading to infarction of nervous tissue [51]. ASAS occurs in approximately 5–8% of acute SCIs [52]. Spinal cord infarctions, which account for 1.2% of all strokes, have an incidence of 3.1 per 100,000 individuals in the United States [53]. ASAS is the most prevalent spinal cord infarction syndrome, reported in up to 87.2% of cases in some studies [31, 54].

Risk factors for ASAS include smoking, hypertension, diabetes mellitus, dyslipidemia, and a personal or family history of ischemic cerebrovascular accidents [55, 56]. Iatrogenic damage to the aorta during surgical procedures, particularly during vascular repairs or prolonged aortic clamping, can also precipitate ASAS. Less common causes include intrinsic arterial occlusion due to emboli or atheroma affecting the anterior spinal artery or its radicular branches, as well as aneurysms, trauma, and syphilitic arteritis [57]. Additionally, hypotensive states, venous infarctions, multiple sclerosis, and spinal cord impingement by fracture fragments are infrequent causes of vascular injury to the anterior cord [58–60].

6.5.2.2 Anatomical Mechanism

The anterior spinal artery supplies the anterior two-thirds of the spinal cord, including crucial motor and sensory pathways. This artery originates from the vertebral arteries at the level of the foramen magnum and extends along the length of the spinal cord, running in the anterior median sulcus up to the conus medullaris. The anterior spinal artery gives rise to several smaller sulcal and penetrating arteries that supply the anterior regions of the spinal cord. The artery of Adamkiewicz, also known as the great anterior radiculomedullary artery, is a significant vessel that often originates from the intercostal arteries between T9 and T12. This artery plays a crucial role in the blood supply of the anterior spinal cord, making it particularly important in the context of ASAS [51, 61].

Ischemia of the anterior spinal artery leads to infarction of the anterior two-thirds of the spinal cord, including the corticospinal tracts and the anterolateral system. The corticospinal tracts, responsible for voluntary motor control, are severely affected, resulting in upper motor neuron weakness and paralysis below the infarction level. Concurrently, the anterolateral system, which conveys pain and temperature sensation, is compromised, leading to the loss of these sensory modalities. The posterior columns, which are supplied by the posterior spinal arteries and mediate proprioception and vibration sense, are spared, thus preserving these functions despite the other deficits. The thoracic segment of the spinal cord is particularly vulnerable to ischemia due to the smaller caliber of the anterior spinal artery in this region and the less extensive network of radiculomedullary arteries, which provide collateral support to the anterior spinal artery. This anatomical vulnerability contributes to the prevalence of anterior spinal artery syndrome in the thoracic region and highlights the critical role of the artery of Adamkiewicz in the pathophysiology of this condition [51, 61].

6.5.2.3 Clinical Presentation

Hallmark symptoms of ASAS typically include acute back pain localized to the level of the SCI, followed by bilateral motor dysfunction and loss of pain and temperature sensation below the level of infarction [51, 61].

The severity of motor impairment can range from paraplegia to quadriplegia, depending on the level of the infarction, with lesions above the C7 level leading to quadriplegia. Involvement of the lateral horns, particularly between T1 and L2, may cause autonomic dysfunction manifesting as neurogenic bladder, bowel issues, hypotension, bradycardia, and sexual dysfunction [62]. In cases where the infarction occurs at high cervical levels, there is a risk of phrenic nerve involvement, potentially resulting in respiratory failure. While bilateral symptoms are most common due to the midline supply from the anterior spinal artery, rare instances of unilateral symptoms may occur due to the occlusion of unilateral sulcal arteries or collateral supply from posterior spinal arteries. The clinical course typically includes both acute symptoms and later manifestations such as spasticity, hyperreflexia, and persistent autonomic dysfunction [60, 63].

6.5.3 Posterior Cord Syndrome (Contusio Cervicalis Posterior)

6.5.3.1 Etiology

Posterior cord syndrome (PCS) is the least common of the SCI incomplete clinical syndromes, with an incidence of about 1% [43, 64]. Common causes include localized tumors in an estimated 78% of patients, followed less frequently by other mass effect-causing lesions such as epidural abscesses, demyelinating disorders, and vascular malformations, including spinal AVMs [65]. Traumatic injuries, though rare, can also result in PCS, typically due to hyperextension injuries that compromise the posterior columns [65, 66]. Furthermore, iatrogenic causes, such as surgical complications or radiation therapy, can lead to PCS [65].

6.5.3.2 Anatomical Mechanism

The posterior spinal cord transmits ipsilateral two-point discrimination, vibration sense, and conscious proprioception from the fasciculus cuneatus and the fasciculus gracilis to the medulla oblongata [66]. Therefore, PCS involves selective dysfunction of proprioception, vibration sense, two-point discrimination, and deep touch and pressure [12]. The damage usually occurs due to compression or occlusion of the posterior spinal artery, leading to ischemia and subsequent neuronal damage. This type of injury is more likely to occur in the cervical region due to the vulnerability of this area to trauma and compression [67].

6.5.3.3 Clinical Presentation

Key clinical signs include a positive Romberg sign, sensory ataxia, and hypotonia. Lhermitte's sign, or the "barber chair phenomenon," may present as electric shock-like sensations radiating down the spine and limbs when the head is flexed or extended [43]. This sign results from nerve fiber irritation. Clinical features often mimic those of tabes dorsalis, a neurosyphilis condition with similar sensory disturbances but distinct from posterior cord syndrome due to its preservation of motor function [43]. Common complications are neuropathic pain (78%), spasticity (44%), neurogenic bladder (78%), neurogenic bowel (33%), and urinary tract infections (33%) [65]. Minimal myelopathic findings are observed, and long-tract abnormalities are rare. Sensory deficits are prominent, while sacral sparing is absent [65].

6.5.4 Central Cord Syndrome

6.5.4.1 Etiology

Central cord syndrome (CCS) accounts for approximately 9.0% of SCIs in adults and 6.6% in children, with an annual incidence total of approximately 11,000 cases in the US, representing the most common form of SCI [43, 68, 69]. The age distribution of patients with CCS is bimodal, affecting both younger and older populations. Neurologic presentations in CCS patients are generally similar, but the traumatic causes differ and appear to be age-dependent, with a notable distinction around the age of 45–50 years.

In individuals under 45–50 years, CCS typically results from high-speed motor vehicle crashes, falls, sports-related injuries, diving accidents, gunshot wounds, and assaults. Conversely, in those over 45–50 years, CCS is more commonly caused by low-energy incidents, including low-speed motor vehicle crashes and falls [70]. This variation in injury patterns is attributed not to age itself but to morphologic and biomechanical differences between younger and older patients, such as the extent of cervical spondylosis, baseline cervical stenosis, and spinal flexibility.

6.5.4.2 Anatomical Mechanism

Within the spinal cord, gray matter is centrally located, surrounded by white matter. The gray matter forms the anterior (ventral), lateral, and posterior (dorsal) horns, which contain neurons responsible for relaying motor, autonomic, and sensory information, respectively. Recent studies have shown that CCS involves injury primarily to the white matter of the lateral corticospinal tracts, with the central gray matter typically spared [71].

CCS is characterized by diffuse axonal injury within the lateral corticospinal tracts [71]. Although hemorrhage was once considered a common feature, it is now rarely observed in modern imaging and autopsy studies. Recent research suggests that the persistent neurological deficits in CCS are likely due to Wallerian degeneration of axons adjacent to the injury site rather than direct axon loss at the epicenter [72].

The biomechanics of injuries producing CCS vary with age. In younger patients (under 45–50 years), high-energy trauma such as fracture dislocations or disc herniations from flexion-compression mechanisms are common causes [73, 74]. In contrast, older patients (over 45–50 years) more frequently experience hyperextension injuries in the presence of chronic spinal stenosis [73, 74]. Schneider's initial 1958 description linked CCS to cervical degenerative disease and hyperextension, causing ligamentum flavum buckling, as demonstrated in cadaver studies using myelography [75, 76]. While CCS can occur without underlying stenosis or radiographic abnormalities, such cases are rare [77, 78]. This is evidenced by whiplash injuries, which have been found not to typically result in CCS in patients with a normal spinal canal diameter [79].

6.5.4.3 Clinical Presentation

CCS is characterized by disproportionately greater motor impairment in the upper extremities compared to the lower extremities. Patients often present with bladder dysfunction, typically urinary retention, and varying degrees of sensory loss below the level of the lesion. Motor weakness is usually more pronounced distally in the upper limbs. Sensory disturbances can vary in severity, and myelopathic findings often include sphincter dysfunction. Sacral sparing is also a notable feature.

The diagnostic criteria for CCS are not universally applied in clinical practice, as evidenced by global surgeon surveys. A proposed enhancement to the diagnostic criteria includes a positive difference of 10 points in the lower extremity motor score compared to the upper extremity motor score on the ASIA scale [80, 81].

However, ongoing debate exists about the required severity of motor deficits for a CCS diagnosis. A variant of CCS, known as burning hands syndrome, specifically affects the lateral spinothalamic tracts, causing a burning sensation in the hands [82].

6.6 Terminal Spinal Cord Lesions

The terminal spinal cord includes the conus medullaris (Fig. 6.1g) and the nerves and nerve roots extending from the conus medullaris, which are known as the cauda equina (Fig. 6.1h).

6.6.1 Conus Medullaris Syndrome

6.6.1.1 Etiology

Conus medullaris syndrome (CMS) is estimated to have an average incidence of 1.5 per million population and a prevalence of 4.5 per 100,000 [83]. CMS represents 1.7% of SCIs [84]. The etiology of CMS is varied, with trauma being a major cause of CMS [85]. Trauma often occurs due to burst or compression fractures of the lumbar spine, leading to retropulsion of bone fragments that compress the conus medullaris [85]. CMS can also result from metastatic cancer or other space-occupying lesions, which can exert pressure on the conus [86]. Spinal infections, such as spinal tuberculosis, may cause inflammation and subsequent compression of this region [87]. Additionally, vascular lesions, including hematomas, can lead to compression of the conus medullaris [88]. Degenerative conditions like spinal stenosis or herniated discs in the thoracolumbar region are also potential causes [89, 90]. Tethered cord syndrome is characterized by stretching and traction on the conus, which can also cause CMS [91].

6.6.1.2 Anatomical Mechanism

The conus medullaris represents the tapering, distal terminus of the spinal cord. The conus medullaris is the structural continuation of the spinal cord's lower segments, transitioning from the epiconus (L4 to S1) to encompass the S2-S5 and coccygeal segments [92]. The pia mater at the conus medullaris extends downward as the filum terminale, a slender fibrous strand approximately 20 cm long. This structure anchors the conus to the coccyx through the coccygeal ligament, thereby stabilizing the spinal cord. The lumbosacral nerve roots extend inferiorly as the cauda equina [93]. Typically, the conus medullaris terminates at the middle third of the L1 vertebra. However, its position can range from as high as the middle third of the T11 vertebra to as low as the middle third of the L3 vertebra. On cross-sectional imaging, the conus medullaris is divided into left and right halves by the ventral median fissure and posterior median sulcus [93]. CMS results from damage to the conus medullaris [94].

6.6.1.3 Clinical Presentation

CMS presents with various symptoms that may vary depending on the underlying etiology and the time since onset. Symptoms can appear acutely or develop gradually. A blend of upper motor neuron (UMN) and lower motor neuron (LMN) signs may affect the perineum and distal lower extremities, with a predominant emphasis on UMN features.

Typically, CMS symptoms include motor and sensory deficits in the saddle region and lower extremities. Key clinical features include localized back pain, which, if present, is usually an early symptom characterized by aching rather than the sharp, sudden pain associated with cauda equina syndrome [95–97]. Motor dysfunction, often a later sign, manifests as varying degrees of weakness, ranging from mild to severe. Lower motor neuron signs are evident due to the involvement of lumbar nerve roots within the thecal sac before their exit at their respective vertebral levels. Diminished or absent bulbocavernosus and anal sphincter reflexes are common indicators of severe spinal cord dysfunction in CMS.

Bladder and bowel dysfunction are notable features, including symptoms such as urinary and/or bowel retention or incontinence. Sensory changes are typically localized to the area around the anus, with a sudden onset affecting both sides of the body. Associated lower motor neuron signs include areflexia (e.g., absent Achilles reflex), hypotonia, and frequent impotence or sexual dysfunction.

The acuity of onset and clinical history are instrumental in differentiating between surgical and non-surgical etiologies. Surgical lesions, such as tumors or vascular malformations, often present with a more insidious onset, while acute processes like traumatic injuries or hemorrhages may require immediate intervention to prevent further neural damage. Autoimmune and inflammatory etiologies, which are more amenable to medical treatment, typically present with acute symptomatology.

Distinguishing CMS from cauda equina syndrome is crucial due to their overlapping symptoms, particularly bowel and bladder dysfunction and lower extremity weakness. CMS often involves more pronounced UMN signs compared to cauda equina syndrome, which predominantly features LMN signs.

6.6.2 Cauda Equina Syndrome

6.6.2.1 Etiology

Cauda equina syndrome (CES) is a rare but severe condition that often manifests as acute lower back pain. Prevalence rates vary between 0.3 and 1 per 100,000 in the general population and 2–6% in patients who have undergone lumbar disc herniation surgery [98]. It represents approximately 5.2% of all SCIs. Obesity and age <50 years are the main risk factors that increase the probability of cauda equina syndrome [99]. The primary etiology, accounting for approximately 45% of cases, is herniation of a lumbar intervertebral disc [100]. Other causes include epidural abscess, spinal epidural hematoma, diskitis, tumors (both metastatic and primary central nervous system tumors), trauma with retropulsion of bone fragments, and spinal stenosis. Additionally, rare cases have been associated with chiropractic manipulation, interspinous device placement, and inferior vena cava thrombosis [101].

6.6.2.2 Anatomical Mechanism

The cauda equina, comprising the lumbosacral nerve roots, coccygeal nerve roots, and the filum terminale, is situated within the thecal sac and is suspended in cerebrospinal fluid. The dura envelops the conus medullaris, cauda equina, and the individual spinal nerve roots as they exit the spinal canal and pass through the intervertebral foramina. Within this sac, the lower sacral (S2-S5) and coccygeal roots are located posteriorly, while the lumbar and first sacral roots descend at an oblique angle. Damage to the cauda equina typically occurs below the level of L1, where the spinal cord terminates and the nerve roots are most vulnerable [102–104]. Damage is more likely to occur in areas where nerve roots are densely packed and traverse confined spaces, such as in the lumbosacral region.

6.6.2.3 Clinical Presentation

CES exhibits a range of clinical manifestations that vary in onset and severity. CES can be incomplete or complete based on the extent of nerve damage and symptomatology. Bladder dysfunction is a prominent feature, with approximately 87.5% of patients experiencing urinary retention or incontinence [105]. In cases of complete CES, urinary retention and incontinence result from extensive nerve damage, while incomplete CES may present with reduced voiding desire or straining during micturition without significant retention [105]. Bowel dysfunction, including retention or incontinence, is less common [106, 107]. Back pain and sensory deficits like sciatica often worsen in the supine position due to nerve root compression [98, 108]. Saddle anesthesia, which involves loss of sensation in the buttocks, inner thighs, and perineal regions, is a notable symptom but lacks high specificity [106, 107]. Motor impairments in CES range from weakness to flaccid paralysis that may be accompanied by decreased or absent reflexes (e.g., patellar and Achilles), hypotonia, and, in chronic cases, muscle atrophy [108]. Erectile dysfunction and sexual dysfunction are less frequent [106, 107].

6.7 Conclusion

Injuries to the spinal cord can occur at any level of the cord and can vary from minimal and transient to complete and permanent. These factors contribute to the many different clinical syndromes and clinical presentations that are seen in patients with SCI. Careful clinical examination is essential to identify the location and severity of injury. The AIS permits classification of SCI in a standardized manner. The AIS also assists with prognostication and with guiding treatment decisions. Accurate assessment of a patient's injury is the first step toward optimizing that patient's outcome.

References

1. University of Alabama at Birmingham. Data from: National Spinal Cord Injury Statistical Center, Facts and Figures at a Glance; 2024.
2. Stein DM, Sheth KN. Management of acute spinal cord injury. Continuum. 2015;21:159–87. https://doi.org/10.1212/01.CON.0000461091.09736.0c.
3. Zohrabian VM, Flanders AE. Imaging of trauma of the spine. Handb Clin Neurol. 2016;136:747–67. https://doi.org/10.1016/B978-0-444-53486-6.00037-5.
4. Ikpeze TC, Mesfin A. Spinal cord injury in the geriatric population: risk factors, treatment options, and long-term management. Geriatr Orthop Surg Rehabil. 2017;8(2):115–8. https://doi.org/10.1177/2151458517696680.
5. Furlan JC, Fehlings MG. The impact of age on mortality, impairment, and disability among adults with acute traumatic spinal cord injury. J Neurotrauma. 2009;26(10):1707–17. https://doi.org/10.1089/neu.2009.0888.
6. Chen Y, Tang Y, Vogel LC, Devivo MJ. Causes of spinal cord injury. Top Spinal Cord Inj Rehabil. 2013;19(1):1–8. https://doi.org/10.1310/sci1901-1.
7. Molinares DM, Gater DR, Daniel S, Pontee NL. Nontraumatic spinal cord injury: epidemiology, etiology and management. J Pers Med. 2022;12(11) https://doi.org/10.3390/jpm12111872.
8. Khadour FA, Khadour YA, Meng L, XinLi C, Xu T. Epidemiology features of traumatic and non-traumatic spinal cord injury in China, Wuhan. Sci Rep. 2024;14(1):1640. https://doi.org/10.1038/s41598-024-52210-4.
9. Alizadeh A, Dyck SM, Karimi-Abdolrezaee S. Traumatic spinal cord injury: an overview of pathophysiology, models and acute injury mechanisms. Front Neurol. 2019;10:282. https://doi.org/10.3389/fneur.2019.00282.
10. van Middendorp JJ, Goss B, Urquhart S, Atresh S, Williams RP, Schuetz M. Diagnosis and prognosis of traumatic spinal cord injury. Global Spine J. 2011;1(1):1–8. https://doi.org/10.1055/s-0031-1296049.
11. Sacino A, Rosenblatt K. Critical care management of acute spinal cord injury-Part II: intensive care to rehabilitation. J Neuroanaesth Crit Care. 2019;6(3):222–35. https://doi.org/10.1055/s-0039-1694686.
12. Al-Chalabi M, Reddy V, Alsalman I. Neuroanatomy, posterior column (Dorsal Column). In: StatPearls. StatPearls Publishing; 2024.
13. Neuroscience. 2nd ed. Sinauer Associates; 2001:681.
14. Emos MC, Agarwal S. Neuroanatomy, upper motor neuron lesion. In: StatPearls. StatPearls Publishing; 2024.
15. Javed K, Reddy V, Lui F. Neuroanatomy, lateral corticospinal tract. In: StatPearls. StatPearls Publishing; 2024.
16. Darby SA, Frysztak RJ. Neuroanatomy of the spinal cord. In: Clinical anatomy of the spine, spinal cord, and ans. Elsevier; 2014. p. 341–412.
17. Roberts TT, Leonard GR, Cepela DJ. Classifications in brief: American spinal injury association (ASIA) impairment scale. Clin Orthop Relat Res. 2017;475(5):1499–504. https://doi.org/10.1007/s11999-016-5133-4.
18. Chafetz RS, Gaughan JP, Vogel LC, Betz R, Mulcahey MJ. The international standards for neurological classification of spinal cord injury: intra-rater agreement of total motor and sensory scores in the pediatric population. J Spinal Cord Med. 2009;32(2):157–61. https://doi.org/10.1080/10790268.2009.11760767.
19. Antao B. Succeeding in paediatric surgery examinations: v: a complete resource for EMQs & a complete resource for MCQs. Radcliffe Pub.; 2012.
20. Bucholz RW, Burkhead WZ. The pathological anatomy of fatal atlanto-occipital dislocations. J Bone Joint Surg Am. 1979;61(2):248–50.

21. Kasliwal MK, Fontes RB, Traynelis VC. Occipitocervical dissociation-incidence, evaluation, and treatment. Curr Rev Musculoskelet Med. 2016;9(3):247–54. https://doi.org/10.1007/s12178-016-9347-6.
22. Traynelis VC, Marano GD, Dunker RO, Kaufman HH. Traumatic atlanto-occipital dislocation. Case report. J Neurosurg. 1986;65(6):863–70. https://doi.org/10.3171/jns.1986.65.6.0863.
23. Dickman CA, Papadopoulos SM, Sonntag VK, Spetzler RF, Rekate HL, Drabier J. Traumatic occipitoatlantal dislocations. J Spinal Disord. 1993;6(4):300–13. https://doi.org/10.1097/00002517-199306040-00004.
24. Martin MD, Bruner HJ, Maiman DJ. Anatomic and biomechanical considerations of the craniovertebral junction. Neurosurgery. 2010;66(3 Suppl):2–6. https://doi.org/10.1227/01.NEU.0000365830.10052.87.
25. Tubbs RS, Hallock JD, Radcliff V, et al. Ligaments of the craniocervical junction. J Neurosurg Spine. 2011;14(6):697–709. https://doi.org/10.3171/2011.1.SPINE10612.
26. Yuksel M, Heiserman JE, Sonntag VK. Magnetic resonance imaging of the craniocervical junction at 3-T: observation of the accessory atlantoaxial ligaments. Neurosurgery. 2006;59(4):888–92; discussion 892–3. https://doi.org/10.1227/01.NEU.0000232661.24547.06.
27. Zampella EJ, Duvall ER, Langford KH. Computed tomography and magnetic resonance imaging in traumatic locked-in syndrome. Neurosurgery. 1988;22(3):591–3. https://doi.org/10.1227/00006123-198803000-00027.
28. Fruin AH, Pirotte TP. Traumatic atlantooccipital dislocation. Case report. J Neurosurg. 1977;46(5):663–6. https://doi.org/10.3171/jns.1977.46.5.0663.
29. Werne S. Studies in spontaneous atlas dislocation. Acta Orthop Scand Suppl. 1957;23:1–150.
30. Hall GC, Kinsman MJ, Nazar RG, et al. Atlanto-occipital dislocation. World J Orthop. 2015;6(2):236–43. https://doi.org/10.5312/wjo.v6.i2.236.
31. Schneider RC, Crosby EC, Russo RH, Gosch HH. Chapter 32. Traumatic spinal cord syndromes and their management. Clin Neurosurg. 1973;20:424–92. https://doi.org/10.1093/neurosurgery/20.cn_suppl_1.424.
32. Daneshi A, Rahimizadeh A, Fattahi A, Darvishnia S, Masoudi O, Mohajeri SMR. Our experiences in patients with atlanto-occipital dislocation: a case series with literature review. J Craniovertebr Junction Spine. 2023;14(1):103–7. https://doi.org/10.4103/jcvjs.jcvjs_152_22.
33. Theodore N, Aarabi B, Dhall SS, et al. The diagnosis and management of traumatic atlanto-occipital dislocation injuries. Neurosurgery. 2013;72 Suppl 2:114–26. https://doi.org/10.1227/NEU.0b013e31827765e0.
34. Inoue T, Morimoto T, Yoshihara T, Tsukamoto M, Hirata H, Mawatari M. Traumatic atlanto-occipital dislocation with successfully bystander resuscitation after cardiopulmonary arrest: a case report. Clin Case Rep. 2024;12(6):e8865. https://doi.org/10.1002/ccr3.8865.
35. Powers B, Miller MD, Kramer RS, Martinez S, Gehweiler JA Jr. Traumatic anterior atlanto-occipital dislocation. Neurosurgery. 1979;4(1):12–7. https://doi.org/10.1227/00006123-197901000-00004.
36. Bellabarba C, Mirza SK, West GA, et al. Diagnosis and treatment of craniocervical dislocation in a series of 17 consecutive survivors during an 8-year period. J Neurosurg Spine. 2006;4(6):429–40. https://doi.org/10.3171/spi.2006.4.6.429.
37. Baliyan V, Shylendran S, Ajay KY, Kumar A, Gamanagatti S, Sinha S. Unusual cord transection in a patient with traumatic spondylolisthesis. Asian J Neurosurg. 2016;11(1):72. https://doi.org/10.4103/1793-5482.165803.
38. Bonner S, Smith C. Initial management of acute spinal cord injury. Cont Educ Anaesth Crit Care Pain. 2013;13(6):224–31. https://doi.org/10.1093/bjaceaccp/mkt021.
39. Eckert MJ, Martin MJ. Trauma: spinal cord injury. Surg Clin North Am. 2017;97(5):1031–45. https://doi.org/10.1016/j.suc.2017.06.008.
40. Hagen E, Rekand T, Grønning M, Færestrand S. Kardiovaskulære følgetilstander etter ryggmargsskade. Tidsskriftet. 2012;132(9):1115–20. https://doi.org/10.4045/tidsskr.11.0551.

41. Bennett J, Das JM, Emmady PD. Spinal cord injuries. In: StatPearls. StatPearls Publishing; 2024.
42. Wang TY, Park C, Zhang H, et al. Management of acute traumatic spinal cord injury: a review of the literature. Front Surg. 2021;8:698736. https://doi.org/10.3389/fsurg.2021.698736.
43. McKinley W, Santos K, Meade M, Brooke K. Incidence and outcomes of spinal cord injury clinical syndromes. J Spinal Cord Med. 2007;30(3):215–24. https://doi.org/10.1080/10790268.2007.11753929.
44. McCarron MO, Flynn PA, Pang KA, Hawkins SA. Traumatic Brown-Séquard–plus syndrome. Arch Neurol. 2001;58(9):1470. https://doi.org/10.1001/archneur.58.9.1470.
45. Kashyap S, Majeed G, Lawandy S. A rare case of Brown-Sequard syndrome caused by traumatic cervical epidural hematoma. Surg Neurol Int. 2018;9(1):213. https://doi.org/10.4103/sni.sni_142_18.
46. Kim SW, Ju CI, Kim HS, Kim YS. Brown-Séquard syndrome caused by a cervical synovial cyst. J Korean Neurosurg Soc. 2014;55(4):215. https://doi.org/10.3340/jkns.2014.55.4.215.
47. Tseng WS, Huang NC, Huang WS, Lee HC. Brown-Séquard syndrome: a rare manifestation of decompression sickness. OCCMED. 2015;65:kqv145. https://doi.org/10.1093/occmed/kqv145.
48. Zhang X-Y, Yang Y-M. Scissors stab wound to the cervical spinal cord at the craniocervical junction. Spine J. 2016;16(6):e403–6. https://doi.org/10.1016/j.spinee.2016.01.189.
49. Roth EJ, Park T, Pang T, Yarkony GM, Lee MY. Traumatic cervical Brown-Sequard and Brown-Sequard-plus syndromes: the spectrum of presentations and outcomes. Spinal Cord. 1991;29(9):582–9. https://doi.org/10.1038/sc.1991.86.
50. Group E-Ss, Pouw MH, Van De Meent H, et al. Relevance of the diagnosis traumatic cervical Brown-Séquard-plus syndrome: an analysis based on the neurological and functional recovery in a prospective cohort of 148 patients. Spinal Cord. 2010;48(8):614–8. https://doi.org/10.1038/sc.2009.189.
51. Peng T, Zf Z. Anterior spinal artery syndrome in a patient with cervical spondylosis demonstrated by CT angiography. Orthop Surg. 2019;11(6):1220–3. https://doi.org/10.1111/os.12555.
52. Jean S, Nguyen B-H, Richard-Denis A, Levy A. Acute anterior spinal artery syndrome in the context of multisystem arterial emboli. Can J Neurol Sci. 2019;46(6):787–9. https://doi.org/10.1017/cjn.2019.279.
53. Qureshi AI, Afzal MR, Suri MFK. A population-based study of the incidence of acute spinal cord infarction. J Vasc Interv Neurol. 2017;9(4):44–8.
54. Pikija S, Mutzenbach JS, Kunz AB, et al. Delayed hospital presentation and neuroimaging in non-surgical spinal cord infarction. Front Neurol. 2017;8 https://doi.org/10.3389/fneur.2017.00143.
55. Müller KI, Steffensen LH, Johnsen SH. Thrombolysis in anterior spinal artery syndrome. BMJ Case Rep. 2012;2012:bcr2012006862. https://doi.org/10.1136/bcr-2012-006862.
56. Pearl NA, Weisbrod LJ, Dubensky L. Anterior cord syndrome (archived). In: StatPearls. StatPearls Publishing; 2024.
57. Ng KS, Abdul HS. Anterior spinal cord syndrome as a rare complication of acute bacterial meningitis in an adult. BMJ Case Rep. 2018:bcr-2018-226082. https://doi.org/10.1136/bcr-2018-226082.
58. Levine A, Hukin J, Dunham C. Pontine embryonal tumor with multilayered rosettes: an autopsy case exhibiting extensive posttreatment glial and neuronal maturation. Pediatr Dev Pathol. 2020;23(4):326–31. https://doi.org/10.1177/1093526620912645.
59. Gomes FC, Larcipretti ALL, Elvir FAR, et al. Early ambulation versus prolonged bed rest for incidental durotomies in spine procedures: a systematic review and meta-analysis. Neurosurg Rev. 2023;46(1):310. https://doi.org/10.1007/s10143-023-02201-2.
60. Sandoval JI, De Jesus O. Anterior spinal artery syndrome. In: StatPearls. StatPearls Publishing; 2024.

61. Gregg L, Gailloud P. Neurovascular anatomy: spine. In: Handbook of clinical neurology. Elsevier; 2021. p. 33–47.
62. Vargas MI, Gariani J, Sztajzel R, et al. Spinal cord ischemia: practical imaging tips, pearls, and pitfalls. AJNR Am J Neuroradiol. 2015;36(5):825–30. https://doi.org/10.3174/ajnr.A4118.
63. Novy J, Carruzzo A, Maeder P, Bogousslavsky J. Spinal cord ischemia: clinical and imaging patterns, pathogenesis, and outcomes in 27 patients. Arch Neurol. 2006;63(8):1113. https://doi.org/10.1001/archneur.63.8.1113.
64. Bosch A, Stauffer ES, Nickel VL. Incomplete traumatic quadriplegia. A ten-year review. JAMA. 1971;216(3):473–8.
65. McKinley W, Hills A, Sima A. Posterior cord syndrome: demographics and rehabilitation outcomes. J Spinal Cord Med. 2021;44(2):241–6. https://doi.org/10.1080/10790268.2019.1585135.
66. Belen JG, Weingarden SI. Posterior central cord syndrome following a hyperextension injury: case report. Spinal Cord. 1988;26(3):209–11. https://doi.org/10.1038/sc.1988.33.
67. Kennamer BT, DelPino BJ, Lettieri SC, Gridley DG, Hollingworth AK, Feiz-Erfan I. Blunt traumatic posterior cord syndrome. Spinal Cord Ser Cases. 2022;8(1):52. https://doi.org/10.1038/s41394-022-00485-y.
68. Brooks NP. Central cord syndrome. Neurosurg Clin N Am. 2017;28(1):41–7. https://doi.org/10.1016/j.nec.2016.08.002.
69. Lo J, Chan L, Flynn S. A systematic review of the incidence, prevalence, costs, and activity and work limitations of amputation, osteoarthritis, rheumatoid arthritis, back pain, multiple sclerosis, spinal cord injury, stroke, and traumatic brain injury in the United States: a 2019 update. Arch Phys Med Rehabil. 2021;102(1):115–31. https://doi.org/10.1016/j.apmr.2020.04.001.
70. Roth TL, Puig-Saus C, Yu R, et al. Reprogramming human T cell function and specificity with non-viral genome targeting. Nature. 2018;559(7714):405–9. https://doi.org/10.1038/s41586-018-0326-5.
71. Quencer RM, Bunge RP, Egnor M, et al. Acute traumatic central cord syndrome: MRI-pathological correlations. Neuroradiology. 1992;34(2):85–94. https://doi.org/10.1007/BF00588148.
72. Jimenez O, Marcillo A, Levi A. A histopathological analysis of the human cervical spinal cord in patients with acute traumatic central cord syndrome. Spinal Cord. 2000;38(9):532–7. https://doi.org/10.1038/sj.sc.3101052.
73. Roth EJ, Lawler MH, Yarkony GM. Traumatic central cord syndrome: clinical features and functional outcomes. Arch Phys Med Rehabil. 1990;71(1):18–23.
74. Shrosbree RD. Acute central cervical spinal cord syndrome—aetiology, age incidence and relationship to the orthopaedic injury. Spinal Cord. 1977;14(4):251–8. https://doi.org/10.1038/sc.1976.42.
75. Schneider RC, Cherry G, Pantek H. The syndrome of acute central cervical spinal cord injury: with special reference to the mechanisms involved in hyperextension injuries of cervical spine. J Neurosurg. 1954;11(6):546–77. https://doi.org/10.3171/jns.1954.11.6.0546.
76. Schneider RC, Thompson JM, Bebin J. The syndrome of acute central cervical spinal cord injury. J Neurol Neurosurg Psychiatry. 1958;21(3):216–27. https://doi.org/10.1136/jnnp.21.3.216.
77. Yamazaki T, Yanaka K, Fujita K, Kamezaki T, Uemura K, Nose T. Traumatic central cord syndrome: analysis of factors affecting the outcome. Surg Neurol. 2005;63(2):95–100. https://doi.org/10.1016/j.surneu.2004.03.020.
78. Guest J, Eleraky MA, Apostolides PJ, Dickman CA, Sonntag VKH. Traumatic central cord syndrome: results of surgical management. J Neurosurg Spine. 2002;97(1):25–32. https://doi.org/10.3171/spi.2002.97.1.0025.
79. Ito S, Panjabi MM, Ivancic PC, Pearson AM. Spinal Canal narrowing during simulated whiplash. Spine. 2004;29(12):1330–9. https://doi.org/10.1097/01.BRS.0000127186.81814.4A.

80. Group E-Ss, Pouw MH, Van Middendorp JJ, et al. Diagnostic criteria of traumatic central cord syndrome. Part 1: a systematic review of clinical descriptors and scores. Spinal Cord. 2010;48(9):652–6. https://doi.org/10.1038/sc.2009.155.
81. EMSCISGC, Van Middendorp JJ, Pouw MH, et al. Diagnostic criteria of traumatic central cord syndrome. Part 2: a questionnaire survey among spine specialists. Spinal Cord. 2010;48(9):657–63. https://doi.org/10.1038/sc.2010.72.
82. Wilberger JE, Abla A, Maroon JC. Burning hands syndrome revisited. Neurosurgery. 1986;19(6):1038–40. https://doi.org/10.1227/00006123-198612000-00025.
83. Podnar S. Epidemiology of cauda equina and conus medullaris lesions. Muscle Nerve. 2007;35(4):529–31. https://doi.org/10.1002/mus.20696.
84. Kingwell SP, Curt A, Dvorak MF. Factors affecting neurological outcome in traumatic conus medullaris and cauda equina injuries. FOC. 2008;25(5):E7. https://doi.org/10.3171/FOC.2008.25.11.E7.
85. Harrop JS, Hunt GE, Vaccaro AR. Conus medullaris and cauda equina syndrome as a result of traumatic injuries: management principles. FOC. 2004;16(6):1–23. https://doi.org/10.3171/foc.2004.16.6.4.
86. Robson P. Metastatic spinal cord compression: a rare but important complication of cancer. Clin Med. 2014;14(5):542–5. https://doi.org/10.7861/clinmedicine.14-5-542.
87. Leowattana W, Leowattana P, Leowattana T. Tuberculosis of the spine. World J Orthop. 2023;14(5):275–93. https://doi.org/10.5312/wjo.v14.i5.275.
88. Moriarty HK, O'Cearbhaill R, Moriarty PD, Stanley E, Lawler LP, Kavanagh EC. MR imaging of spinal haematoma: a pictorial review. BJR. 2019;92(1095):20180532. https://doi.org/10.1259/bjr.20180532.
89. Huang Y-L, Chang S-T. High-riding conus medullaris syndrome: a case report and literature review—its comparison with cauda equina syndrome. Tomography. 2023;9(6):1999–2005. https://doi.org/10.3390/tomography9060156.
90. Chaudhary K, Bapat M. Conus medullaris syndrome due to an intradural disc herniation: a case report. Indian J Orthop. 2008;42(1):94. https://doi.org/10.4103/0019-5413.38590.
91. Lew SM, Kothbauer KF. Tethered cord syndrome: an updated review. Pediatr Neurosurg. 2007;43(3):236–48. https://doi.org/10.1159/000098836.
92. Liu A, Yang K, Wang D, et al. Level of conus medullaris termination in adult population analyzed by kinetic magnetic resonance imaging. Surg Radiol Anat. 2017;39(7):759–65. https://doi.org/10.1007/s00276-017-1813-3.
93. Nene Y, Jilani TN. Neuroanatomy, conus medullaris. In: StatPearls. StatPearls Publishing; 2024.
94. Brouwers E, Van De Meent H, Curt A, Starremans B, Hosman A, Bartels R. Definitions of traumatic conus medullaris and cauda equina syndrome: a systematic literature review. Spinal Cord. 2017;55(10):886–90. https://doi.org/10.1038/sc.2017.54.
95. Laasonen EM, Kivioja A. Delayed diagnosis of extremity injuries in patients with multiple injuries. J Trauma. 1991;31(2):257–60.
96. Kostuik JP, Harrington I, Alexander D, Rand W, Evans D. Cauda equina syndrome and lumbar disc herniation. J Bone Joint Surg Am. 1986;68(3):386–91.
97. Ahn UM, Ahn NU, Buchowski JM, Garrett ES, Sieber AN, Kostuik JP. Cauda equina syndrome secondary to lumbar disc herniation: a meta-analysis of surgical outcomes. Spine (Phila Pa 1976). 2000;25(12):1515–22. https://doi.org/10.1097/00007632-200006150-00010.
98. Gardner A, Gardner E, Morley T. Cauda equina syndrome: a review of the current clinical and medico-legal position. Eur Spine J. 2011;20(5):690–7. https://doi.org/10.1007/s00586-010-1668-3.
99. Miller JK, West J, Khawar H, Middleton R. Cauda equina syndrome. Br J Hosp Med. 2023;84(11):1–7. https://doi.org/10.12968/hmed.2023.0012.
100. Korse NS, Pijpers JA, Van Zwet E, Elzevier HW, Vleggeert-Lankamp CLA. Cauda Equina Syndrome: presentation, outcome, and predictors with focus on micturition,

defecation, and sexual dysfunction. Eur Spine J. 2017;26(3):894–904. https://doi.org/10.1007/s00586-017-4943-8.

101. Lavy C, James A, Wilson-MacDonald J, Fairbank J. Cauda equina syndrome. BMJ. 2009;338(mar31 1):b936. https://doi.org/10.1136/bmj.b936.
102. Yanez ML, Miller JJ, Batchelor TT. Diagnosis and treatment of epidural metastases. Cancer. 2017;123(7):1106–14. https://doi.org/10.1002/cncr.30521.
103. Babu JM, Patel SA, Palumbo MA, Daniels AH. Spinal emergencies in primary care practice. Am J Med. 2019;132(3):300–6. https://doi.org/10.1016/j.amjmed.2018.09.022.
104. Will JS, Bury DC, Miller JA. Mechanical low back pain. Am Fam Physician. 2018;98(7):421–8.
105. Domen PM, Hofman PA, Van Santbrink H, Weber WEJ. Predictive value of clinical characteristics in patients with suspected cauda equina syndrome. Euro J Neurology. 2009;16(3):416–9. https://doi.org/10.1111/j.1468-1331.2008.02510.x.
106. Mukherjee S, Thakur B, Crocker M. Cauda equina syndrome: a clinical review for the frontline clinician. Br J Hosp Med. 2013;74(8):460–4. https://doi.org/10.12968/hmed.2013.74.8.460.
107. Korse NS, Jacobs WCH, Elzevier HW, Vleggeert-Lankamp CLAM. Complaints of micturition, defecation and sexual function in cauda equina syndrome due to lumbar disk herniation: a systematic review. Eur Spine J. 2013;22(5):1019–29. https://doi.org/10.1007/s00586-012-2601-8.
108. Kavanagh M, Walker J. Assessing and managing patients with cauda equina syndrome. Br J Nurs. 2013;22(3):134–7. https://doi.org/10.12968/bjon.2013.22.3.134.

Neuroradiological Imaging: Techniques and Prognostication

7

Elio Mazzapicchi, Nicola Montemurro, Mirco Cosottini, Etrusca Brogi, Elaheh Foroughi, Federico Coccolini, and Francesco Acerbi

7.1 Introduction

Traumatic spine cord injury (TSCI) represents a significant cause of morbidity and mortality worldwide, with potential long-term physical, psychological, and economic consequences [1]. Indeed, traumatic spinal cord injury (SCI) remains one of the most devastating conditions, often leading to permanent disability and profound quality of life impairment [2]. These injuries often result from high-energy mechanisms, such as motor vehicle accidents, falls, and sports-related trauma, and they demand a multidisciplinary approach for effective management [3]. Accurate assessment and timely intervention are crucial to mitigate complications and

E. Mazzapicchi
Neurosurgery Unit, Pisa University Hospital, Pisa, Italy

University of Milano, Milan, Italy

N. Montemurro
Neurosurgery Unit, Pisa University Hospital, Pisa, Italy

M. Cosottini
Neuroradiology Department, Pisa University Hospital, Pisa, Italy

E. Brogi (✉)
Neuroscience Intensive Care Unit, ASST Grande Ospedale Metropolitano Niguarda, Milan, Italy

E. Foroughi
Isfahan University of Medical Sciences, Isfahan, Iran

F. Coccolini
General, Emergency and Trauma Surgery Department, Pisa University Hospital, Pisa, Italy

F. Acerbi
Neurosurgery Unit, Pisa University Hospital, Pisa, Italy

Department of Translational Research and New Technology in Medicine, University of Pisa, Pisa, Italy

E. Brogi et al. (eds.), *Traumatic Spinal Cord Injury*, Hot Topics in Acute Care Surgery and Trauma, https://doi.org/10.1007/978-3-031-99890-4_7

optimize outcomes. Neuroradiological imaging plays a pivotal role in the evaluation, diagnosis, and prognostication of TSCI, providing critical information about the nature and extent of injury, including the involvement of neural and vascular structures [4].

The complex pathophysiology of TSCI involves mechanical damage to the spinal cord, subsequent secondary injury mechanisms such as ischemia, inflammation, and cellular apoptosis, which can lead to further neuronal and axonal damage [5]. Recent advances in imaging technology have revolutionized the approach to spine trauma, enabling more precise and comprehensive assessments [4]. These modalities range from traditional radiographs to advanced techniques such as computed tomography (CT), magnetic resonance imaging (MRI), and functional imaging [6]. In order to guide clinicians to decide the best imaging technique and to the judiciously use imaging resources and enhance patient care, a set of clinical decision rules was designed to determine the necessity of cervical spine imaging in patients who have experienced trauma. Indeed, the "National Emergency X-Radiography Utilization Study (NEXUS) Low-Risk Criteria (NLC)" and the "Canadian C-Spine Rule (CCR)" represent widely validated approach to cervical spine injury evaluation in trauma settings [7–9] (Table 7.1 and Fig. 7.1). These criteria aim to reduce unnecessary imaging in patients with a low risk of cervical spine injury (CSI) while ensuring that patients with clinically significant injuries are identified and appropriately managed. They are widely used in emergency departments worldwide as a standard guideline for evaluating trauma patients [10]. However, like all clinical decision tools, they should be applied in conjunction with clinical judgment, especially in atypical cases or special populations.

Radiography remains an essential initial screening tool in certain settings, particularly for suspected cervical spine injuries. CT imaging is often the first-line modality in acute trauma settings due to its rapid acquisition, superior spatial resolution, and ability to detect fractures, bony abnormalities, and subtle osseous lesions [11]. MRI, on the other hand, provides incomparable soft-tissue contrast, making it invaluable for evaluating spinal cord injuries, ligamentous disruptions, and associated haemorrhage or edema, as well as detecting non-osseous injuries that are otherwise missed by CT [12]. Functional imaging techniques, including diffusion tensor imaging (DTI) and magnetic resonance spectroscopy (MRS), are emerging as promising tools for assessing neural integrity and predicting recovery potential [13]. These modalities offer the ability to visualize microstructural damage and biochemical changes within the spinal cord, providing insights that go beyond conventional imaging. Additionally, advancements in three-dimensional imaging and

Table 7.1 NEXUS criteria for C-spine imaging

Variable	No	Yes
Focal neurologic deficit present	0	1
Midline spinal tenderness present	0	1
Altered level of consciousness present	0	1
Intoxication present	0	1
Distracting injury present	0	1

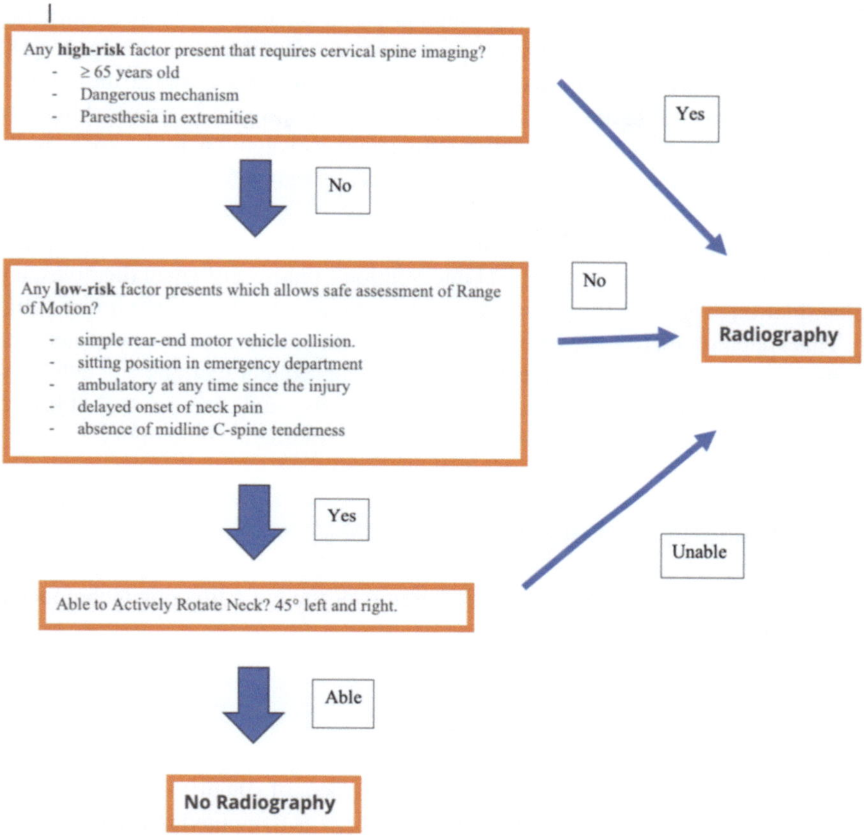

Fig. 7.1 Canadian C-spine rules

image fusion techniques have improved preoperative planning and intraoperative navigation, further enhancing patient outcomes [14]. However, their routine clinical adoption is currently limited.

The role of neuroradiological imaging extends beyond diagnosis to include prognostication [15]. Early and accurate neuroprognostication and the prediction of the potential functional recovery of patients with TSCI, are critical in guiding clinical decisions, determining the likelihood of neurological recovery, and shaping rehabilitation strategies [16]. Overall, neuroimaging stands as an indispensable tool in neuroprognostication for traumatic spinal cord injury, offering both quantitative and qualitative insights into the injury's extent, underlying mechanisms, and potential for recovery. By improving our understanding of TSCI at both the macroscopic and microscopic levels, neuroimaging continues to play a pivotal role in enhancing clinical outcomes and fostering the development of novel therapies [17]. Imaging findings, such as the presence and severity of spinal cord compression, edema, and haemorrhage, are critical markers for predicting neurological recovery and functional outcomes. Advanced imaging findings, derived from techniques like DTI, have shown potential in stratifying patients based on injury severity, estimating recovery trajectories, and guiding personalized rehabilitation strategies [18]. Emerging evidence suggests that integrating these imaging findings into clinical scoring systems could refine prognostic models and improve decision-making. The integration of neuroimaging findings with clinical evaluation tools, such as the American Spinal Injury Association (ASIA) scale, can refine prognostic predictions, helping clinicians to better understand the long-term consequences of the injury [19]. These combined approaches allow for personalized treatment plans, including the optimization of surgical interventions, pharmacological therapies, and rehabilitation protocols, based on a more precise understanding of the injury [20].

This chapter aimed to provide an overview of the indispensable role of neuroradiological imaging in the management of TSCI. Subsequent sections will delve into the specific imaging modalities, their applications, and their contributions to improving prognostic accuracy and patient care in traumatic spine injury.

7.2 Imaging Techniques: An Overview

Indications, limitations, and prognostic features of the main imaging techniques in TSCI is presented in Table 7.2.

7.2.1 Plain Radiography (X-Ray)

X-rays are a fundamental tool in the initial assessment of spinal cord injuries (SCI), especially in settings where advanced imaging such as computed tomography (CT) or magnetic resonance imaging (MRI) is unavailable. While their sensitivity is significantly lower than CT, X-rays are widely used for their accessibility and cost-effectiveness [21]. Guidelines recommend that asymptomatic, alert patients without neurological deficits or distracting injuries may not require imaging and can be cleared clinically using decision rules such as the Canadian C-Spine Rule (CCR) or the NEXUS criteria [21–25]. Conversely, symptomatic patients with neck pain or tenderness are better served by high-resolution CT imaging, but a three-view X-ray series (anteroposterior, lateral, and odontoid views) may suffice when CT is unavailable [21]. Radiographic "surveillance" is warranted for thoracic and lumbar spine injuries in patients with blunt trauma if specific risk factors are present, such as back pain, a fall from over 10 feet, ejection from a vehicle traveling ≥50 mph, a Glasgow Coma Scale (GCS) score ≤8, or neurological deficits [26]. The NEXUS criteria, validated in over 34,000 patients, aim to rapidly exclude cervical spine injury in low-risk trauma cases and reduce unnecessary imaging costs [9, 10]. Similarly, the CCR, which has been tested in nearly 9000 cases, is tailored for alert (GCS = 15), stable trauma patients and has demonstrated superior sensitivity and specificity compared to NEXUS [22]. Despite their utility, X-rays underestimate the extent of

Table 7.2 Indication, uses/role, limitations, and prognostic features

Technique	Indication	Role	Limitations	Prognostic feature
Plain radiography (X-ray)	Minor trauma	Useful for assessing bone injuries or vertebral alignment issues	Some fractures may be missed It does not provide detailed information about the spinal cord itself	Limited
Computed tomography (CT)	Major trauma Polytrauma	Useful for assessing bony injuries and vertebral fractures or dislocations in a more accurate way	In some patients (e.g., those with metal implants) imaging artifacts may occur that compromise image quality	Identify instability risks and need for interventions
Magnetic resonance imaging (MRI)	Minor or major trauma in patients with neurological deficit	Preferred for visualizing soft tissue, spinal cord edema, hemorrhage, and injury to the cord itself	In some patients (e.g., those with metal implants) imaging artifacts may occur that compromise image quality. MRI may not be considered in patients with old pacemakers or old prostheses	Evaluate lesion severity
Functional and advanced MRI	Diagnosis of post-trauma microstructural damage	Assess axonal and myelin integrity	Complex data, nonspecific interpretation challenges	Predict neurological recovery after SCI

traumatic spinal injuries. Studies show they detect only 50–62% of cervical spine fractures, leaving a significant number of hairline fractures, non-displaced injuries, and subluxations undiagnosed even with three-view imaging [21, 27]. Paediatric cases require additional caution due to their heightened susceptibility to radiation risks. While X-rays are often the initial choice in children, CT is preferred for cases with high clinical suspicion of significant injury [28]. For soporous or unevaluable patients, X-rays serve as a secondary option when CT is unavailable, though their limitations in identifying subtle or complex injuries are well-documented [21]. Multidetector CT (MDCT), due to its precision and efficiency, has become the primary imaging modality in many trauma centres for high-risk cases [23]. However, in resource-limited environments, X-rays remain a valuable diagnostic tool. Integrating clinical decision rules, imaging technologies, and clinical expertise ensures timely and accurate management of SCI while minimizing unnecessary radiation exposure and healthcare costs.

7.2.2 Computed Tomography (CT)

Multidetector computed tomography (MDCT) has become an indispensable tool in the evaluation of spinal injuries in trauma patients, offering unparalleled sensitivity and specificity compared to traditional radiography. Its ability to rapidly acquire high-resolution images and perform multiplanar reconstructions makes it the gold standard for initial imaging in moderate-to-severe trauma cases. Key radiological features include cortical disruptions, vertebral height loss, and retropulsed fragments in burst fractures (Fig. 7.2). CT also reveals subtle misalignments in dislocations and associated pathologies like epidural hematomas. MDCT has demonstrated superior diagnostic performance in detecting spinal fractures. Studies report a sensitivity of 97–100% for cervical spine fractures compared to 63–70% for plain lateral radiographs [29–31]. In a prospective analysis of 100 severely injured patients, MDCT identified unstable fractures with a sensitivity of 97.2% and achieved excellent interobserver agreement ($\kappa = 0.951$), significantly outperforming conventional radiography, which had a sensitivity of 33.3% and a lower interobserver agreement ($\kappa = 0.368$) [30]. Furthermore, MDCT detected 146 additional traumatic lesions that were missed by plain radiography [30].

For thoracolumbar spine fractures, MDCT has similarly shown superior sensitivity. In one comparative study, MDCT identified 34 out of 34 fractures (100%),

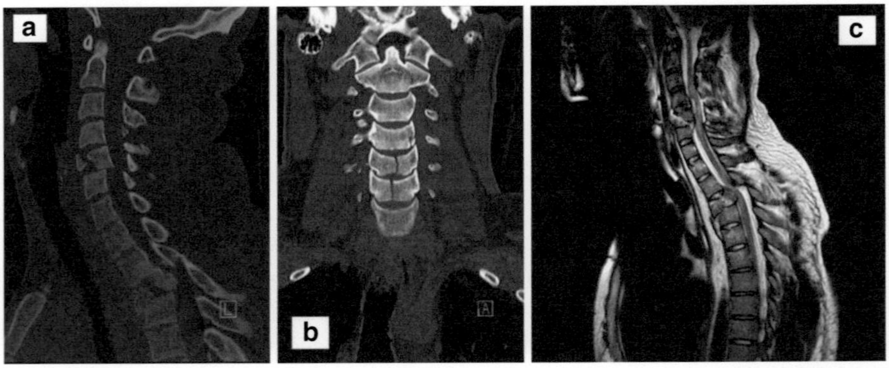

Fig. 7.2 Sagittal (**a**) and coronal (**b**) tomographic view of multifragmentary fracture of the body of C5 and C6. The sagittal view shows fractures of the laminae and of the spinosa of C5 with migration of the posterior ruptured fragment, with consequent compression of the dural sac. Diastasis of the C5-C6 articular facets on both sides. Multifragmentary fracture of the body of D3 with migration of the posterior fragment in the right paramedian-lateral area with consequent compression of the dural sac. Multifragmentary fracture also of the pedicle, the right facet joint, the left facet joint, and the left lamina. Sagittal (**c**) RMN view showing the fracture of the body of C5 with migration of the posterior wall with compression of the dural sac. T2 shows the relevance of intramedullary hyperintense signal alteration referable to microhaemorrhages. Multifragmentary fractures of the body of D3 with migration of the posterior wall in the right paramedian area, with consequent marked compression on the medulla, which presents a hyperintense signal alteration in T2 due to suffering of the nervous tissue; signal alteration of the posterior arch in the presence of known fractures. Anteriorly from C6 to T2. It is possible to observe a slight epidural hyperintense collection on T2 referable to a thin blood collection

whereas plain radiography detected only 14 out of 20 fractures (70%) [32]. The ability to provide detailed characterization of fracture morphology and stability further underscores its diagnostic utility. MDCT significantly reduces the time required for radiologic evaluation, facilitating quicker clinical decision-making. A retrospective study found that the average time spent in the radiology department during initial imaging was 1.0 h for MDCT compared to 1.9 h for plain radiography ($p < 0.001$) [32]. This efficiency is critical in trauma settings, where timely diagnosis impacts patient outcomes.

Although MDCT is more costly per scan than plain radiography, it has been shown to reduce overall institutional costs. A cost-minimization analysis reported that MDCT costs $554 per patient, compared to $2142 for plain radiographs, when factoring in costs associated with missed injuries and subsequent complications such as paralysis [31, 33]. By improving diagnostic accuracy, MDCT minimizes the risk of medicolegal consequences and reduces the need for additional imaging [21]. Concerns regarding radiation exposure have been addressed in recent studies. For cervical spine imaging, MDCT delivers higher doses (26 msv vs. 4 msv for plain radiography). However, for thoracolumbar imaging, MDCT exposes patients to less radiation (13 msv vs. 26 msv for plain radiography) [32]. These findings suggest that MDCT achieves a balance between diagnostic performance and radiation safety. Despite its strengths, MDCT has limitations. It is less effective in detecting ligamentous injuries and spinal cord lesions, which require complementary imaging modalities such as magnetic resonance imaging (MRI) [29]. Additionally, image interpretation can be challenging in patients with severe degenerative disease. MDCT has revolutionized the evaluation of spinal trauma by providing rapid, accurate, and cost-effective diagnostic capabilities. Its high sensitivity and specificity, combined with reduced time for imaging and improved resource utilization, make it the preferred modality for initial spinal assessment in trauma patients. While supplementary imaging is necessary for comprehensive evaluation of soft tissue and ligamentous injuries, MDCT remains the cornerstone of modern trauma imaging protocols.

7.2.3 Magnetic Resonance Imaging (MRI)

Magnetic resonance imaging (MRI) is increasingly recognized as an indispensable tool in the evaluation of spinal trauma patients, offering critical advantages in the visualization of soft tissue and spinal cord injuries. Unlike plain radiographs or computed tomography (CT), MRI excels in its superior contrast resolution, enabling precise detection of occult injuries and soft tissue lesions, including ligamentous and intervertebral disc abnormalities [34, 35] (Fig. 7.2). For cervical spine trauma with negative radiographs but suspected occult injuries, MRI is invaluable, as demonstrated by studies revealing ligamentous damage in approximately 7.8% of such cases [36]. Furthermore, MRI protocols, including sagittal T1-weighted, gradient-recalled T2*, and short-tau inversion recovery (STIR) sequences, enhance the visibility of ligamentous edema and other subtle soft tissue changes [37, 38].

Studies indicate MRI's sensitivity for injuries to the posterior longitudinal ligament, interspinous soft tissues, and intervertebral discs approaches 93–100%, although sensitivity for anterior longitudinal ligament and ligamentum flavum injuries remains lower, at 71% and 67%, respectively [35]. This underscores the critical role of MRI not only in identifying spinal instability but also in informing surgical decision-making. For instance, in acute trauma settings, MRI findings directly influenced surgical interventions in 2.2% of cases among patients with ligamentous injuries [36] (Fig. 7.3).

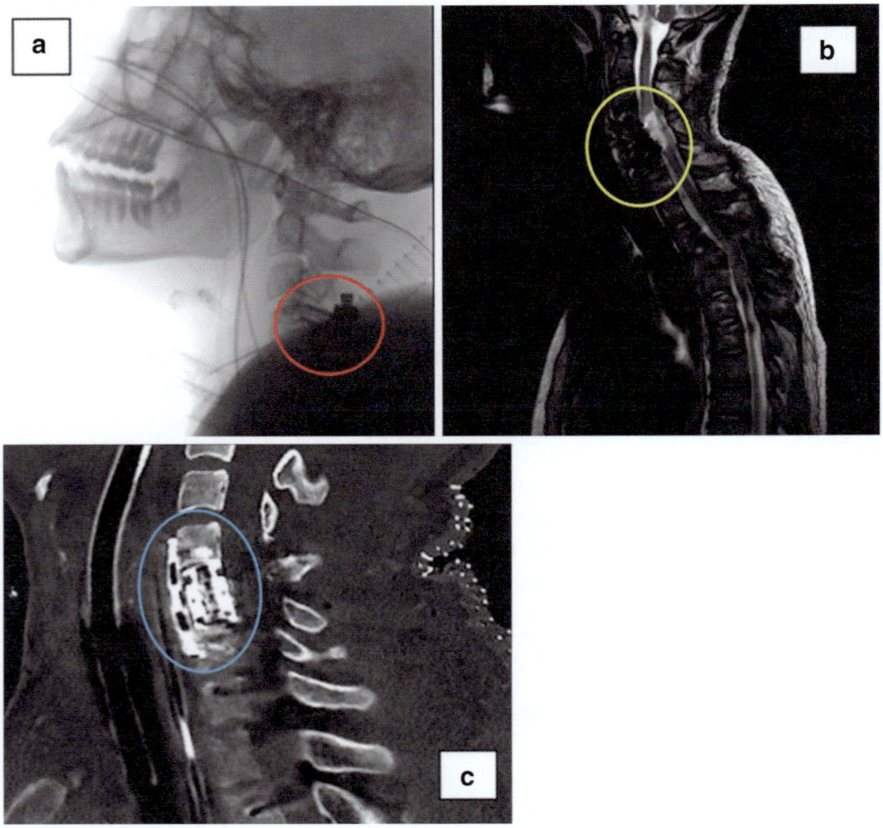

Fig. 7.3 C5 vertebrectomy and C4-5 and C5-6 discectomy. Intraoperative imaging of radioscopic control (**a**) after the insertion of an expanding mesh and a plate, fixed with somatic screws at C4 and C6. The procedure was performed under radioscopic control. RMN control (**b**) for suspected CSF collection after myelic cervical trauma and Anterior fixation C3-D6. RMN image shows heterogeneous hyperintense signal alteration in T2 of contusive significance affecting the cervical cord, currently extended cranio-caudally from C2-C3 to C7 with consensual greater spinal swelling. TC control (**c**) after cervical arthrodesis performed from an anterior approach, showing the positioning of interbody metal prosthesis, of plate and pairs of metal screws at C4 and C6. The tomographic control shows the restored alignment between C4 and C6 with intact means of synthesis

MRI is also pivotal for patients with suspected spinal cord injuries. It delineates the severity and location of lesions, reveals causes of cord compression such as hematomas or bone fragments, and assists in predicting neurological recovery. Evidence from studies highlights poor recovery in cases of intramedullary haemorrhage, while edema and contusions show a more favourable prognosis [35]. Furthermore, novel imaging modalities, such as diffusion-weighted MRI, augment prognostic capabilities by detecting cellular-level disruptions not visible on conventional sequences [39]. Additionally, the utility of MRI extends to detecting bone marrow changes, such as contusions or edema, which often accompany spinal trauma and may not be apparent on radiographs or CT. MR imaging sequences like STIR and T2-weighted imaging with fat suppression are especially effective in these scenarios. Notably, in patients undergoing procedures such as vertebroplasty, follow-up MR imaging shows a correlation between changes in bone marrow edema and clinical outcomes [40].

The concept of spinal cord injury without radiological abnormality (SCIWORA) further illustrates the indispensability of MRI. This entity, generally observed in paediatric populations, highlights the limitations of conventional imaging in detecting subtle spinal cord pathologies [37]. In such cases, MRI is not only diagnostic but also prognostic, guiding early therapeutic interventions such as the use of methylprednisolone to improve outcomes [41].

In conclusion, MRI's unparalleled ability to detect soft tissue and spinal cord injuries, combined with its role in surgical planning and prognostication, firmly establishes it as the imaging modality of choice in the comprehensive evaluation of spinal trauma.

7.2.4 Functional and Advanced MRI

Traumatic spinal cord injury (SCI) presents significant diagnostic and prognostic challenges due to its complex pathophysiology and diverse clinical manifestations. While diffusion tensor imaging (DTI) has shown potential in identifying microstructural damage in the spinal cord, its routine clinical adoption is limited [42]. The primary barriers include difficulty in acquiring high-quality, reliable data, a lack of robust automated processing tools, and challenges in interpreting DTI metrics in relation to the underlying biological changes associated with SCI [23]. Recent advancements in MRI technology aim to improve the diagnostic performance in SCI. Optimized coil designs and ultra-high-field MRI systems enhance signal-to-noise ratios and image resolution [43–45]. Additionally, new pulse sequences specifically tailored to spinal cord imaging, dynamic shimming, and retrospective corrections for motion artifacts are being developed to reduce distortions caused by patient movement and respiratory fluctuations [43–45]. Traditional pulsed-field gradient designs remain the standard, but emerging methods like double diffusion encoding and nonlinear diffusion models offer promising avenues to capture the complexity of spinal cord microstructures, potentially improving the accuracy of SCI assessments [46]. DTI metrics, such as axial and radial diffusivity, are commonly used to infer axonal and myelin integrity in SCI. However, these measures are nonspecific, as they reflect a mix of factors like axonal density, myelination, and fibre orientation [47]. Advanced models, such as neurite orientation dispersion and density imaging (NODDI) and the composite hindered and restricted model of diffusion (CHARMED), provide more targeted insights into microstructural changes. For example, NODDI has been used to detect reduced intra-axonal volume fractions in SCI, correlating with the severity of neurological dysfunction and recovery potential [48, 49]. However, these models require high-quality data and longer acquisition times, making their integration into routine clinical workflows challenging [50]. Other advanced MRI techniques complement DTI by providing additional insights into the pathological changes in SCI. Magnetization transfer imaging (MTI) and Myelin water fraction (MWF) imaging directly assess myelin integrity, which is often compromised in SCI. MTI quantifies macromolecular content, while MWF measures the proportion of myelin-associated water in the spinal cord [51, 52]. Magnetic resonance spectroscopy (MRS) has shown metabolic changes in SCI, such as reduced N-acetylaspartate levels, indicative of neuronal damage, and increased myoinositol, reflecting neuroinflammation [53]. The development of automated segmentation tools and normalization techniques has streamlined the analysis of spinal cord imaging. Tools like the PAM50 spinal cord template facilitate tissue-specific and tract-based analyses, enhancing reproducibility and enabling multicentre studies. These innovations reduce the variability of manual segmentation, making it easier to extract meaningful metrics from imaging studies and apply them to clinical decision-making [54]. The integration of advanced imaging technologies and processing techniques is transforming the assessment of SCI. By improving the accuracy of microstructural and metabolic evaluations, these innovations have the potential to enhance diagnostic precision, prognostic evaluations, and therapeutic planning for patients with SCI [55]. While challenges in clinical adoption remain, these advancements represent a crucial step forward in the management of spinal cord injuries.

7.3 Prognostication

TSCI can lead to significant motor, sensory, and autonomic dysfunctions, with the severity of impairment varying widely depending on the level and completeness of the injury. Prognosis for neurological recovery following TSCI is influenced by various factors, including the severity and level of injury, the mechanism of injury, and the time to treatment. Several prognosticators can help predict outcomes for recovery, although no single predictor can provide a definitive forecast due to the complex nature of SCI recovery.

The ASIA impairment scale is one of the most important tools used to assess the severity of SCI. The higher the grade of injury (A and B score), the worse the prognosis for neurological recovery [56]. For the same reason, early motor function assessment and the degree of voluntary movement can predict long-term outcomes. Significant motor recovery within the first few weeks of injury is generally associated with better outcomes [56]. In addition, the duration and extent of spinal shock (a condition that often occurs immediately after SCI) are critical for predicting recovery. A shorter duration of spinal shock is generally associated with better functional outcomes [57]. Age and comorbidities seem to affect the overall functional outcome, too. Younger patients typically have better chances of recovery compared to older patients due to greater plasticity and reserve capacity in the nervous system. Similarly, patients with fewer comorbid conditions tend to have better recovery prospects, whereas pre-existing conditions like diabetes and cardiovascular disease can complicate recovery [57]. Furthermore, the level of the injury (cervical, thoracic, lumbar, or sacral) significantly influences recovery outcomes. Generally, the higher the injury (i.e., cervical or upper thoracic), the more severe the motor and sensory loss, and the worse the prognosis for recovery [16, 58].

Neuroradiological imaging plays a critical role in both the acute management and long-term prognostication of SCI. The main techniques used for evaluating TSCI include X-ray, CT scans, and MRI, with each providing unique and complementary information. X-ray is the initial imaging modality used in trauma settings to rule out fractures or dislocations of the spine. X-rays are fast, widely available, and relatively cheap; however, they do not provide detailed information about the spinal cord itself. They are mainly useful for assessing bone injuries, such as fractures or vertebral alignment issues. CT scan plays a very important role in imaging techniques, as it is highly sensitive in detecting bone fractures, dislocations, and bony abnormalities of the spine [59]. It is particularly useful in evaluating complex fractures, subluxations, and vertebral instability, also in patients with polytrauma. It offers rapid and detailed assessment of bone structures, often in cases where plain X-rays are insufficient; however, it does not visualize the spinal cord well, making it less useful for assessing soft tissue damage, including the spinal cord and nerve roots. MRI is very useful for assessing spinal cord and soft tissue injuries [59]. It provides high-resolution images of the spinal cord, discs, ligaments, and surrounding tissues. For all these reasons, it is the best modality for detecting spinal cord contusions, haemorrhage, edema, and compression. It can identify the extent of damage to the cord, both in acute and chronic phases. It is also useful for monitoring SCI progression and healing. Some limitations are the fact that it cannot be performed in all patients (e.g., those with old implants and old pacemakers), and it is more time-consuming and less widely available than CT.

An early restoration of the spinal canal diameter and reduction in bone fragments or hematoma is a good indicator of potential recovery. A CT scan can assess the bone vertebral alignment, whereas radiological evidence of stable vertebral alignment following trauma, that is, with no significant displacement or subluxation, correlates with better prognosis [23].

MRI probably represents the gold standard for assessing the extent of the lesion and predicting its outcome, as well as for assessing some important neuroprognostication. First, complete transection or significant disruption of the spinal cord's continuity, visualized on MRI, often predicts a poor outcome [23]. Second, severe cord edema, hemorrhage, or contusion seen on MRI suggests more extensive injury and is associated with poor recovery [60]. T2-weighted images are commonly used to assess the level of injury and presence of edema, haemorrhage, or necrosis in the spinal cord. The extent and location of lesions (e.g., contusion or transection) can help predict functional recovery. An MRI that shows less edema or hemorrhage in the spinal cord is generally associated with better outcomes. A large area of hyperintensity (often seen in T2 imaging) following SCI is associated with a more severe injury and worse prognosis. Preservation of normal spinal cord signal or less severe cord contusion indicates better potential for functional recovery [60]. The extent and severity of spinal cord edema, as seen on MRI, are related to poor outcomes. Severe cord edema or haemorrhage on MRI is typically linked to less favourable prognoses [61]. Patients with incomplete (ASIA score grade B to D) generally show a better prognosis compared to patients with complete (ASIA score grade A), where a better recovery is often associated with imaging findings such as partial preservation of the spinal cord's integrity [61]. Third, severe spinal canal compression due to vertebral fractures or dislocations, especially when associated with a high degree of compression on the cord, as reported on CT scan or MRI, is associated with poor prognosis [62].

Imaging is essential for guiding the acute management of SCI, including the decision to proceed with surgical intervention (e.g., decompression, stabilization), but also to assess the success of surgical decompression and the stability of spinal instrumentation at post-surgical time, as also to evaluate for long-term complications (e.g., post-traumatic syringomyelia, infection, scar tissue formation or hardware failure) and assess potential for functional recovery over time.

Advanced imaging modalities such as DTI and MRS are increasingly used in patients with TSCI. DTI has shown promise in early-stage prognosis, helping to predict motor recovery potential and neural regeneration [63], whereas MRS is often correlated with motor and sensory function recovery, with more severe metabolic changes being associated with poorer functional outcomes.

The extent of secondary damage caused by inflammatory processes following spinal cord injury has been shown to influence recovery [64]. Efforts to modulate this inflammation with drugs may play a role in improving outcomes, as proper modulation of inflammation may improve recovery outcomes. Factors such as inflammatory cytokines, reactive oxygen species, and glial activation contribute to secondary damage and functional impairments [65].

Imaging studies, especially MRI and CT, are essential for determining the extent of injury and predicting recovery in TSCI patients. MRI plays a crucial role in predicting the prognosis of patients with TSCI. Prognostic indicators such as the degree of spinal cord edema and or contusion, preservation of cord integrity, and the presence of significant spinal cord compression or transection are critical in determining outcomes. These MRI findings, along with clinical assessments (ASIA scale), help in prognostication and guiding treatment strategies. In addition to these imaging prognostic indicators, early restoration of the spinal canal diameter and stabilization of the vertebral alignment are associated with a better outcome.

7.4 Conclusions

Imaging plays a pivotal role in the diagnosis of TSCI by providing detailed insights into the nature and extent of the injury. MRI remains the cornerstone, with advanced techniques like DTI and quantitative imaging offering enhanced prognostic performance. Combining imaging data with clinical assessments and emerging functional imaging holds the promise of personalized, accurate predictions for patients with TSCI. Neuroradiological imaging not only aids in diagnosing TSCI but also provides critical prognostic information, enabling tailored therapeutic strategies to improve patient outcomes.

References

1. McDaid D, Park AL, Gall A, Purcell M, Bacon M. Understanding and modelling the economic impact of spinal cord injuries in the United Kingdom. Spinal Cord. 2019;57(9):778–88.
2. van Den Hauwe L, Sundgren PC, Flanders AE. IDKD springer series spinal trauma and spinal cord injury (SCI). In: Hodler J, Kubik-Huch RA, von Schulthess GK, editors. Diseases of the brain, head and neck, spine 2020–2023: diagnostic imaging. Cham: Springer; 2020. p. 231–40.
3. Kumar R, Lim J, Mekary RA, Rattani A, Dewan MC, Sharif SY, et al. Traumatic spinal injury: global epidemiology and worldwide volume. World Neurosurg. 2018;113:e345–e63.
4. Shah LM, Ross JS. Imaging of spine trauma. Neurosurgery. 2016;79(5):626–42.
5. Zhang Y, Al Mamun A, Yuan Y, Lu Q, Xiong J, Yang S, et al. Acute spinal cord injury: pathophysiology and pharmacological intervention (Review). Mol Med Rep. 2021;23(6)
6. Wolf M, Weber MA. Neuroimaging of the traumatic spine. Magn Reson Imaging Clin N Am. 2016;24(3):541–61.
7. Stiell IG, Wells GA, Vandemheen KL, Clement CM, Lesiuk H, De Maio VJ, et al. The Canadian C-spine rule for radiography in alert and stable trauma patients. JAMA. 2001;286(15):1841–8.
8. Stiell IG, Clement CM, McKnight RD, Brison R, Schull MJ, Rowe BH, et al. The Canadian C-spine rule versus the NEXUS low-risk criteria in patients with trauma. N Engl J Med. 2003;349(26):2510–8.
9. Hoffman JR, Wolfson AB, Todd K, Mower WR. Selective cervical spine radiography in blunt trauma: methodology of the National Emergency X-radiography utilization study (NEXUS). Ann Emerg Med. 1998;32(4):461–9.
10. Hoffman JR, Mower WR, Wolfson AB, Todd KH, Zucker MI. Validity of a set of clinical criteria to rule out injury to the cervical spine in patients with blunt trauma. National Emergency X-radiography utilization study group. N Engl J Med. 2000;343(2):94–9.
11. Hussain O, Kaushal M, Agarwal N, Kurpad S, Shabani S. The role of magnetic resonance imaging and computed tomography in spinal cord injury. Life (Basel). 2023;13(8)
12. Shah LM, Flanders AE. Update on new imaging techniques for trauma. Neurosurg Clin N Am. 2017;28(1):1–21.
13. Zhu F, Wang Y, Kong X, Liu Y, Zeng L, Jing X, et al. Assessment of acute traumatic cervical spinal cord injury using conventional magnetic resonance imaging in combination with diffusion tensor imaging-tractography: a retrospective comparative study. Eur Spine J. 2022;31(7):1700–9.
14. O'Brien S, Darwish N. 3D visualisation of the spine. Adv Exp Med Biol. 2023;1406:139–68.
15. Lammertse D, Dungan D, Dreisbach J, Falci S, Flanders A, Marino R, et al. Neuroimaging in traumatic spinal cord injury: an evidence-based review for clinical practice and research: report of the National Institute on Disability and Rehabilitation Research spinal cord injury measures meeting. J Spinal Cord Med. 2007;30(3):205–14.

16. Mahanes D, Muehlschlegel S, Wartenberg KE, Rajajee V, Alexander SA, Busl KM, et al. Guidelines for neuroprognostication in adults with traumatic spinal cord injury. Neurocrit Care. 2024;40(2):415–37.
17. van Middendorp JJ, Goss B, Urquhart S, Atresh S, Williams RP, Schuetz M. Diagnosis and prognosis of traumatic spinal cord injury. Global Spine J. 2011;1(1):1–8.
18. Tulsky DS, Boulton AJ, Kisala PA, Heinemann AW, Charlifue S, Kalpakjian CZ, et al. Physical function recovery trajectories after spinal cord injury. Arch Phys Med Rehabil. 2022;103(2):215–23.
19. Spiess MR, Müller RM, Rupp R, Schuld C, van Hedel HJ. Conversion in ASIA impairment scale during the first year after traumatic spinal cord injury. J Neurotrauma. 2009;26(11):2027–36.
20. Suthar PP, Jhaveri MD, Kounsal A, Pierce LD, Singh JS. Role of clinical and multimodality neuroimaging in the evaluation of brain death/death by neurologic criteria and recent highlights from 2023 updated guidelines. Diagnostics (Basel). 2024;14(12)
21. Ryken TC, Hadley MN, Walters BC, Aarabi B, Dhall SS, Gelb DE, et al. Radiographic assessment. Neurosurgery. 2013;72(Suppl 2):54–72.
22. Ghelichkhani P, Shahsavarinia K, Gharekhani A, Taghizadieh A, Baratloo A, Fattah FHR, et al. Value of Canadian C-spine rule versus the NEXUS criteria in ruling out clinically important cervical spine injuries: derivation of modified Canadian C-spine rule. Radiol Med. 2021;126(3):414–20.
23. Fehlings MG, Tetreault LA, Wilson JR, Kwon BK, Burns AS, Martin AR, et al. A clinical practice guideline for the management of acute spinal cord injury: introduction, rationale, and scope. Global Spine J. 2017;7(3 Suppl):84s–94s.
24. Diaz JJ Jr, Cullinane DC, Altman DT, Bokhari F, Cheng JS, Como J, et al. Practice management guidelines for the screening of thoracolumbar spine fracture. J Trauma. 2007;63(3):709–18.
25. Como JJ, Diaz JJ, Dunham CM, Chiu WC, Duane TM, Capella JM, et al. Practice management guidelines for identification of cervical spine injuries following trauma: update from the eastern association for the surgery of trauma practice management guidelines committee. J Trauma. 2009;67(3):651–9.
26. Frankel HL, Rozycki GS, Ochsner MG, Harviel JD, Champion HR. Indications for obtaining surveillance thoracic and lumbar spine radiographs. J Trauma. 1994;37(4):673–6.
27. Holmes JF, Akkinepalli R. Computed tomography versus plain radiography to screen for cervical spine injury: a meta-analysis. J Trauma. 2005;58(5):902–5.
28. Hale AT, Alvarado A, Bey AK, Pruthi S, Mencio GA, Bonfield CM, et al. X-ray vs. CT in identifying significant C-spine injuries in the pediatric population. Childs Nerv Syst. 2017;33(11):1977–83.
29. Platzer P, Jaindl M, Thalhammer G, Dittrich S, Wieland T, Vecsei V, et al. Clearing the cervical spine in critically injured patients: a comprehensive C-spine protocol to avoid unnecessary delays in diagnosis. Eur Spine J. 2006;15(12):1801–10.
30. Wintermark M, Mouhsine E, Theumann N, Mordasini P, van Melle G, Leyvraz PF, et al. Thoracolumbar spine fractures in patients who have sustained severe trauma: depiction with multi-detector row CT. Radiology. 2003;227(3):681–9.
31. Griffen MM, Frykberg ER, Kerwin AJ, Schinco MA, Tepas JJ, Rowe K, et al. Radiographic clearance of blunt cervical spine injury: plain radiograph or computed tomography scan? J Trauma. 2003;55(2):222–6; discussion 6–7.
32. Antevil JL, Sise MJ, Sack DI, Kidder B, Hopper A, Brown CV. Spiral computed tomography for the initial evaluation of spine trauma: a new standard of care? J Trauma. 2006;61(2):382–7.
33. Grogan EL, Morris JA Jr, Dittus RS, Moore DE, Poulose BK, Diaz JJ, et al. Cervical spine evaluation in urban trauma centers: lowering institutional costs and complications through helical CT scan. J Am Coll Surg. 2005;200(2):160–5.
34. Voormolen MH, van Rooij WJ, van der Graaf Y, Lohle PN, Lampmann LE, Juttmann JR, et al. Bone marrow edema in osteoporotic vertebral compression fractures after percutaneous vertebroplasty and relation with clinical outcome. AJNR Am J Neuroradiol. 2006;27(5):983–8.

35. Goradia D, Linnau KF, Cohen WA, Mirza S, Hallam DK, Blackmore CC. Correlation of MR imaging findings with intraoperative findings after cervical spine trauma. AJNR Am J Neuroradiol. 2007;28(2):209–15.
36. Geck MJ, Yoo S, Wang JC. Assessment of cervical ligamentous injury in trauma patients using MRI. J Spinal Disord. 2001;14(5):371–7.
37. Kalra V, Gulati S, Kamate M, Garg A. SCIWORA-spinal cord injury without radiological abnormality. Indian J Pediatr. 2006;73(9):829–31.
38. Wilmink JT. MR imaging of the spine: trauma and degenerative disease. Eur Radiol. 1999;9(7):1259–66.
39. Shen H, Tang Y, Huang L, Yang R, Wu Y, Wang P, et al. Applications of diffusion-weighted MRI in thoracic spinal cord injury without radiographic abnormality. Int Orthop. 2007;31(3):375–83.
40. Baur A, Stäbler A, Brüning R, Bartl R, Krödel A, Reiser M, et al. Diffusion-weighted MR imaging of bone marrow: differentiation of benign versus pathologic compression fractures. Radiology. 1998;207(2):349–56.
41. Adams JM, Cockburn MI, Difazio LT, Garcia FA, Siegel BK, Bilaniuk JW. Spinal clearance in the difficult trauma patient: a role for screening MRI of the spine. Am Surg. 2006;72(1):101–5.
42. Seif M, David G, Huber E, Vallotton K, Curt A, Freund P. Cervical cord neurodegeneration in traumatic and non-traumatic spinal cord injury. J Neurotrauma. 2020;37(6):860–7.
43. Barry RL, Vannesjo SJ, By S, Gore JC, Smith SA. Spinal cord MRI at 7T. NeuroImage. 2018;168:437–51.
44. Setsompop K, Fan Q, Stockmann J, Bilgic B, Huang S, Cauley SF, et al. High-resolution in vivo diffusion imaging of the human brain with generalized slice dithered enhanced resolution: simultaneous multislice (gSlider-SMS). Magn Reson Med. 2018;79(1):141–51.
45. Cohen-Adad J. Functional magnetic resonance imaging of the spinal cord: current status and future developments. Semin Ultrasound CT MR. 2017;38(2):176–86.
46. Yang G, Tian Q, Leuze C, Wintermark M, McNab JA. Double diffusion encoding MRI for the clinic. Magn Reson Med. 2018;80(2):507–20.
47. Jensen JH, Helpern JA, Ramani A, Lu H, Kaczynski K. Diffusional kurtosis imaging: the quantification of non-gaussian water diffusion by means of magnetic resonance imaging. Magn Reson Med. 2005;53(6):1432–40.
48. Zhang H, Schneider T, Wheeler-Kingshott CA, Alexander DC. NODDI: practical in vivo neurite orientation dispersion and density imaging of the human brain. NeuroImage. 2012;61(4):1000–16.
49. Assaf Y, Basser PJ. Composite hindered and restricted model of diffusion (CHARMED) MR imaging of the human brain. NeuroImage. 2005;27(1):48–58.
50. Okita G, Ohba T, Takamura T, Ebata S, Ueda R, Onishi H, et al. Application of neurite orientation dispersion and density imaging or diffusion tensor imaging to quantify the severity of cervical spondylotic myelopathy and to assess postoperative neurologic recovery. Spine J. 2018;18(2):268–75.
51. MacKay A, Whittall K, Adler J, Li D, Paty D, Graeb D. In vivo visualization of myelin water in brain by magnetic resonance. Magn Reson Med. 1994;31(6):673–7.
52. Helms G, Dathe H, Kallenberg K, Dechent P. High-resolution maps of magnetization transfer with inherent correction for RF inhomogeneity and T1 relaxation obtained from 3D FLASH MRI. Magn Reson Med. 2008;60(6):1396–407.
53. Wyss PO, Huber E, Curt A, Kollias S, Freund P, Henning A. MR spectroscopy of the cervical spinal cord in chronic spinal cord injury. Radiology. 2019;291(1):131–8.
54. De Leener B, Fonov VS, Collins DL, Callot V, Stikov N, Cohen-Adad J. PAM50: unbiased multimodal template of the brainstem and spinal cord aligned with the ICBM152 space. NeuroImage. 2018;165:170–9.
55. Cadotte DW, Fehlings MG. Will imaging biomarkers transform spinal cord injury trials? Lancet Neurol. 2013;12(9):843–4.
56. Kirshblum S, Snider B, Eren F, Guest J. Characterizing natural recovery after traumatic spinal cord injury. J Neurotrauma. 2021;38(9):1267–84.

57. Wang TY, Park C, Zhang H, Rahimpour S, Murphy KR, Goodwin CR, et al. Management of Acute Traumatic Spinal Cord Injury: a review of the literature. Front Surg. 2021;8:698736.
58. Scivoletto G, Tamburella F, Laurenza L, Torre M, Molinari M. Who is going to walk? A review of the factors influencing walking recovery after spinal cord injury. Front Human Neurosci. 2014;8:141. (1662–5161 (Print)).
59. Picetti E, Demetriades AK, Catena F, Aarabi B, Abu-Zidan FM, Alves OL, et al. Early management of adult traumatic spinal cord injury in patients with polytrauma: a consensus and clinical recommendations jointly developed by the World Society of Emergency Surgery (WSES) & the European Association of Neurosurgical Societies (EANS). World J Emerg Surg. 2024;19(1):4.
60. Magu S, Singh D, Yadav RK, Bala M. Evaluation of traumatic spine by magnetic resonance imaging and correlation with neurological recovery. Asian Spine J. 2015;9(5):748–56.
61. Parashari UC, Khanduri S, Bhadury S, Kohli N, Parihar A, Singh R, et al. Diagnostic and prognostic role of MRI in spinal trauma, its comparison and correlation with clinical profile and neurological outcome, according to ASIA impairment scale. J Craniovertebr Junction Spine. 2011;2(1):17–26.
62. Sharwood LN, King V, Ball J, Varma D, Stanford RW, Middleton JW. The influence of initial spinal cord haematoma and cord compression on neurological grade improvement in acute traumatic spinal cord injury: a prospective observational study. J Neurol Sci. 2022;443:120453.
63. Rutman AM, Peterson DJ, Cohen WA, Mossa-Basha M. Diffusion tensor imaging of the spinal cord: clinical value, investigational applications, and technical limitations. Curr Probl Diagn Radiol. 2018;47(4):257–69.
64. Sterner RC, Sterner RM. Immune response following traumatic spinal cord injury: pathophysiology and therapies. Front Immunol. 2022;13:1084101.
65. Ramer LM, Ramer MS, Bradbury EJ. Restoring function after spinal cord injury: towards clinical translation of experimental strategies. Lancet Neurol. 2014;13(12):1241–56.

Traumatic Spinal Cord Injury: Principles and Timing of the Surgical Management of Traumatic Spinal Cord Injury

8

Vikas N. Vattipally, Oludotun Ogunsola, A. Daniel Davidar, Kelly Jiang, Carly Weber-Levine, Tej D. Azad, and Nicholas Theodore

8.1 Introduction

Traumatic spinal cord injury (SCI) affects nearly one million patients globally each year, including approximately 18,000 new cases in the United States [1, 2]. Most cases of SCI in the United States are caused by motor vehicle collisions or falls and have been associated with significant population burden as measured by disability-adjusted life years and direct healthcare spending [3–5]. Patients with traumatic SCI may experience deficits across multiple body systems, often contributing to a poor prognosis for complete functional recovery. In-hospital mortality rates range from 4% to 17% [3]. In the acute setting, operative management of traumatic SCI typically involves decompressive measures in order to relieve pressure and increase blood flow to affected cord tissue [6].

Despite the proven efficacy of surgical decompression for SCI, there is limited consensus about its optimal timing. Clinical practice guidelines for the timing of acute SCI decompression, sponsored by AO Spine and the American Association of Neurological Surgeons (AANS)/Congress of Neurological Surgeons (CNS) Joint Section on Neurotrauma and Critical Care, were published in 2017 [7]. The authors "suggest" based on weak evidence that early surgery, defined as occurring within 24 hours of injury, should always be offered to patients with acute SCI. In 2024, AO Spine and the Praxis Spinal Cord Institute published updated clinical practice guidelines, based on a rigorous review of evidence published in the interim, strengthening this position by "recommending" decompression within 24 hours instead of merely suggesting it [8]. In response to this, the AANS/CNS Joint Sections for spine and

V. N. Vattipally · A. D. Davidar · K. Jiang · C. Weber-Levine · T. D. Azad · N. Theodore (✉)
Department of Neurosurgery, Johns Hopkins University School of Medicine, Baltimore, MD, USA
e-mail: theodore@jhmi.edu

O. Ogunsola
Department of Neurosurgery, University of Michigan Medical School, Ann Arbor, MI, USA

E. Brogi et al. (eds.), *Traumatic Spinal Cord Injury*, Hot Topics in Acute Care Surgery and Trauma, https://doi.org/10.1007/978-3-031-99890-4_8

neurotrauma most recently stated that much of the current evidence for early decompression is limited by experimental design, especially as there is currently no class I evidence supporting early decompression [9]. Their position statement concluded that there is minimal ability to define the role of early decompression from the current body of research. Moreover, some clinical studies have posited that associations between early decompression and positive clinical outcomes may be confounded by other factors, such as the intramedullary lesion length [10] (Fig. 8.1).

The lack of consensus surrounding the timing of decompression has contributed to variability in the surgical management of traumatic SCI across the world [11]. This chapter details surgical principles in the management of traumatic SCI, then explores current evidence related to the timing of decompression and discusses common barriers to early decompression.

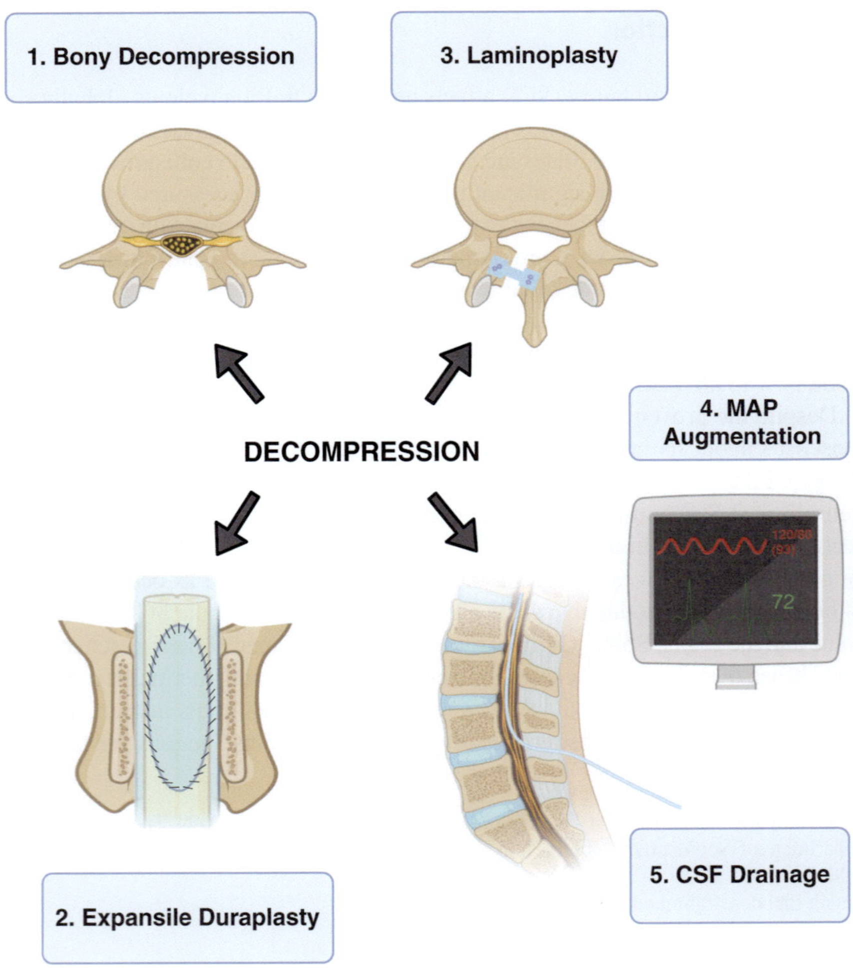

Fig. 8.1 Strategies for surgical spinal cord decompression after traumatic SCI

8.2 Principles of Surgical Management

8.2.1 Initial Assessment

The initial assessment of a patient with suspected spine trauma follows the principles of Advanced Trauma Life Support [12]:

8.2.1.1 Primary Survey

The primary survey encompasses assessment of airway patency, breathing, circulation, neurological status, and exposure/environment control.

8.2.1.2 Neurological Examination

Performance of a detailed neurological examination to assess motor and sensory function should incorporate the American Spinal Injury Association (ASIA) Impairment Scale (AIS). This scale uses clinical examination findings to classify patients with SCI into grades E (preservation of intact sensation and motor function), D (incomplete injury where more than half of the muscle groups below the level of injury have a strength grade greater than or equal to 3), C (incomplete injury where more than half of the key muscles below the level of injury have a maximum strength score of 2), B (incomplete injury with sensory preservation but no motor function preservation), or A (complete injury without sensory or motor function preservation) [13]. Importantly, in cases of spinal shock with absence of the bulbocavernosus reflex, an AIS grade cannot be assigned until the reflex returns. However, a recent study challenged the utility of the bulbocavernosus reflex in the acute assessment of spinal shock [14].

8.2.1.3 Imaging

Completion and interpretation of imaging studies, including X-rays, computed tomography (CT), and magnetic resonance imaging (MRI), can help clinicians evaluate the extent of bony and soft tissue injuries. An initial assessment via radiograph must include both anterior-posterior and lateral films to assess the structural aspects of the spine, including locus of injury, vertebral column height, spinal alignment, fractures, presence of prior instrumentation, and interpedicular widening. Meanwhile, a total spine CT scan can help in detecting any bone fragmentation into the vertebral canal along with fracture classification at every affected spinal level. In many settings, postoperative MRI is obtained immediately after surgery to ensure that adequate decompression has been achieved. Thus, thorough imaging assessment remains an important first step for detecting and classifying spinal injuries as well as guiding subsequent treatment.

8.2.2 Evaluation of Spinal Column Injury

The presence of spinal fractures in a patient with spinal trauma may be an indication for decompression, especially if fracture fragments impinge upon the spinal cord. The following fracture classification systems may help guide treatment decisions.

8.2.2.1 Denis Three-Column Theory

The Denis model describes injuries based on involvement of the anterior (anterior longitudinal ligament and anterior half of the vertebral column and intervertebral disc), middle (posterior half of the vertebral column and posterior longitudinal ligament [PLL]), and posterior (all structures posterior to the PLL) columns [30]. The spinal column is deemed to be unstable if two or more columns are affected. Of note, the Denis classification does not associate neurologic recovery with the pattern of fracture and oversimplifies injuries based on the number of columns involved. As a result, other classifiers, such as the AO Spine classification, have been developed for surgical decision-making in spinal trauma.

8.2.2.2 AO Spine Classification

This system provides a comprehensive classification of a spinal fracture based on morphology, neurological status, and clinical modifiers. It classifies these into compression fractures, burst fractures, distraction injuries, and translational injuries in a manner that highlights the severity of injury [15].

8.2.2.3 Thoracolumbar Injury Classification Score (TLICS)

The TLICS is used alongside AO Spine Classification in surgical decision-making as it integrates fracture morphology, posterior ligamentous injury, and neurologic deficits to predict the utility of surgical intervention [16]. However, several studies, including one published by Park et al., emphasize the utility of TLICS in conservative management and recognize the importance of MRI for the assessment of posterior ligamentous complex injury [17]. The TLICS score suggests that surgical intervention is warranted if a patient's injury scores greater than 5, and there has been a recent push to perform this intervention within 24 hours of injury. Surgical options include vertebroplasty or kyphoplasty, percutaneous fixation, long-segment fixation with or without laminectomy, or a corpectomy with posterior fixation.

8.2.2.4 Subaxial Cervical Injury Classification System (SLICS)

The SLICS provides a standardized method for evaluating and classifying injuries to the subaxial cervical spine (C3-C7). This CT-based system uses three main parameters to assess the injury: morphology (compression, burst, distraction, and translation/rotation), discoligamentous complex integrity (intact, indeterminate, and disrupted), and neurological status (intact, root injury, complete cord injury, incomplete cord injury, and continuous cord compression). Scores of 5 or greater indicate the need for surgical intervention to decompress neural elements and stabilize the spinal column [18].

8.2.3 Indications for Surgery

Absolute indications for surgical intervention in a spinal trauma patient include the following:

Progressive or complete neurological deficits that require decompression.
Mechanical instability that poses a risk of further neurological injury or deformity.
Severe pain not responsive to conservative measures.

Relative indications for surgical intervention include:

Persistent instability or pain despite conservative management.
Significant deformity that may cause long-term functional impairment or aesthetic concerns.

8.2.4 Surgical Management

Surgical management of traumatic SCI often involves decompression of the spinal canal to relieve pressure on the spinal cord and reduce the risk of permanent injury. A multifaceted approach to the surgical treatment of traumatic SCI may include decompression procedures, mean arterial pressure and spinal cord perfusion pressure management, and postoperative care.

8.2.5 Spinal Cord Decompression

Spinal cord decompression procedures are performed to address cytotoxic and vasogenic edema with a focus on ameliorating secondary injury following traumatic SCI. Spinal cord decompression includes a variety of techniques, including bony decompression, duraplasty, and spinal cord pressure optimization.

8.2.5.1 Bony Decompression

Bony decompression involves partial or complete removal of bony tissue to aid decompression by improving spinal cord perfusion and flow of cerebrospinal fluid (CSF). Various techniques for bony decompression are discussed below.

Conventional decompressive laminectomy involves complete removal of the lamina while sparing the facet joint and is a commonly performed procedure for both acute and chronic SCI. A study comparing various methods of decompression indicated that laminectomy was the only significant predictor of adequate decompression on postoperative MRI images of traumatic cervical SCI compared to other procedures [19]. Laminectomies can be performed through either open or minimally invasive endoscopic approaches. However, in the setting of acute SCI, the endoscopic approach is not commonly performed. Laminectomy is usually performed with the patient prone and with localization of levels with intraoperative X-ray imaging. After a posterior midline incision is made, subperiosteal dissection is carried out to reach the lamina. In a classical laminectomy, care is taken not to damage the pars interarticularis or facet joint, but in case of traumatic injury, surgical planning based on preoperative imaging may require a facetectomy in conjunction with fusion. A foraminotomy can be performed along with a laminectomy to address any foraminal stenosis. An adequate laminectomy will result in sufficient CSF volume in the subarachnoid space, both dorsal and ventral to the spinal cord. This is visible on intraoperative ultrasound (IOUS) or postoperative MRI/CT myelogram [20]. Recently, Chryssikos et al. demonstrated that the use of IOUS allowed for higher sensitivity for the detection of adequate decompression as compared to postoperative MRI/CT myelogram, indicating that IOUS is a useful adjunctive imaging modality in the surgical management of traumatic SCI [21]. Postoperative clinical improvement may also be an indicator of adequate decompression.

Minimally invasive laminectomy via an endoscopic approach involves a paramedian incision followed by dissection and placement of tubular retractors. Once the level is radiographically verified, a high-speed drill is used to perform an ipsilateral laminectomy and/or medial facetectomy. Resection of ligamentum flavum and visualization of spinal structures is followed by contralateral decompression [22]. Advantages of minimally invasive procedures include decreased postoperative pain due to avoidance of paraspinal musculature dissection. However, a steep learning curve, technical complexity, minimal visualization, and potentially increased rates of durotomy prevent it from being performed commonly in traumatic SCI [23].

Laminoplasty is another potential option for a decompressive procedure, especially in the cervical region. Several techniques for performing laminoplasty have been reported. These generally involve the use of a burr to remove the lamina on the ipsilateral side or create a hinge on the contralateral side by removing the lamina but preserving the ventral cortex (open-door laminoplasty) [24]. Laminoplasty plates are used to fix the lamina in position and prevent destabilization. While laminoplasty has been described for the treatment of acute SCI, it is not commonly performed for this indication [25, 26].

8.2.5.2 Duraplasty

Laminectomy is routinely performed to relieve extrinsic and intrinsic spinal cord pressure, but some studies monitoring intraspinal pressure noted that a laminectomy alone was insufficient to attain complete decompression [27, 28]. In these patients, expansile duraplasty assisted in restoring patency of the subarachnoid space and maintaining spinal cord perfusion pressure, spinal perfusion reactivity index, and autoregulation. This procedure involves making a longitudinal incision on the post-laminectomy dura, followed by the placement of a suitable dural graft, which is sutured onto the dura. While this technique is an established procedure, its efficacy in treating SCI remains under investigation.

Several clinical prospective trials have explored the efficacy of duraplasty for treating SCI, including a prospective trial in 21 patients undergoing either bony decompression alone or bony decompression with duraplasty [29]. Improvement was seen in intradural space, intraspinal perfusion, spinal cord pressure, and vascular pressure reactivity in the duraplasty group. Another study in 17 patients divided into decompression with or without duraplasty demonstrated the relative efficacy of both procedures [30]. Ongoing prospective phase III multicenter clinical trials, such as the DISCUS study, aim to conclusively evaluate the efficacy of duraplasty by dividing patients into two study arms: bony decompression and bony decompression with laminoplasty [31]. The trial recruited 222 AIS grade A-C traumatic cervical SCI patients and assessed outcome at 6 and 12 months. An additional subgroup underwent monitoring of intraspinal pressure and spinal cord perfusion pressure as well as monitoring of chemical metabolites with a microdialysis catheter. A management algorithm that would indicate which patients would require expansile duraplasty in addition to bony decompression has been proposed [27].

8.2.6 Spinal Cord Pressures

Pressure dynamics have long been known to impact the prognosis of SCI. Spinal cord perfusion pressure (SCPP) is calculated as the difference between mean arterial pressure (MAP) and intraspinal pressure (ISP):

$$\text{SCPP} = \text{MAP} - \text{ISP}$$

After traumatic SCI, ISP rises due to swelling of the cord and loss of CSF buffer around the cord [32]. This in turn produces intraspinal hypertension, which may lead to spinal cord ischemia and neuronal cell death. In this section, we will discuss interventions to manage both MAP and ISP.

8.2.6.1 MAP Augmentation

An elevated MAP has been recommended to improve outcomes after SCI. Primary SCI leads to localized white and grey matter injury and ischemia, and several secondary mechanisms contribute to further injury [33]. A recommendation to maintain MAP between 85 and 90 mm Hg for 7 days after injury is the current standard of care [34]. Several vasopressors may be used to raise MAP, including phenylephrine, dopamine, and norepinephrine, with studies showing variable efficacy of these agents. One study of patients with traumatic central cord syndrome demonstrated that, compared to phenylephrine, dopamine had a significantly greater rate of complications in patients older than 55 years [35]. Another study recommended the use of norepinephrine rather than dopamine for reducing intraspinal pressure [36]. Norepinephrine also demonstrated superior blood flow restoration and oxygenation in traumatic SCI compared to phenylephrine. Another consideration is the location of the spinal cord injury. Cervical and upper thoracic SCI may require inotropic and chronotropic support of the heart and vasculature with dopamine and norepinephrine because of their effects on α_1 and β_1 receptors. In lower thoracic and lumbar SCI, peripheral vasoconstrictors acting only on α_1 receptors, such as phenylephrine are recommended [37].

8.2.6.2 CSF Drainage and Spinal Cord Perfusion Pressure

Another method to augment spinal cord perfusion pressure is to alter the ISP through CSF drainage. CSF drainage has been used in thoracoabdominal aneurysm repair to decrease intrathecal pressure. Recent evidence indicates the potential utility of CSF drainage in the treatment of traumatic SCI. A class 2B randomized controlled trial of patients with C4-C7 AIS grade A-C SCI was recently conducted, aiming for MAP maintenance of 85–90 mm Hg for five days [38]. In total, 11 patients were divided into an experimental group of seven patients, who had a lumbar catheter placed with CSF drainage and a target intrathecal pressure (ITP) of <10 mm Hg, and a control group of 4 patients who had the lumbar catheter placed but without CSF drainage. The study revealed that the mean ITP was significantly lower and the SCPP was significantly higher in the experimental group compared to the control group. While further research is needed, the strategy of CSF drainage shows promise for improving SCPP and perhaps outcomes for patients with traumatic SCI.

8.2.7 Postoperative Care

The immediate postoperative care of patients with SCI requires careful monitoring of patient stability and management of pain and other symptoms.

Continuous monitoring of neurological status, hemodynamics, and respiratory function is necessary in the post-operative period. As stated above, maintaining MAP between 85 and 90 mm Hg MAP for 7 days postinjury has become standard practice [34]. An association has been demonstrated between higher MAP and neurologic recovery for patients with AIS grades A-C after SCI, but not for those with AIS grade D injury, highlighting the need for elevated MAP after more severe SCI [39].

Multimodal analgesia is commonly required to control pain and maximize patient comfort.

Early mobilization with appropriate bracing should be pursued to prevent such complications as venous thromboembolism, decubitus ulcers, and pneumonia.

Later phases of postoperative care should focus on the recovery of function and assessment of procedural success.

Tailored rehabilitation programs in the inpatient and outpatient settings can help patients maximize function and mobility.

Occupational therapists can help patients perform activities of daily living and adapt to any residual neurologic deficits.

Periodic imaging should be performed to assess for adequacy of fusion and alignment after surgery.

8.2.8 Potential Complications

As with most surgical procedures, operative interventions for spinal trauma carry inherent intraoperative risks.

Risk of hemorrhage can be reduced with meticulous surgical technique and the use of hemostatic agents.

Suspected or confirmed leaks should urgently be repaired with sutures and/or sealants to prevent persistent CSF leakage.

Other complications from CSF leaks may present in the immediate postoperative or later recovery periods.

Perioperative prophylactic antibiotics and sterile surgical technique must be used to reduce infection risk. Preoperative administration of prophylactic antibiotics is widely accepted. Dosing antibiotics for only the first postoperative day (as opposed to much longer durations) is effective for preventing surgical site infections for non-instrumented lumbar spine procedures, and one study suggests that postoperative antibiotic prophylaxis does not significantly reduce the incidence of surgical site infections compared to not receiving postoperative prophylaxis [40, 41].

Regular follow-up with imaging is necessary to detect potential hardware failure.

Bony non-union may require revision surgery and enhanced fusion techniques.

8.3 Timing of Surgery

8.3.1 Findings from Animal Studies

Use of animal models of traumatic SCI allows researchers to create consistent injuries across subjects and isolate the effects of different interventions. One early study employing a rodent SCI model demonstrated greater histological evidence of severe spinal cord damage with increasing spinal canal narrowing and time to decompression [42]. The authors further reported a negative dose-response relationship between delay to decompression (0 hours, 2 hours, 6 hours, 24 hours, or 72 hours) and improvement in motor scores after six weeks. Later synthesis of preclinical SCI research indicated that a complex interplay exists between the severity and duration of the compression and its effect on motor outcomes [43]. Specifically, less compression created greater tolerance for a longer time to decompression, whereas a greater degree of compression necessitated earlier decompression in order to achieve the same outcome. Using analogous compression parameters to those found in typical human SCI, the authors estimated that decompression earlier than 12 hours postinjury may lead to more favorable motor outcomes than those observed after later intervention [43]. Another review notes that while some studies suggest there is little to no effect of decompression prior to 24 hours in animal SCI models, the majority of evidence suggests that reduced time to intervention improves outcomes [44].

Overall, the results of animal studies of the timing of decompression after experimental acute SCI suggest a benefit to early intervention, often with improving outcomes as the duration of delay shortens from greater than 24 hours to less than 24 hours to even less than 12 hours. Nevertheless, it is important to note several limitations to these data. In the clinical setting, patients often present with multifocal injuries, especially after motor vehicle collisions, falls, or gunshot wounds. SCI treatment or recovery may be complicated by concomitant injuries to other parts of the body or by delays to medical stabilization. Similarly, patients often have various medical and surgical comorbidities that may affect the safety or efficacy of surgical intervention for SCI. Findings from animal studies are also limited because researchers cannot elicit reports of pain, paresthesias, or other key subjective complaints that are often very troubling for patients after SCI. In addition, animals are not able to fully perform complex functions like those required for human activities of daily living or for work-related tasks. For these reasons, simple assessments of motor improvement after surgical intervention in animals may not correspond to holistic recovery trajectories in humans with SCI.

8.3.2 Findings from Human Studies

Although human studies are limited by patient and injury heterogeneity, a substantial amount of information has accumulated about the value of early intervention for traumatic SCI. The most recent data from a systematic review and meta-analysis of 21 human studies suggest that decompression within 24 hours of injury in acute SCI patients is associated with clinical benefit [45]. Specifically, the authors reported that for patients decompressed within 24 hours, 6- and 12-month AIS grades were twice as likely to improve by two or more grades when compared to later-decompressed patients (> 24 hours). AIS scores represent an assessment of a patient's motor function and pinprick sensation at the time of examination, and scores have been demonstrated to possess significant prognostic value for long-term functional outcomes like ambulation [46, 47]. These findings, which are supported by randomized controlled trials and multicenter prospective cohort studies such as the STASCIS trial [48–50], indicate that decompression within 24 hours of injury may significantly improve functional outcome during the recovery period. To this point, time to decompression for patients with acute SCI has even been demonstrated to exhibit a dose-response relationship with functional outcome measures. Modeling time to decompression as a continuous variable against total AIS motor score changes during one year of postinjury follow-up, Badhiwala et al. found an inverse relationship between treatment delay and improvements in motor scores [51]. This effect plateaued at 36 hours of delay, further suggesting that early intervention after injury maximizes patient benefit. Overall, the contemporary literature offers a significant body of evidence supporting early decompression across a wide population of SCI patients.

However, the positive effect of early decompression has not been universally reported. One recent controlled trial found no effect of the timing of surgery on total motor recovery in patients with traumatic cervical SCI and pre-existing cervical spinal stenosis, although early surgery was associated with accelerated recovery [52]. Another study found that intramedullary lesion length in SCI patients, but not timing of surgery, was associated with neurological outcome in patients with traumatic cervical SCI [10]. Other data suggest that the benefit of early decompression may be confined to AIS grade A patients, with minimal benefit to AIS grade B-D patients [53].

Because logistical and ethical issues may arise when designing a multicenter trial with sufficient power to definitively determine the benefit of early surgery [54], the current evidence base should be considered in the context of potential risks and benefits. Risks of early decompression for traumatic SCI are rarely reported, whereas numerous studies report the benefits of this practice. Although each patient presents with unique circumstances that should be considered in the clinical decision-making process, current evidence suggests that earlier surgical decompression after traumatic SCI, especially within the first 24 hours after injury, is associated with more favorable long-term neurological outcomes. Even though, as the 2024 AANS/CNS statement notes, there is currently no class I evidence that early decompression is causally related to improved outcome after SCI [9], the volume and consistency of contemporary research strongly suggest that the benefits of early decompression outweigh the risks. Patients with traumatic SCI would more likely than not experience a reduced burden of functional impairment if early decompression were to be pursued as often as possible.

8.3.3 Challenges to Performing Early Decompression

Despite the benefits of early decompression discussed above, its practical implementation may be limited by a variety of clinical and logistical factors. Delays in patient presentation after injury are common and can be due to concerns about cost, low health literacy, and lack of transportation to the hospital [55]. Many patients do not live near a facility that is equipped to perform decompression, introducing further delays in transport and potentially necessitating transfers [6]. Upon arrival to the hospital, patients with suspected SCI often require an MRI before the care team can develop a management plan and decide if surgery should be pursued [56]. Acquiring and interpreting MRI results may be slowed in the acute setting due to understaffing, high patient volume, technical difficulties, or other logistical factors, leading to further surgical delays. The presence of concomitant traumatic brain injury has also been associated with delayed decompression for patients with acute SCI, partly because of potential challenges in obtaining informed consent or relevant patient history due to altered mental status [57]. Because acute traumatic SCI commonly occurs in combination with other injuries, surgery for SCI may have to be delayed until immediately life-threatening conditions have been stabilized. A thorough analysis of the acute SCI care continuum should be performed to identify areas of delay between injury and surgery, and process improvement efforts should be undertaken with input from clinicians, patient advocates, and hospital administration.

8.4 Conclusion

This chapter provides an overview of current management strategies for the surgical management of traumatic SCI. Bony decompression via laminectomy or laminoplasty is often performed to rapidly decompress the spinal canal. Further decompression may be pursued via duraplasty, which is currently being investigated for its efficacy in improving patient outcomes. Management of patients' mean arterial pressure via pharmacological agents and spinal cord perfusion pressure via cerebrospinal fluid drainage are potentially beneficial adjunctive strategies that are under investigation. Controversy surrounds the optimal timing of decompression for patients with traumatic SCI. Numerous studies suggest that surgical decompression within 24 hours of injury is associated with more favorable long-term neurological outcomes, but significant logistical and injury barriers may often limit the feasibility of performing early decompression.

References

1. Ding W, Hu S, Wang P, et al. Spinal cord injury: the global incidence, prevalence, and disability from the global burden of disease study 2019. Spine (Phila Pa 1976). 2022;47(21):1532–40. https://doi.org/10.1097/BRS.0000000000004417.
2. National Spinal Cord Injury Statistical Center. Traumatic Spinal Cord Injury Facts and Figures at a Glance. Published 2024. Accessed 21 June 2024. https://www.nscisc.uab.edu/public/Facts%20and%20Figures%202024%20-%20Final.pdf
3. Ahuja CS, Wilson JR, Nori S, et al. Traumatic spinal cord injury. Nat Rev Dis Primers. 2017;3:17018. https://doi.org/10.1038/nrdp.2017.18.
4. Hall OT, McGrath RP, Peterson MD, et al. The burden of traumatic spinal cord injury in the United States: disability-adjusted life years. Arch Phys Med Rehabil. 2019;100(1):95–100. https://doi.org/10.1016/j.apmr.2018.08.179.
5. Bennett J, Das JM, Emmady PD. Spinal cord injuries. 2024.
6. Ahuja CS, Badhiwala JH, Fehlings MG. "Time is spine": the importance of early intervention for traumatic spinal cord injury. Spinal Cord. 2020;58(9):1037–9. https://doi.org/10.1038/s41393-020-0477-8.
7. Fehlings MG, Tetreault LA, Wilson JR, et al. A clinical practice guideline for the management of patients with acute spinal cord injury and central cord syndrome: recommendations on the timing (≤24 hours versus >24 hours) of decompressive surgery. Global Spine J. 2017;7(3 Suppl):195S–202S. https://doi.org/10.1177/2192568217706367.
8. Kwon BK, Tetreault LA, Evaniew N, Skelly AC, Fehlings MG. AO spine/praxis clinical practice guidelines for the management of acute spinal cord injury: an introduction to a focus issue. Global Spine J. 2024;14(3_suppl):5S–9S. https://doi.org/10.1177/21925682231189928.
9. AANS/CNS Joint Section on Disorders of the Spine and Peripheral Nerves, AANS/CNS Joint Section on Neurotrauma and Critical Care. Position Statement on the AO Spine/PRAXIS Clinical Practice Guidelines for the Management of Acute Spinal Cord Injury; 2024.
10. Aarabi B, Akhtar-Danesh N, Chryssikos T, et al. Efficacy of ultra-early (<12 h), early (12–24 h), and late (>24–138.5 h) surgery with magnetic resonance imaging-confirmed decompression in American Spinal Injury Association Impairment Scale Grades A, B, and C cervical spinal cord injury. J Neurotrauma. 2020;37(3):448–57. https://doi.org/10.1089/neu.2019.6606.
11. Ramakonar H, Fehlings MG. "Time is spine": new evidence supports decompression within 24 h for acute spinal cord injury. Spinal Cord. 2021;59(8):933–4. https://doi.org/10.1038/s41393-021-00654-0.
12. Schmidt OI, Gahr RH, Gosse A, Heyde CE. ATLS(R) and damage control in spine trauma. World J Emerg Surg. 2009;4:9. https://doi.org/10.1186/1749-7922-4-9.
13. Kirshblum SC, Burns SP, Biering-Sorensen F, et al. International standards for neurological classification of spinal cord injury (revised 2011). J Spinal Cord Med. 2011;34(6):535–46. https://doi.org/10.1179/204577211X13207446293695.

14. Mansoor Ali D, Sivaganesan A, Neal CJ, et al. Bulbocavernosus reflex has no prognostic features during the acute evaluation of spinal cord injuries. J Neurotrauma. 2023;40(17–18):1970–5. https://doi.org/10.1089/neu.2022.0412.
15. Magerl F, Aebi M, Gertzbein SD, Harms J, Nazarian S. A comprehensive classification of thoracic and lumbar injuries. Eur Spine J. 1994;3(4):184–201. https://doi.org/10.1007/BF02221591.
16. Lee JY, Vaccaro AR, Lim MR, et al. Thoracolumbar injury classification and severity score: a new paradigm for the treatment of thoracolumbar spine trauma. J Orthop Sci. 2005;10(6):671–5. https://doi.org/10.1007/s00776-005-0956-y.
17. Park CJ, Kim SK, Lee TM, Park ET. Clinical relevance and validity of TLICS system for thoracolumbar spine injury. Sci Rep. 2020;10(1):19494. https://doi.org/10.1038/s41598-020-76473-9.
18. Vaccaro AR, Hulbert RJ, Patel AA, et al. The subaxial cervical spine injury classification system: a novel approach to recognize the importance of morphology, neurology, and integrity of the disco-ligamentous complex. Spine (Phila Pa 1976). 2007;32(21):2365–74. https://doi.org/10.1097/BRS.0b013e3181557b92.
19. Aarabi B, Olexa J, Chryssikos T, et al. Extent of spinal cord decompression in motor complete (American spinal injury association impairment scale grades a and B) traumatic spinal cord injury patients: post-operative magnetic resonance imaging analysis of standard operative approaches. J Neurotrauma. 2019;36(6):862–76. https://doi.org/10.1089/neu.2018.5834.
20. Tat J, Tat J, Yoon S, Yee AJM, Larouche J. Intraoperative ultrasound in spine decompression surgery: a systematic review. Spine (Phila Pa 1976). 2022;47(2):E73–85. https://doi.org/10.1097/BRS.0000000000004111.
21. Chryssikos T, Stokum JA, Ahmed AK, et al. Surgical decompression of traumatic cervical spinal cord injury: a pilot study comparing real-time intraoperative ultrasound after laminectomy with postoperative MRI and CT myelography. Neurosurgery. 2023;92(2):353–62. https://doi.org/10.1227/neu.0000000000002207.
22. Rahman M, Summers LE, Richter B, Mimran RI, Jacob RP. Comparison of techniques for decompressive lumbar laminectomy: the minimally invasive versus the "classic" open approach. Minim Invasive Neurosurg. 2008;51(2):100–5. https://doi.org/10.1055/s-2007-1022542.
23. Phan K, Mobbs RJ. Minimally invasive versus open laminectomy for lumbar stenosis: a systematic review and meta-analysis. Spine (Phila Pa 1976). 2016;41(2):E91–E100. https://doi.org/10.1097/BRS.0000000000001161.
24. Weinberg DS, Rhee JM. Cervical laminoplasty: indication, technique, complications. J Spine Surg. 2020;6(1):290–301. https://doi.org/10.21037/jss.2020.01.05.
25. Uribe J, Green BA, Vanni S, Moza K, Guest JD, Levi AD. Acute traumatic central cord syndrome—experience using surgical decompression with open-door expansile cervical laminoplasty. Surg Neurol. 2005;63(6):505–10.; discussion 510. https://doi.org/10.1016/j.surneu.2004.09.037.
26. Lee HJ, Kim HS, Nam KH, Han IH, Cho WH, Choi BK. Neurologic outcome of laminoplasty for acute traumatic spinal cord injury without instability. Korean J Spine. 2013;10(3):133–7. https://doi.org/10.14245/kjs.2013.10.3.133.
27. Aarabi B, Chixiang C, Simard JM, et al. Proposal of a management algorithm to predict the need for expansion duraplasty in American spinal injury association impairment scale grades A–C traumatic cervical spinal cord injury patients. J Neurotrauma. 2022;39(23–24):1716–26. https://doi.org/10.1089/neu.2022.0218.
28. Hogg FRA, Gallagher MJ, Chen S, Zoumprouli A, Papadopoulos MC, Saadoun S. Predictors of intraspinal pressure and optimal cord perfusion pressure after traumatic spinal cord injury. Neurocrit Care. 2019;30(2):421–8. https://doi.org/10.1007/s12028-018-0616-7.
29. Phang I, Werndle MC, Saadoun S, et al. Expansion duroplasty improves intraspinal pressure, spinal cord perfusion pressure, and vascular pressure reactivity index in patients with traumatic spinal cord injury: injured spinal cord pressure evaluation study. J Neurotrauma. 2015;32(12):865–74. https://doi.org/10.1089/neu.2014.3668.

30. Telemacque D, Zhu F, Chen K, et al. Method of decompression by durotomy and duroplasty for cervical spinal cord injury in patients without fracture or dislocation. J Neurorestoratol. 2018;6(1):158–64. https://doi.org/10.26599/JNR.2018.9040017.
31. Saadoun S, Grassner L, Belci M, et al. Duroplasty for injured cervical spinal cord with uncontrolled swelling: protocol of the DISCUS randomized controlled trial. Trials. 2023;24(1):497. https://doi.org/10.1186/s13063-023-07454-2.
32. Varsos GV, Werndle MC, Czosnyka ZH, et al. Intraspinal pressure and spinal cord perfusion pressure after spinal cord injury: an observational study. J Neurosurg Spine. 2015;23(6):763–71. https://doi.org/10.3171/2015.3.SPINE14870.
33. Hadley MN, Walters BC, Grabb PA, et al. Blood pressure management after acute spinal cord injury. Neurosurgery. 2002;50(3 Suppl):S58–62. https://doi.org/10.1097/00006123-200203001-00012.
34. Ryken TC, Hurlbert RJ, Hadley MN, et al. The acute cardiopulmonary management of patients with cervical spinal cord injuries. Neurosurgery. 2013;72(Suppl 2):84–92. https://doi.org/10.1227/NEU.0b013e318276ee16.
35. Readdy WJ, Whetstone WD, Ferguson AR, et al. Complications and outcomes of vasopressor usage in acute traumatic central cord syndrome. J Neurosurg Spine. 2015;23(5):574–80. https://doi.org/10.3171/2015.2.SPINE14746.
36. Streijger F, So K, Manouchehri N, et al. A direct comparison between norepinephrine and phenylephrine for augmenting spinal cord perfusion in a porcine model of spinal cord injury. J Neurotrauma. 2018;35(12):1345–57. https://doi.org/10.1089/neu.2017.5285.
37. Ploumis A, Yadlapalli N, Fehlings MG, Kwon BK, Vaccaro AR. A systematic review of the evidence supporting a role for vasopressor support in acute SCI. Spinal Cord. 2010;48(5):356–62. https://doi.org/10.1038/sc.2009.150.
38. Theodore N, Martirosyan N, Hersh AM, et al. Cerebrospinal fluid drainage in patients with acute spinal cord injury: a multi-center randomized controlled trial. World Neurosurg. 2023;177:e472–9. https://doi.org/10.1016/j.wneu.2023.06.078.
39. Catapano JS, John Hawryluk GW, Whetstone W, et al. Higher mean arterial pressure values correlate with neurologic improvement in patients with initially complete spinal cord injuries. World Neurosurg. 2016;96:72–9. https://doi.org/10.1016/j.wneu.2016.08.053.
40. Shawky Abdelgawaad A, El Sadik MHM, Hassan KM, El-Sharkawi M. Perioperative antibiotic prophylaxis in spinal surgery. SICOT J. 2021;7:31. https://doi.org/10.1051/sicotj/2021029.
41. Abola MV, Lin CC, Lin LJ, et al. Postoperative prophylactic antibiotics in spine surgery. J Bone Joint Surg. 2021;103(3):219–26. https://doi.org/10.2106/JBJS.20.00934.
42. Dimar JR, Glassman SD, Raque GH, Zhang YP, Shields CB. The influence of spinal canal narrowing and timing of decompression on neurologic recovery after spinal cord contusion in a rat model. Spine (Phila Pa 1976). 1999;24(16):1623–33. https://doi.org/10.1097/00007632-199908150-00002.
43. Batchelor PE, Wills TE, Skeers P, et al. Meta-analysis of pre-clinical studies of early decompression in acute spinal cord injury: a battle of time and pressure. PLoS One. 2013;8(8):e72659. https://doi.org/10.1371/journal.pone.0072659.
44. Furlan JC, Noonan V, Cadotte DW, Fehlings MG. Timing of decompressive surgery of spinal cord after traumatic spinal cord injury: an evidence-based examination of pre-clinical and clinical studies. J Neurotrauma. 2011;28(8):1371–99. https://doi.org/10.1089/neu.2009.1147.
45. Fehlings MG, Hachem LD, Tetreault LA, et al. Timing of decompressive surgery in patients with acute spinal cord injury: systematic review update. Global Spine J. 2024;14(3_suppl):38S–57S. https://doi.org/10.1177/21925682231197404.
46. Roberts TT, Leonard GR, Cepela DJ. Classifications in brief: American spinal injury association (ASIA) impairment scale. Clin Orthop Relat Res. 2017;475(5):1499–504. https://doi.org/10.1007/s11999-016-5133-4.
47. van Middendorp JJ, Hosman AJF, Donders ART, et al. A clinical prediction rule for ambulation outcomes after traumatic spinal cord injury: a longitudinal cohort study. Lancet. 2011;377(9770):1004–10. https://doi.org/10.1016/S0140-6736(10)62276-3.

48. Haghnegahdar A, Behjat R, Saadat S, et al. A randomized controlled trial of early versus late surgical decompression for thoracic and thoracolumbar spinal cord injury in 73 patients. Neurotrauma Rep. 2020;1(1):78–87. https://doi.org/10.1089/neur.2020.0027.
49. Rahimi-Movaghar V, Niakan A, Haghnegahdar A, Shahlaee A, Saadat S, Barzideh E. Early versus late surgical decompression for traumatic thoracic/thoracolumbar (T1-L1) spinal cord injured patients. Primary results of a randomized controlled trial at one year follow-up. Neurosciences (Riyadh). 2014;19(3):183–91.
50. Fehlings MG, Vaccaro A, Wilson JR, et al. Early versus delayed decompression for traumatic cervical spinal cord injury: results of the Surgical Timing in Acute Spinal Cord Injury Study (STASCIS). PLoS One. 2012;7(2):e32037. https://doi.org/10.1371/journal.pone.0032037.
51. Badhiwala JH, Wilson JR, Witiw CD, et al. The influence of timing of surgical decompression for acute spinal cord injury: a pooled analysis of individual patient data. Lancet Neurol. 2021;20(2):117–26. https://doi.org/10.1016/S1474-4422(20)30406-3.
52. Badhiwala JH, Wilson JR, Harrop JS, et al. Early vs late surgical decompression for central cord syndrome. JAMA Surg. 2022;157(11):1024–32. https://doi.org/10.1001/jamasurg.2022.4454.
53. Yousefifard M, Hashemi B, Forouzanfar MM, Khatamian Oskooi R, Madani Neishaboori A, Jalili Khoshnoud R. Ultra-early spinal decompression surgery can improve neurological outcome of complete cervical spinal cord injury; a systematic review and meta-analysis. Arch Acad Emerg Med. 2022;10(1):e11. https://doi.org/10.22037/aaem.v10i1.1471.
54. Silber JS, Vaccaro AR. Summary statement: the role and timing of decompression in acute spinal cord injury: evidence-based guidelines. Spine (Phila Pa 1976). 2001;26(24S). https://journals.lww.com/spinejournal/fulltext/2001/12151/summary_statement__the_role_and_timing_of.18.aspx
55. Azad TD, Nair SK, Kalluri AL, et al. Delays in presentation after traumatic spinal cord injury-a systematic review. World Neurosurg. 2023;169:e121–30. https://doi.org/10.1016/j.wneu.2022.10.086.
56. Chandra J, Sheerin F, Lopez de Heredia L, et al. MRI in acute and subacute post-traumatic spinal cord injury: pictorial review. Spinal Cord. 2012;50(1):2–7. https://doi.org/10.1038/sc.2011.107.
57. Azad TD, Raj D, Ran KR, et al. Concomitant traumatic brain injury delays surgery in patients with traumatic spinal cord injury. Neurosurgery. Published online January 10, 2024. https://doi.org/10.1227/neu.0000000000002816

Anesthetic Considerations for Traumatic Spinal Cord Injuries

9

Emily Anne Smith Bergbower, Elizabeth Cox-Williams, and Samuel Galvagno

9.1 Introduction

With an estimated incidence of over 17,000 traumatic spinal cord injury (SCI) cases per year in the United States and nearly one million cases worldwide annually, clinicians working in the acute care, perioperative, and critical care settings will inevitably have a direct role in managing patients with these injuries [18, 63]. Moreover, with an aging population at higher risk for SCI due to conditions such as osteoporosis, cervical spondylosis, and other risk factors, the incidence of these devastating injuries is not predicted to decrease. Older adults have been noted to be particularly susceptible to SCI, with a rising number of occurrences, 66% of which are attributable to falls [34]. Hence, potential SCI remains a significant issue for clinicians tending to patients in the acute care setting because improper management of the spine after traumatic injury can lead to disastrous neurological outcomes. In this chapter, we discuss anesthetic considerations for the management of adult patients with traumatic SCI, including airway management, anesthetic techniques, hemodynamic stabilization, and intraoperative monitoring.

9.2 Spinal Motion Restriction

Approximately 1.5–4% of all trauma patients may have an undiagnosed cervical SCI; hence, cervical immobilization is obligatory [24]. Spinal motion restriction (SMR) specifically refers to limiting the motion of the spine in patients at risk of

E. A. S. Bergbower (✉) · E. Cox-Williams · S. Galvagno
Department of Anesthesiology, University of Maryland School of Medicine, Baltimore, MD, USA
e-mail: Emily.Bergbower@som.umaryland.edu; Elizabeth.Williams@som.umaryland.edu; sgalvagno@som.umaryland.edu

E. Brogi et al. (eds.), *Traumatic Spinal Cord Injury*, Hot Topics in Acute Care Surgery and Trauma, https://doi.org/10.1007/978-3-031-99890-4_9

displacement of an unstable spinal injury. This term has largely replaced the phrase "spinal immobilization" in the care of trauma patients with potential acute spinal cord injuries. The *American College of Surgeons 2022 Best Practice Guidelines: Spine Injury* recommends that SMR should be applied to the entire spinal column for patients with any of the following indications after blunt trauma: an acutely altered level of consciousness, midline neck or back pain/tenderness, focal neurologic symptoms, anatomic spinal deformity, or "distracting circumstances" (e.g., degloving or crush injuries, long bone fractures, communication barriers) that prevent reliable examination [1]. If patients meet these criteria, clinicians should ensure that the head, neck, and torso are kept in alignment through the use of an appropriately sized cervical collar (c-collar) in conjunction with either a long backboard, ambulance cot, or scoop stretcher depending on resource availability. These restrictions serve to minimize flexion, extension, and rotation of the spine [17].

While motion restriction is necessary for management of a patient with potential or confirmed SCI, it is important to consider that these interventions are not without risk in a hospital setting. Spinal motion restriction has been associated with poor laryngoscopy views, deep venous thrombosis, aspiration, increased intracranial pressure, local pressure injuries, and pain [1, 66]. The overall goal should be to clear the spine as soon as possible through either interview and examination or appropriate radiographic assessment as recommended by the Congress of Neurological Surgeons in their 2013 Guidelines for the Management of Acute Cervical and Spinal Cord Injuries [27, 57]. If SCI is confirmed or cannot yet be ruled out, precautions and restrictions should be maintained. This is particularly pertinent for the cervical spine, in which the hard c-collar must be sustained throughout the process of airway preparation, preoxygenation, and eventual induction.

9.3 Preoxygenation and Preparation for Airway Management

Before induction, preoxygenation can be performed passively by face mask or high-flow nasal cannula with the stretcher or operating room bed positioned in reverse Trendelenburg. This is the ideal position for preoxygenation in SCI patients as it optimizes respiratory mechanics without the risk of sitting the patient upright [5, 59, 69]. If the patient is able to protect the airway without a jaw thrust, clinicians may consider application of high-flow nasal oxygen for pre- and periprocedural oxygenation. While data supporting the use of high-flow nasal cannula oxygen delivery in patients with SCI are lacking, some studies in other populations of patients requiring emergency intubation have demonstrated increased safe apnea time, greater first pass success rates, and less hypoxemia [3, 25].

During preoxygenation, the patient should be assessed for secretions, bronchospasm, and the use of accessory respiratory muscles. Respiratory failure may occur abruptly after direct SCI, or insidiously if edema or bleeding progresses. Cervical nerve roots (C3-C5) that comprise the phrenic nerve may be compromised, inhibiting diaphragmatic movement. Increased production of secretions may occur within one hour of injury and is likely caused by autonomic dysfunction with unopposed vagal activity. Treatment with anticholinergic agents such as glycopyrrolate may help optimize airway conditions for induction and intubation. Bronchospasm, frequently seen with cervical spine injuries, is also caused by autonomic dysfunction and should be aggressively treated with inhaled bronchodilators prior to induction [8, 23].

9.4 Airway Management

Patients with a cervical SCI often require airway management in the emergency department, trauma bay, or operating room. While airway management is required for every patient undergoing surgery for SCI, this discussion is focused on management of patients with a cervical SCI because these injuries are traditionally thought to either increase a preexisting injury or cause a new one [70].

In a published international airway management guideline, nine recommendations were made for airway management in patients with cervical SCI. These recommendations are summarized in Table 9.1.

9.4.1 Airway Maneuvers

Prior to securing the airway, several airway maneuvers are recommended to minimize movement of the cervical spine [70, 71]. Face mask ventilation is often required prior to intubation, and use of a jaw thrust maneuver is recommended (rather than chin-tilting) to prevent cervical spine movement [29]. Supraglottic airway devices (SAD) should be readily available, and the device the clinician is most familiar with should be used. Intubation through an SAD is possible, though other definitive techniques should be attempted first. No SAD has been shown to be superior in terms of limiting cervical spinal motion during intubation or improving intubation success [70].

The anterior portion of the rigid or semi-rigid c-collar should be removed prior to securing the airway, with a dedicated assistant subsequently providing manual in-line stabilization. Semi-rigid c-collars have been shown to reduce inter-incisor distance and unpredictably restrict mouth opening, which can impede definitive airway placement [26, 30]. Furthermore, rigid neck immobilization can worsen laryngoscopy views [30]. However, the act of both placing and subsequently removing the c-collar may also exacerbate cervical spine displacement, so the careful

Table 9.1 Recommendations from the Difficult Airway Society, Association of Anaesthetists, British Society of Orthopaedic Anaesthetists, Intensive Care Society, Neuro Anaesthesia and Critical Care Society, and Faculty of Prehospital Care and Royal College of Emergency Medicine for airway management in patients with cervical SCI

	Recommendation	Level of evidence
1	Attempts should be made to minimize cervical spine movement during preoxygenation and face mask ventilation	Grade D, weak recommendation
2	When a simple maneuver is required to maintain an airway, the jaw thrust should be used rather than head tilt plus chin lift	Grade D, weak recommendation
3	If tracheal intubation through a supraglottic airway device (SAD) is indicated, there is no specific device that is clearly superior in reducing cervical spine movement or successful tracheal intubation. Clinicians should use the SAD that they are most familiar with	Grade D, strong recommendation
4	Second generation SADs should be considered in preference to first generation SADs	Grade D, strong recommendation
5	Where possible, videolaryngoscopy should be used for tracheal intubation in patients with suspected or confirmed cervical SCI	Grade A, moderate recommendation
6	Clinicians who perform tracheal intubation in patients with suspected or confirmed SCI should receive regular training in the use of videolaryngoscopy with cervical spine immobilization	Grade D, weak recommendation
7	Clinicians should consider using an adjunct such as a stylet or bougie when performing tracheal intubation in a patient whose cervical spine is immobilized	Grade D, weak recommendation
8	During tracheal intubation attempts, a semirigid or rigid cervical collar should be removed, which can be done most easily by only removing the anterior part of the collar. This will help minimize any movement to the cervical spine	Grade D, weak recommendation
9	Multidisciplinary planning, preparation, and optimization of human factors should be considered before airway management in patients with suspected or confirmed cervical SCI	Grade D, weak recommendation

Source: Wiles et al. [70]

application of manual in-line stabilization becomes essential [50]. For this maneuver to be successful, the assistant will generally stand at the patient's head or off to the side and use the palms of the hands to support the occiput and mandible, reducing movement and counteracting the motion associated with airway manipulation. However, it should be noted that this technique worsens the laryngoscopic view when compared to the traditional sniffing position and increases the amount of pressure applied by the laryngoscope blade [47, 60].

The simple jaw thrust maneuver, when uncoupled from head lift and chin tilt, minimizes cervical spine displacement and can be a key intervention for maintaining airway patency in an emergency. Prasarn et al. demonstrated that in the presence of an unstable C1-C2 injury, jaw thrust alone produces less angular motion in all planes as well as less axial displacement [52]. Sawada et al. noted only a slight change in the cervical vertebral angle at C0-C4 when mandibular advancement and mouth opening are used to maintain airway patency in a neutral neck position [61]. Cricoid pressure is occasionally used to theoretically compress the esophagus to prevent aspiration of gastric contents during emergency intubation. When coupled with manual support, cricoid pressure causes minimal displacement of the cervical spine when used as an accessory technique for securing an airway [31, 51]. In the IRIS trial of over 3400 patients receiving rapid sequence intubation, cricoid pressure failed to show any benefit in terms of preventing pulmonary aspiration; hence, in many systems, this technique has been abandoned [9, 24].

9.4.2 Endotracheal Intubation Techniques

Once a patient has been appropriately positioned, prepared, and stabilized, there are three general pathways for definitive airway management for patients with SCI: direct laryngoscopy, video laryngoscopy, and awake fiberoptic intubation. Awake fiberoptic intubation has historically been regarded as the "gold standard" for cervical SCI patients. This technique may be an ideal choice for a cooperative patient in a controlled or semi-urgent situation because it is the most time-consuming technique and requires the most skill. This method allows for flexible manipulation with minimal cervical motion and provides excellent views [10, 14, 19]. It should be noted that among experienced anesthesiologists, there was no difference in time to intubation between awake fiberoptic and video laryngoscopy [55]. Thus, clinician experience should be an active factor in case-by-case decision making. A suggested technique for awake fiberoptic intubation is listed in Table 9.2.

Similar to the technique used for awake fiberoptic intubation, indirect visualization of the glottis via video laryngoscopy is thought to decrease the overall movement of the cervical spine during intubation and provide better views of the glottis compared to traditional direct laryngoscopy [20, 41, 49, 54, 71]. Thus, video laryngoscopy may reduce the risk of secondary damage to the cervical spine during intubation. However, the data are not completely consistent. Some investigators have observed no significant difference in the degree of movement when compared to direct laryngoscopy [53]. Clinician skill and experience with individual techniques are again noted to be an important factor, as experienced anesthesiologists displayed a reduced angle of deviation of the cervical spine compared to those less experienced when securing airways by video laryngoscopy [41]. In some cases, a hybrid technique may be used, utilizing topicalization of the airway as described in Table 9.2. Following topicalization, a video laryngoscope may be introduced in a spontaneously breathing patient followed by either placement of the endotracheal tube or use of a fiberoptic scope as a guide.

Direct laryngoscopy (DL) is the traditional method of intubation and is available in resource-limited locations. While both convenient and a standard of general practice, this method causes the most deviation of the cervical spine and produces the worst views, especially when coupled with cervical spine precautions and manual in-line stabilization [6, 28, 49, 53, 54]. While laryngoscope insertion has been shown to result in minimal movement, Sawin et al. demonstrated that blade elevation significantly extends all segments of the cervical spine, especially the atlanto-occipital and atlanto-axial joints [62]. Another cadaveric study revealed that when compared to video laryngoscopy, DL caused a 1.6 mm reduction in the dural sac

Table 9.2 Procedure for awake fiberoptic intubation

Preparation
Glycopyrrolate (0.2–0.4 mg IV) may be considered to decrease secretions. Sedation should be accomplished with either low-dose opioids or titration of benzodiazepines (i.e., incremental doses of midazolam, 0.5 mg IV). Opioids and benzodiazepines should not be combined to prevent apnea. Dexmedetomidine is an alternative. Suggested dosing: 10-minute loading infusion (0.5–1.0 mcg/kg) followed by a 0.2–0.7 mcg/kg/hr continuous infusion. Effects should be evident within 5–10 minutes
Equipment
1% and 4% lidocaine The drug totals for this technique are: 3 mL of 5% lidocaine = approximately 150 mg of lidocaine 5–10 mL of 4% lidocaine = 200–400 mg of lidocaine 1–2 mL of 1% lidocaine = 10–20 mg of lidocaine The total amount used is approximately 350 mg, but much of the lidocaine may be swallowed and rapidly metabolized by first pass hepatic metabolism Adult vs. pediatric fiberoptic scope 8.5 or 7.5 endotracheal tube Surgical lubricant or silicone solution (for scope lubrication) Suction tubing and working suction Gauze pads: 4 × 4 or 4.8 cm Right angle tonsil holder or Magill forceps (Magill forceps are more readily available) Nasal cannula (or high flow nasal cannula), preferably with end-tidal CO_2 monitoring capability (regular nasal cannula tubing can be perforated with a 14 g intravenous catheter for end-tidal CO_2 monitoring connection)
Procedure
Apply nasal cannula and monitors Administer sedation as above Maintain meaningful contact with the patient at all times; the goal is amnesia, not apnea (maintain spontaneous ventilation at all times) Apply 2–3% lidocaine ointment generously to the back of the tongue. This anesthetizes the glossopharyngeal nerve Soak two gauze pads with 4% lidocaine. The gauze pads should be "dripping wet" Wrap the lidocaine-soaked gauze around the forceps and gently introduce the forceps into the pyriform sinus (deep past the base of the tongue). Hold the forceps in place for 60–90 seconds. Repeat on the opposite side. The patient will report that their "throat feels numb." A few initial coughs may be expected; provide reassurance. This technique anesthetizes the superior laryngeal nerves Place an oral airway. This prevents the patient from biting the scope and assures that the gag reflexes are suppressed Ensure the endotracheal tube is placed over the fiberoptic scope Introduce the fiberoptic scope with suction attached to clear secretions as necessary Once the glottis (vocal cords) is visualized, inject 1–2 mL of 1% lidocaine into the fiberoptic scope to spray the cords. The patient will usually cough with this. This technique anesthetizes the recurrent laryngeal nerve Place the endotracheal tube and ensure proper placement with fiberoptic visualization Confirm placement with end-tidal capnography Initiate general anesthesia with a sedative (i.e., propofol, opioids) and neuromuscular blocking agent

width, reflecting an increased risk of spinal cord impingement during intubation [43]. While there are significant drawbacks to consider, DL is the most readily available method and may be required in resource-limited areas.

9.4.3 Supraglottic Airways

Supraglottic airways (SGAs) may be required when endotracheal intubation is not possible and a temporary airway is necessary. The laryngeal mask airway (LMA) is a widely available SGA that can be used safely in cervical spine injury but may be difficult to place in the presence of spine restrictions and can exert some degree of negative force on the cervical spine [40, 45]. Kihara et al. have demonstrated that the intubating LMA produces segmental movement of the cervical spine even in the presence of manual in-line stabilization [39]. Similarly, Keller et al. found that the LMA exerted greater pressures against the cervical spine, producing posterior displacement [38]. However, as an airway rescue device, the LMA is a critical part of the American Society of Anesthesiologists' (ASA) difficult airway practice guidelines and would be required as an emergent intervention in this patient population, regardless [4]. As with other methods discussed, the risks and benefits should always be weighed and plans determined on a case-by-case basis through assessment of the patient as a whole.

9.5 General Anesthesia

The primary clinical objectives of anesthesia for surgery after acute SCI are to maintain hemodynamic and pulmonary stability, manage postoperative pain, prevent further neurologic injury, ensure optimal operating conditions, and facilitate accurate neuromonitoring.

9.5.1 Hemodynamic Monitoring

From a hemodynamic perspective, hypotension following SCI worsens neurologic outcomes and must be aggressively treated [57]. In addition, augmentation of mean arterial pressure (MAP) to 85–90 mm Hg for a period of 7 days likely improves neurologic outcome by ensuring spinal cord perfusion, although the data for this recommendation is not conclusive [15, 42, 58, 67, 68]. A MAP target of 85–90 mm Hg assumes intact baseline autoregulation. Patients with chronic, poorly controlled hypertension may require even higher MAP goals, balancing the risk of intraoperative and postoperative hemorrhage from elevated MAP. Consequently, arterial line monitoring during surgery for acute SCI is required to ensure accurate blood pressure measurement and enable prompt intervention.

Volume resuscitation to treat and prevent hypotension is an essential aspect of anesthetic care following SCI. Volume resuscitation must be balanced against the risk of pulmonary edema that could worsen respiratory injury. In addition, when prone positioning is necessary, excessive volume administration could worsen facial and airway edema.

Neurogenic shock must be considered, particularly when the SCI is at T6 or above [12, 72]. The bradycardia and hypotension caused by the disruption of normal sympathetic nervous system function should be treated with a thoughtful combination of volume resuscitation and pressor support [12, 72]. While no vasopressor is clearly superior in the treatment of neurogenic shock, norepinephrine may be preferred as its dual α and β activity effectively treats both vasodilatory hypotension and bradycardia. Central venous access, while not required for anesthesia for SCI surgery, may be helpful if vasopressor use is likely.

9.5.2 Respiratory Considerations

Respiratory complications following SCI are a leading cause of morbidity and mortality in these patients [57]. While there is no conclusive evidence of its benefit in neurosurgical patients [44], pursuing lung-protective ventilation intraoperatively may improve pulmonary outcomes and is unlikely to cause harm based on data from other major surgeries [22]. During lung-protective ventilation, hypercapnia and increased $PaCO_2$ must be avoided to prevent increased spinal cord pressure that could worsen underlying injury.

9.5.3 Induction and Maintenance

Regarding choice of induction agent, as long as oxygenation, ventilation, blood pressure and heart rate are maintained at goal, any standard anesthetic medication can be utilized. Representative induction agents are listed in Table 9.3.

Neuromuscular blockade can be used for intubation, although prompt return of full muscle strength will be necessary for neuromonitoring purposes during surgery. Caution must be exercised with succinylcholine because upregulation of acetylcholine receptors can occur following SCI. Receptor upregulation usually begins 3–4 days following injury, but the timing is variable [36].

The selected anesthetic must be compatible with neuromonitoring (discussed later in this chapter). While inhaled anesthetics at a concentration of 0.5 MAC or less should be compatible with neuromonitoring, many anesthesiologists elect for total intravenous anesthesia to ensure that anesthesia medications are not a cause of abnormal intraoperative neuromonitoring signals.

Propofol may have neuroprotective effects [2, 7], and these features may be beneficial in patients with SCI [37, 64]. However, there is no clear correlation between the choice of anesthetic and postoperative cognitive outcomes in other surgical fields [16].

Table 9.3 Induction agents used for patients requiring anesthesia for traumatic SCI surgery

Agent	Initial dose	Onset	Duration of action	SCI Considerations
Propofol	1–3 mg/kg	10–30 s	8–10 min	If the patient has hypotension or other traumatic injuries, the dose must be reduced, sometimes by as much as 1/10 the recommended induction dose (due to decreases in systemic vascular resistance)
Ketamine	1–2 mg/kg IV 2–4 mg/kg IM	30–60 s	5–20 min	Direct myocardial depressant but has indirect stimulatory effects (usually avoided in patients with coronary artery disease)
Etomidate	0.2–0.3 mg/kg	30–45 s	10–20 min	A single dose may cause adrenocortical suppression
Remifentanil	1 mcg/kg	30–60 s	<10 min	250 times more potent than morphine; may cause hypotension; not a reliable amnestic; does not accumulate; metabolized by non-specific esterases
Midazolam	0.3–0.6 mg/kg	2–3 min	20–30 min	When combined with opioids, may cause marked hypotension and respiratory depression

A propofol infusion is usually combined with an opioid infusion during spine surgery. Remifentanil is a popular choice as it is easily titratable, accommodating changes in hemodynamics and surgical stimulus. It is also rapidly metabolized. Alfentanil, sufentanil, and fentanyl are also excellent choices if context-sensitive half times are taken into account.

9.6 Intraoperative Neurophysiological Monitoring

In many centers, intraoperative neurophysiological monitoring (IONM) is used during surgery for spinal cord injuries. While there is no universal guideline that dictates the use of IONM, techniques are available to detect potential ischemia or secondary direct physical damage to the spinal cord during surgical procedures, including the placement of pedicle screws for spinal fixation [11, 32, 46]. IONM may also help inform targets for blood pressure augmentation, thereby serving as a guide for titration of fluids and vasopressors to maintain or enhance spinal cord perfusion.

Both the sensory and motor tracts of the spinal cord may be monitored using somatosensory evoked potentials (SSEPs) and transcranial motor evoked potentials (MEPs), respectively (Fig. 9.1). Spontaneous or triggered electromyography (EMG) may also be employed to monitor muscles innervated by spinal roots that might be at risk of damage during surgery [21]. Decreases in the amplitude or prolongation of the latency of SSEP or MEP signals, especially during or after a surgical intervention, may help decrease complications by over 50% in nontraumatic spinal cord surgeries, though the ability of IONM to prevent additional complications in

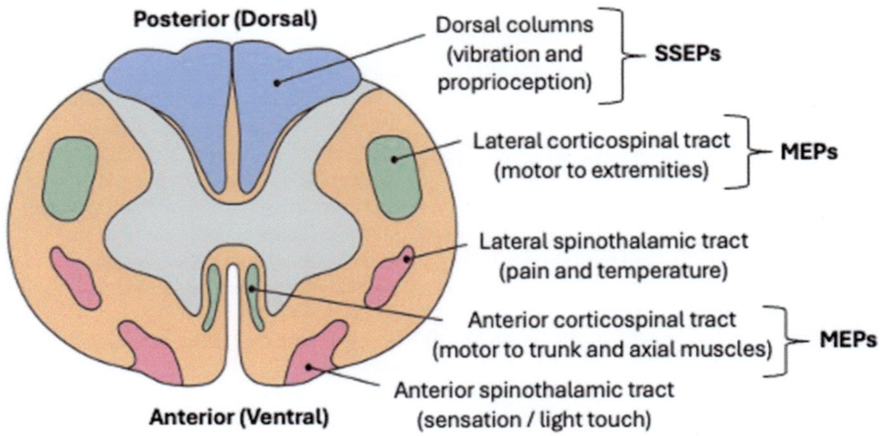

Fig. 9.1 General overview of spinal cord tracts and pathways assessed during IONM

traumatic SCI surgery remains understudied [33, 48, 56, 65]. While a comprehensive discussion of IONM is beyond the scope of this chapter, a brief overview is presented, followed by a discussion regarding anesthetic effects that may enhance or suppress IONM signals.

9.6.1 Monitoring Modalities

SSEPs monitor sensory pathways located along the dorsal (posterior) and lateral portions of the spinal cord. Sensory fibers responsible for position and vibration sensation occupy the posterior (dorsal) portion of the spinal cord, ascending ipsilateral to the brain stem in two fasciculi. The fasciculus gracilis receives fibers from the lower extremities, and the fasciculus cuneatus receives fibers from the upper extremities. In the brainstem, these dorsal tracts cross to the opposite side, terminating in the thalamus and synapsing in the ventral posterolateral nucleus. SSEPs involve the application of electrical stimuli by needles positioned near the median or ulnar nerve (upper extremity monitoring) or the posterior tibial nerve (lower extremity monitoring). Electrodes placed on the scalp detect afferent signals from the stimulated nerves. A decrease in amplitude of at least 50% or a 10% increase in latency from baseline may suggest an injury to the dorsal tracts [21].

Afferent (sensory) pathways use unmyelinated or small myelinated sensory fibers to detect temperature and pain via the spinothalamic tract. This tract is located in the anterior and lateral aspects of the spinal cord and is not reliably monitored by SSEPs. Damage to the ventral aspect of the spinal cord is also not reliably detected by SSEPs. Clinically, damage to the dorsal columns manifests as ipsilateral impairment of vibration and proprioception when an injury occurs before the point of decussation (i.e., point where fibers cross) and contralateral impairment when an injury occurs above the point of decussation.

MEPs are used to monitor efferent (motor) pathways, including the corticospinal tract. The corticospinal tract is the largest descending tract in humans and is divided into anterior and lateral components [35]. The lateral corticospinal tract sends fibers predominantly to the extremity muscles, and the cortical innervation is contralateral (i.e., the left motor cortex controls the right extremities). The anterior corticospinal tract sends fibers mainly to the trunk or axial muscles [35]. MEPs provide data primarily on the lateral corticospinal tract [21]. Electrodes placed along the cranium provide stimulation, and electrical activity at the peripheral muscle groups is then monitored. At the epidural level, D waves may be recorded. For upper extremity monitoring, the adductor pollicis brevis muscle is monitored; the lower extremities are monitored by placing electrode needles at the gastrocnemius, tibialis anterior, or abductor hallucis muscles. MEPs are sensitive and specific for identifying SCI and poor spinal cord perfusion [21].

With trauma to the spinal cord, the arterial supply may be disrupted. The anterior spinal artery arises from the subclavian and vertebral arteries superiorly and from two radicular arteries in the cervical and upper thoracic region [32]. In the lower thoracic and upper lumbar region, the anterior spinal artery is supplied by the arteria radicularis magna (ARM), also known as the artery of Adamkiewicz. The two posterior spinal arteries receive blood primarily from the vertebral arteries, with contributions in the cervical region from deep cervical and subclavian radicular branches. Posterior intercostal, lumbar, and sacral arteries supply the posterior arteries in the thoracic, lumbar, and sacral regions. Hence, based on clinical examination and radiological findings, clinicians may ascertain anatomical areas of risk during spinal cord surgery, thereby informing the choice of IONM techniques that may be used.

9.6.2 Anesthetic Considerations

Anesthetics affect IONM. In particular, inhalation anesthetics may affect IONM signals, especially MEPs. MEPs may not be detectable when the minimal alveolar concentration (MAC) of volatiles is greater than 0.5% [32]. SSEPs are less sensitive to volatiles than MEPs. Historically, total intravenous anesthesia, using combinations of agents such as propofol, opioids, or other sedatives, has been recommended as a technique of choice when using IONM. However, there is a paucity of data to inform choices about the ideal anesthetic [13]. Some institutions use high-concentration nitrous oxide with opioids, whereas others use hybrid techniques that combine sedatives, opioids, and volatiles. At our institution, a common hybrid approach is to use sevoflurane titrated to a MAC of ≤0.5% with additional infusions of propofol (25–75 mcg/kg/minute) and remifentanil (0.05 to 2 mcg/kg/minute). Both ketamine and etomidate may enhance SSEP and MEP signals, with etomidate increasing the amplitude of motor responses at low doses [32]. As with all anesthetics, high doses of ketamine and etomidate can suppress the amplitude of signals [46]. Neuromuscular blocking drugs do not affect SSEPs but should be avoided when MEPs are used, unless only D waves from MEPs are being monitored, as D waves are not affected by these agents [46].

9.7 Conclusion

Anesthetic considerations in SCI patients focus on preventing exacerbation of injuries and optimizing conditions for recovery. Specific actions that meet these goals include maintaining spinal motion restriction, avoiding hypotension and hypoxia during surgical procedures, and administering anesthetic agents that are compatible with the use of IONM. Helping patients get through the perioperative period safely is the first step in their path to recovery.

Acknowledgments None.

Competing Interests The authors have no competing financial or non-financial interests in relation to the content of this work.

References

1. ACS-TQIP 2022: https://www.facs.org/media/k45gikqv/spine_injury_guidelines.pdf
2. Adembri C, Venturi L, Pellegrini-Giampietro DE. Neuroprotective effects of propofol in acute cerebral injury. CNS Drug Rev. 2007;13(3):333–51.
3. Ahmad I, El-Boghadadly K, Bhagrath R, et al. Difficult airway society guidelines for awake tracheal intubation (ATI) in adults. Anaesthesia. 2020;75:509–28.
4. Apfelbaum JL, Hagberg CA, Connis RT, et al. 2022 American Society of Anesthesiologists Practice Guidelines for management of the difficult airway. Anesthesiology. 2022;136:31–81.
5. Azam D. Preoxygenation and anesthesia: a detailed review. Cureus. 2021;13:e13240.
6. Bathory I, Frascarlolo P, Kern C, et al. Evaluation of the GlideScope for tracheal intubation in patients with cervical spine immobilisation by a semi-rigid collar. Anaesthesia. 2009;64:1337–41.
7. Bayona NA, Gelb AW, Jiang Z, et al. Propofol neuroprotection in cerebral ischemia and its effects on low-molecular-weight antioxidants and skilled motor tasks. Anesthesiology. 2004;100:1151–9.
8. Berlly M, Shem K. Respiratory management during the first five days after spinal cord injury. J Spinal Cord Med. 2007;30:309–18.
9. Birenbaum A, Hajage D, Roche S, et al. Effect of cricoid pressure compared with a sham procedure in the rapid sequence induction of anesthesia: the IRIS randomized clinical trial. JAMA Surg. 2019;154(1):9–17.
10. Brimacombe J, Keller C, Kunzel K, et al. Cervical spine motion during airway management: a cinefluoroscopic study of the posteriorly destabilized third cervical vertebrae in human cadavers. Anesth Analg. 2000;91:1274–8.
11. Bible JE, Goss M. To use or not use intraoperative neuromonitoring: utilization of neuromonitoring during spine surgeries and associated conflicts of interest, a cross-sectional survey study. J Am Acad Orthop Surg Glob Res Rev. 2022;6(3):e21.00273.
12. Dave S, Dahlstrom JJ, Weisbrod LJ. Neurogenic shock. In: StatPearls [Internet]. Treasure Island (FL): StatPearls Publishing; 2024 Jan; 2023. Available from: https://www.ncbi.nlm.nih.gov/books/NBK459361/.
13. Deiner S. Highlights of anesthetic considerations for intraoperative neuromonitoring. Semin Cardiothorac Vasc Anesth. 2010;14(1):51–3.
14. Dutta K, Sriganesh K, Chakrabarti D, et al. Cervical spine movement during awake orotracheal intubation with fiberoptic scope and McGrath videolaryngoscope in patients undergoing surgery for cervical spine instability: a randomized control trial. J Neurosurg Anesthesiol. 2020;32:249–55.

15. Evaniew N, Mazlouman SJ, Belley-Côté EP, et al. Interventions to optimize spinal cord perfusion in patients with acute traumatic spinal cord injuries: a systematic review. J Neurotrauma. 2020;37:1127–39.
16. Evered LA, Silbert BS. Postoperative cognitive dysfunction and noncardiac surgery. Anesth Analg. 2018;127(2):496–505.
17. Fischer PE, Perina DG, Delbridge TR, et al. Spinal motion restriction in the trauma patient—a joint position statement. Prehosp Emerg Care. 2018;22:659–61.
18. Fitzharris M, Cripps RA, Lee BB. Estimating the global incidence of traumatic spinal cord injury. Spinal Cord. 2014;52:117–22.
19. Ford P, Nolan J. Cervical spine injury and airway management. Curr Opin Anaesthesiol. 2002;15:193–201.
20. Foulds L, McGuire BE, Shippey BJ. A randomised cross-over trial comparing the McGrath((R)) series 5 videolaryngoscope with the Macintosh laryngoscope in patients with cervical spine immobilisation. Anaesthesia. 2016;71:437–42.
21. Furlan D, Deana C, Orso D, et al. Perioperative management of spinal cord injury: the anesthesiologist's point of view. Minerva Anestesiol. 2021;87(12):1347–58.
22. Futier E, Constantin JM, Paugam-Burtz C, for the IMPROVE Study Group, et al. A trial of intraoperative low-tidal-volume ventilation in abdominal surgery. N Engl J Med. 2021;369(5):428–37.
23. Galeriras-Vazquez R, Rascado-Sedes P, Mourelo FM, et al. Respiratory management in the patient with spinal cord injury. Biomed Res Int. 2013;2013:168757.
24. Galvagno SM, Scalea TM. Airway management in the trauma patient. In: Cameron J, Cameron A, editors. Cameron's current surgical therapy. New York: Elsevier; 2022. p. 22–9.
25. Gleason JM, Christian BR, Barton ED. Nasal cannula apneic oxygenation prevents desaturation during endotracheal intubation: an integrative literature review. West J Emerg Med. 2018;19(2):403–11.
26. Goutcher CM, Lochhead V. Reduction in mouth opening with semi-rigid cervical collars. Br J Anaesth. 2005;95:344–8.
27. Hadley MN, Walters BC, Aarabi B, et al. Clinical assessment following acute cervical spinal cord injury. Neurosurgery. 2013;72(Suppl 2):40–53.
28. Hansel J, Rogers AM, Lewis SR, et al. Videolaryngoscopy versus direct laryngoscopy for adults undergoing tracheal intubation: a Cochrane systematic review and meta-analysis update. Br J Anaesth. 2022;129:612–23.
29. Hauswald M, Sklar DP, Tandberg D, et al. Cervical spine movement during airway management: cinefluoroscopic appraisal in human cadavers. Am J Emerg Med. 1991;9:535–8.
30. Heath KJ. The effect of laryngoscopy of different cervical spine immobilisation techniques. Anaesthesia. 1994;49:843–5.
31. Helliwell V, Gabbott DA. The effect of single-handed cricoid pressure on cervical spine movement after applying manual in-line stabilisation—a cadaver study. Resuscitation. 2001;49:53–7.
32. Husain AM. Neurophysiologic intraoperative monitoring (second edition). New York: Demos Medical; 2015. p. 106–26.
33. Ibrahim T, Mrowczynski O, Zalatimo O, et al. The impact of neurophysiological intraoperative monitoring during spinal cord and spine surgery: a critical analysis of 121 cases. Cureus. 2017;9:e1861.
34. Jain NB, Ayers GD, Peterson EN, et al. Traumatic spinal cord injury in the United States, 1993–2012. JAMA. 2015;313:2236–43.
35. Javed K, Reddy V, Lui F. Neuroanatomy, lateral corticospinal tract. In: StatPearls [Internet]. Treasure Island (FL): StatPearls Publishing; 2024 Jan; 2023. Available from: https://www.ncbi.nlm.nih.gov/books/NBK534818.
36. Julien F, Biebuyck JAJ, Martyn D, et al. Up-and-down regulation of skeletal muscle acetylcholine receptors effects on neuromuscular blockers. Anesthesiology. 1992;78:822–43.

37. Kaur J, Flores-Gutiérrez J, Nistri A. Neuroprotective effect of propofol against excitotoxic injury to locomotor networks of the rat spinal cord in vitro. Eur J Neurosci. 2016;44(7):2418–30.
38. Keller C, Brimacombe J, Keller K. Pressures exerted against the cervical vertebrae by the standard and intubating laryngeal mask airways: a randomized, controlled, cross-over study in fresh cadavers. Anesth Analg. 1999;89:1296–300.
39. Kihara S, Watanabe S, Brimacombe J, et al. Segmental cervical spine movement with the intubating laryngeal mask during manual in-line stabilization in patients with cervical pathology undergoing cervical spine surgery. Anesth Analg. 2000;91:195–200.
40. Kilic T, Goksu E, Durmaz D, et al. Upper cervical spine movement during intubation with different airway devices. Am J Emerg Med. 2013;31:1034–6.
41. Kill C, Risse J, Wallot P, et al. Videolaryngoscopy with glidescope reduces cervical spine movement in patients with unsecured cervical spine. J Emerg Med. 2013;44:750–6.
42. Lee YS, Kim KT, Kwon BK. Hemodynamic management of acute spinal cord injury: a literature review. Neurospine. 2021;18(1):7–14. https://doi.org/10.14245/ns.2040144.072.
43. Liao S, Schneider NRE, Weilbacher F, et al. Spinal movement and dural sac compression during airway management in a cadaveric model with atlanto-occipital instability. Eur Spine J. 2018;27:1295–302.
44. Longhini F, Pasin L, Montagnini C, et al. Intraoperative protective ventilation in patients undergoing major neurosurgical interventions: a randomized clinical trial. BMC Anesthesiol. 2021;21:184. https://doi.org/10.1186/s12871-021-01404-8.
45. Malik M, Subramaniam R, Churasia S, et al. Tracheal intubation in patients with cervical spine immobilization: a comparison of the Airwayscope, LMA CTrach, and the Macintosh laryngoscopes. Br J Anaesth. 2009;102:654–61.
46. Moller AR. Intraoperative neurophysiological monitoring (third edition). New York: Springer; 2011. p. 207–34.
47. Nolan JP, Wilson ME. Orotracheal intubation in patients with potential cervical spine injuries. An indication for the gum elastic bougie. Anaesthesia. 1993;48:630–3.
48. Nuwer MR, Dawson EG, Carlson LG. Somatosensory evoked potential spinal cord monitoring reduces neurologic deficits after scoliosis surgery: results of a large multicenter study. Electroencephalogr Clin Neurophysiol. 1995;96:6–11.
49. Paik H, Park HP. Randomized crossover trial comparing cervical spine motion during tracheal intubation with a Macintosh laryngoscope versus a C-MAC D-blade videolaryngoscope in a simulated immobilized cervical spine. BMC Anesthesiol. 2020;20:201.
50. Prasarn ML, Conrad B, Del Rossi G, et al. Motion generated in the unstable cervical spine during the application and removal of cervical immobilization collars. J Trauma Acute Care Surg. 2012;72:1609–13.
51. Prasarn ML, Horodyski M, Schneider P, et al. The effect of cricoid pressure on the unstable cervical spine. J Emerg Med. 2016;50:427–32.
52. Prasarn ML, Horodyski M, Scott N, et al. Motion generated in the unstable upper cervical spine during head tilt-chin lift and jaw thrust maneuvers. Spine J. 2014;14:609–14.
53. Robaitaille A, Williams SR, Tremblay MH, et al. Cervical spine motion during tracheal intubation with manual in-line stabilization: direct laryngoscopy versus GlideScope videolaryngoscopy. Anesth Analg. 2008;106:935–41.
54. Romito JW, Riccio CA, Bagley CA, et al. Cervical spine movement in a cadaveric model of severe spinal instability: a study comparing tracheal intubation with 4 different laryngoscopes. J Neurosurg Anesthesiol. 2020;32:57–62.
55. Rosenstock CV, Thorgersen B, Afshari A, et al. Awake fiberoptic or awake video laryngoscopic tracheal intubation in patients with anticipated difficult airway management: a randomized clinical trial. Anesthesiology. 2012;116:1210–6.
56. Raynor BL, Bright JD, Lenke LG, et al. Significant change or loss of intraoperative monitoring data: a 25-year experience in 12,375 spinal surgeries. Spine. 2013;38:E101–8.
57. Ryken TC, Hadley MN, Walters BC, et al. Radiographic assessment. Neurosurgery. 2013a;72(Suppl 2):54–72.

58. Ryken TC, Hurlbert RJ, Hadley MN, et al. The acute cardiopulmonary management of patients with cervical spinal cord injuries. Neurosurgery. 2013b;72:84–92.
59. Sacino A, Rosenblatt K. Early management of acute spinal cord injury-part I: initial injury to surgery. J Neuroanaesth Crit Care. 2019;6:213–21.
60. Santoni BG, Hindman BJ, Puttlitz CM, et al. Manual in-line stabilization increases pressures applied by the laryngoscope blade during direct laryngoscopy and orotracheal intubation. Anesthesiology. 2009;110:24–31.
61. Sawada A, Ochiai G, Yamakage M. A two-handed airway maneuver of mandibular advancement and mouth opening in the neutral neck position for immobilization of the cervical spine. J Anesth. 2021;35:811–7.
62. Sawin PD, Todd MM, Traynelis VC, et al. Cervical spine motion with direct laryngoscopy and orotracheal intubation. An in vivo cinefluoroscopic study of subjects without cervical abnormality. Anesthesiology. 1996;85:26–36.
63. Spinal Cord Injury Facts and Figures at a Glance: 2021 SCI data sheet. National Spinal Cord Injury Statistical Center. https://www.nscisc.uab.edu/Public/Facts%20and%20Figures%20-%202021.pdf
64. Sun C, Liu D, Gao S, et al. Propofol ameliorates spinal cord injury process by mediating miR-672-3p/TNIP2 Axis. Biochem Genet. Epub ahead of print. 2024;62 https://doi.org/10.1007/s10528-024-10718-4.
65. Sutter M, Eggspuehler A, Jeszenszky D, et al. The impact and value of uni- and multimodal intraoperative neurophysiological monitoring (IONM) on neurological complications during spine surgery: a prospective study of 2728 patients. Eur Spine J. 2019;28:599–610.
66. Velopulos CG, Shihab HM, Lottenberg L, et al. Prehospital spine immobilization/spinal motion restriction in penetrating trauma: A practice management guideline from the eastern Association for the Surgery of trauma (EAST). J Trauma Acute Care Surg. 2018;84:736–44.
67. Walters BC, Hadley MN, Hurlbert RJ, et al. Guidelines for the management of acute cervical spine and spinal cord injuries: 2013 update. Neurosurgery. 2013;60:82–91.
68. Weinberg JA, Farber S, Harrison MD, et al. Mean arterial pressure maintenance following spinal cord injury: does meeting the target matter? J Trauma Acute Care Surg. 2021;90(1):97–106.
69. Weingart SD, Levitan RM. Preoxygenation and prevention of desaturation during emergency airway management. Ann Emerg Med. 2012;59:165–75 e1.
70. Wiles MD, Iliff HA, Brooks K, et al. Airway management in patients with suspected or confirmed cervical spine injury: Guidelines from the Difficult Airway Society (DAS), Association of Anaesthetists (AoA), British Society of Orthopaedic Anaesthetists (BSOA), Intensive Care Society (ICS), Neuro Anaesthesia and Critical Care Society (NACCS), Faculty of Prehospital Care and Royal College of Emergency Medicine (RCEM). Anaesthesia. 2024;79 https://doi.org/10.1111/anae.16290.
71. Wiles MD. Airway management in patients with suspected or confirmed traumatic spinal cord injury: a narrative review of current evidence. Anaesthesia. 2022;77(10):1120–8.
72. Ziu E, Weisbrod LJ, Mesfin FB. Spinal Shock. [Updated 2024 Feb 12]. In: StatPearls [Internet]. Treasure Island (FL): StatPearls Publishing; 2025 Jan-. Available from: https://www.ncbi.nlm.nih.gov/books/NBK448163/

Neuroprotection and Pharmacological Treatment of Spinal Cord Injury

10

Tetsuhiko Mimura, Karlo Pedro, François Dantas, Peyton Lawrence, and Michael G. Fehlings

10.1 Introduction

The spinal cord facilitates the transmission of information through electrochemical transduction from the brain to the rest of the body. A spinal cord injury (SCI) disrupts this conduction by damaging the nerve tracts responsible for conveying information. The pathophysiology of SCI can be divided into acute, subacute, intermediate, and chronic phases of injury. SCI can result in long-term consequences, including paralysis, loss of sensation, difficulties with urinary and bowel control, respiratory compromise, and neuropathic pain. SCI can be further classified as complete, where there is a total loss of nerve communication below the injury site, or incomplete, where some signaling pathways are preserved in the spinal cord.

T. Mimura
Division of Genetics and Development, Krembil Brain Institute, University Health Network, Toronto, ON, Canada

K. Pedro · F. Dantas · P. Lawrence
Division of Neurosurgery, Krembil Neuroscience Centre, Toronto Western Hospital, University Health Network, Toronto, ON, Canada

Division of Neurosurgery and Spine Program, Department of Surgery, University of Toronto, Toronto, ON, Canada

M. G. Fehlings (✉)
Division of Genetics and Development, Krembil Brain Institute, University Health Network, Toronto, ON, Canada

Division of Neurosurgery, Krembil Neuroscience Centre, Toronto Western Hospital, University Health Network, Toronto, ON, Canada

Division of Neurosurgery and Spine Program, Department of Surgery, University of Toronto, Toronto, ON, Canada
e-mail: Michael.Fehlings@uhn.ca

E. Brogi et al. (eds.), *Traumatic Spinal Cord Injury*, Hot Topics in Acute Care Surgery and Trauma, https://doi.org/10.1007/978-3-031-99890-4_10

Current treatment options for SCI are mainly focused on managing symptoms or on surgical decompression. However, there remains a high demand for pharmaceutical interventions to treat SCI. This chapter discusses novel and emerging pharmacological candidates for the treatment of traumatic SCI, synthesizing a common base of knowledge for clinicians and researchers.

10.2 Pharmaceuticals Currently in Preclinical Studies

10.2.1 Fibroblast Growth Factor 22

Fibroblast growth factor 22 (FGF22; Fig. 10.1) plays a crucial role in the development of new excitatory synapses and the enhancement of synaptic organization. Preclinical studies have demonstrated FGF22's ability to reduce endoplasmic reticulum stress and apoptotic protein expression, leading to significant improvement in the survival of anterior horn neurons. This, in turn, manifests as improved motor function, as evidenced by improved Basso-Beattie-Bresnahan scores and plantar step indices in treated rodents. Notably, higher doses (10 μg/ml) show more substantial effects than lower doses (5 μg/ml) [1].

Additionally, targeted FGF22 gene therapy, specifically in long propriospinal neurons (LPSN), has demonstrated the capacity to promote synaptogenesis, particularly augmenting connections between the hindlimb corticospinal tract and LPSNs, while concurrently boosting motoneuron survival [2]. This therapy has also facilitated the recruitment of spinal interneurons into circuit remodeling processes, indicating its potential to effectively rewire neuronal circuits. However, the timing of FGF22 application is critical, with optimal benefits primarily observed when it is

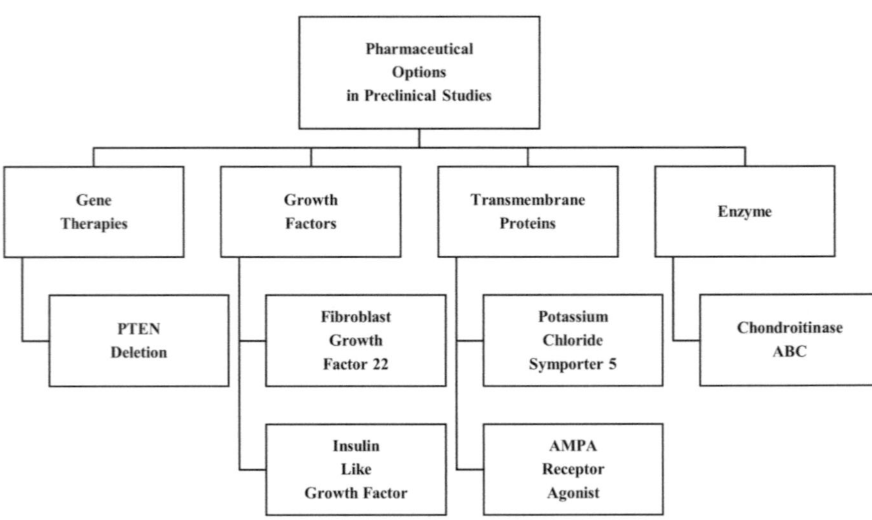

Fig. 10.1 Pharmaceutical options for SCI are currently being examined in preclinical studies

administered within 24 hours of traumatic SCI [2]. Although promising, these preclinical findings are still in the early stages.

10.2.2 Insulin-like Growth Factor 1

Insulin-like growth factor 1 (IGF-1; Fig. 10.1) promotes bone and tissue growth through such pathways as JAK2-STAT, PI3K/Akt, and RAS/MAPK, ultimately leading to mTOR activation [3]. Elevated levels of IGF-1 have been correlated with improved neurological recovery in SCI patients [4]. In experimental settings, IGF-1 has been found to promote neurogenesis, reduce apoptosis, and improve neuronal survival, particularly under stress conditions [5, 6]. Additionally, when combined with neural stem cell therapies, IGF-1 promotes differentiation and integration of new neural circuits [7, 8]. This underscores its potential in SCI regenerative medicine.

10.2.3 Potassium Chloride Symporter 5 (KCC2)

KCC2 is essential for chloride balance in neurons, and its downregulation after SCI contributes to the development of spasticity and neuropathic pain [9, 10]. Increasing KCC2 expression using specific enhancers like CLP257 and CLP290 has shown promise in preclinical models, effectively reducing spasticity and improving motor function in rats [10, 11]. These treatments also normalized neuronal activity patterns, suggesting its potential for restoring function in SCI patients. Additionally, increased KCC2 expression has been associated with the alleviation of pain and bladder overactivity, indicating broader therapeutic implications beyond motor function [12, 13]. These findings underscore the potential of KCC2 as a promising agent for SCI treatment.

10.2.4 PTEN Deletion

PTEN, a negative regulator of mTOR, impacts cell growth signaling and axonal regeneration after injury, particularly within the corticospinal tract [14, 15]. Studies have shown that PTEN deletion post-SCI can significantly enhance axonal regrowth and motor function recovery in mice [16]. However, despite its promising role in promoting neuronal growth, long-term consequences such as neuronal hypertrophy have been observed, indicating the potential for adverse outcomes [17]. These findings suggest PTEN deletion could be a valuable therapeutic target for SCI, although further research is needed to fully elucidate its implications.

10.2.5 Chondroitinase ABC Enzyme

Chondroitinase ABC (ChABC; Fig. 10.1) degrades chondroitin sulfate proteoglycan, enhancing axonal regeneration after SCI by increasing neurite growth and axonal plasticity [18, 19]. Numerous studies have shown that ChABC promotes nerve growth, facilitates nerve graft integration, and improves motor and sensory nerve functions in various animal models [20–22]. However, its clinical application is hindered by thermal instability and the associated risks related to current delivery methods [23, 24], underscoring the need for further research to develop effective administration techniques.

10.2.6 AMPA Receptor Agonists

Following SCI, excitotoxicity and oxidative stress lead to significant neuronal and tissue damage that impair motor and respiratory functions [25, 26]. AMPA receptors (AMPAR; Fig. 10.1) show therapeutic promise for these secondary issues. Studies have shown that ampakines like CX546, which modulate AMPARs, enhance the survival and proliferation of neural stem/progenitor cells (NSPCs), improving motor outcomes and promoting neuroprotection through mechanisms like the pCREB pathway [27]. Additionally, AMPAR modulation has been linked to improved respiratory neuroplasticity, suggesting broader benefits for SCI recovery [25, 26].

10.2.7 Mannitol

Currently, there is limited preclinical evidence demonstrating the benefit of mannitol over placebo. The exact mechanism of neuroprotection remains uncertain. However, it may be related to a combination of several factors [28, 29]. The osmotic effect is based on the increase in serum tonicity, which draws edema fluid away from the neuraxis. The onset of action via creation of osmolar gradients across the blood-brain barrier (BBB) is about 15–30 minutes. The effective duration of action varies from approximately 1.5–6 hours, depending on the clinical condition of the BBB [30, 31]. Another important mechanism may be improved rheology, whereby the immediate plasma expansion supports microcirculation by reducing hematocrit and blood viscosity. This improves oxygen-carrying capacity, especially when tissue perfusion pressures exceed 70 mm Hg. Free radical scavenging also seems to play a role in preventing cellular injury and subsequent cell death. Mannitol appears to have lipophilic scavenging capabilities, enabling it to cross the BBB and exert its effect on the neuraxis [29, 32].

10.3 Pharmaceutical Agents Currently in Clinical Trials

10.3.1 Anti-RGMa

SCI upregulates the expression of repulsive guidance molecule A (RGMa), which inhibits axonal growth [33] (Fig. 10.2). Inhibition of RGMa has shown promise in promoting axonal regrowth and synapse formation, significantly aiding recovery. For instance, monoclonal antibodies targeting RGMa have improved neuronal survival, axonal regeneration, and motor function in animal models, with effects such as improved locomotion as well as reduced inflammation and microgliosis [34–37]. These antibodies have also shown potential for crossing the blood-spinal cord barrier and maintaining effectiveness over time [37]. Currently, a phase II clinical trial is assessing the efficacy of this therapeutic approach, with results expected by 2026 (NCT04295538, NCT04278235). Another group is also conducting a phase II clinical trial in the USA, Canada, and Japan (NCT04683848).

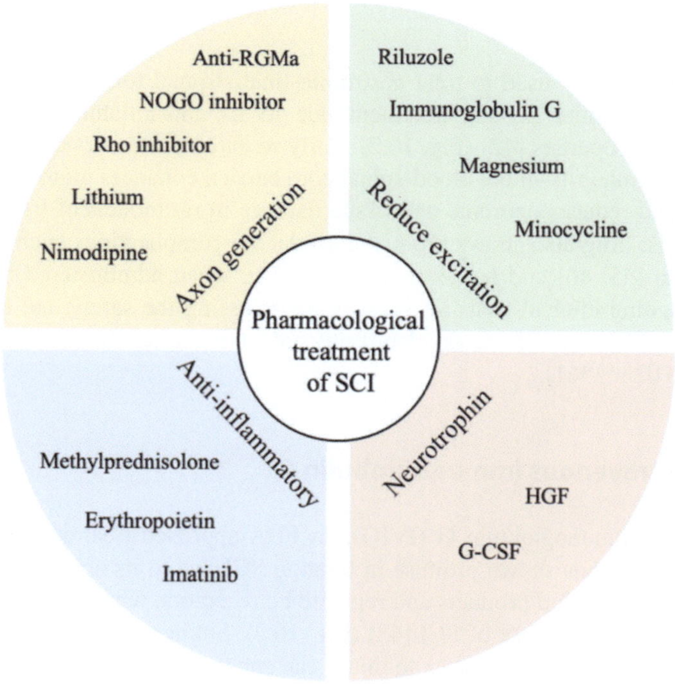

Fig. 10.2 Pharmacological treatments currently being examined in clinical trials and their pharmacological actions

10.3.2 NOGO Inhibitor

NOGO inhibitors target Nogo-A, a protein that inhibits neurite outgrowth and plasticity in the adult CNS [38, 39, 73] (Fig. 10.2). The underlying mechanism by which Nogo-A exerts its inhibitory effects involves its interaction with specific receptors on neurons, which activate downstream signaling pathways that limit neurite outgrowth. By blocking these interactions, Nogo inhibitors promote the intrinsic growth capacity of neurons and facilitate the reconnection of disrupted neural circuits. Animal studies have demonstrated that blocking Nogo-A enhances axonal regeneration and improves functional outcomes after SCI [40, 41]. These studies showed increased plasticity and collateral sprouting of axons in rodents with SCIs. The Nogo Inhibition in Spinal Cord Injury (NISCI) trial is a notable ongoing phase II clinical trial investigating the effects of NG-101, an anti-Nogo-A antibody, in patients with acute cervical SCI (NCT03935321). The results of this randomized controlled trial (RCT) are expected to be published in late 2024.

10.3.3 Imatinib

Imatinib, commonly used to treat gastrointestinal stromal tumors and leukemias, has shown potential in SCI treatment due to its anti-inflammatory and anti-hemorrhagic properties [42] (Fig. 10.2). Early research demonstrated that imatinib improves the integrity of the blood-spinal cord barrier, enhances motor and sensory function, and reduces neuronal and tissue damage in rat models of traumatic SCI [42–44]. The drug also shows promise in reducing complications such as bladder dysfunction [45, 46] and has been effective even when administered hours after injury. Ongoing clinical trials in Sweden are assessing the safety and efficacy of imatinib for SCI, with a focus on identifying potential markers for its bioavailability ([47], NCT02363361).

10.3.4 Intravenous Immunoglobulin G

Intravenous Immunoglobulin G (IVIG), an FDA-approved treatment for autoimmune disorders, has shown promise in treating SCI due to its ability to neutralize complement activation products and regulate Fc receptors, which are crucial in the secondary injury response of SCI [48] (Fig. 10.2). Studies have demonstrated that IVIG administration shortly after an injury can enhance tissue preservation, myelin preservation, and neurobehavioral and locomotor recovery in various models of SCI [49, 50]. Currently, a phase 1/2a clinical trial in Australia (ACTRN12616001385437) is underway to evaluate the pharmacokinetics and efficacy of IVIG in SCI. This trial is aiming to further establish the therapeutic potential of IVIG as a treatment option for individuals with SCI, potentially paving the way for its broader clinical use in the future.

10.3.5 Riluzole

Riluzole, a sodium channel-blocking anticonvulsant approved for use in patients with amyotrophic lateral sclerosis, has demonstrated potential benefits in SCI, as evidenced by both preclinical and clinical studies (Fig. 10.2). Research indicates that riluzole can improve motor function, somatosensory evoked potentials, and tissue preservation in SCI models [51–53]. It has also been observed to reduce neuropathic pain and spasticity, enhancing the survival and function of neurons and motor neurons across various SCI models [54–57]. In vitro studies showed that the neuroprotective mechanism of action appears to be multifaceted, involving the stimulation of neurotrophic factors such as GDNF and BDNF, as well as enhancement of transporter-mediated glutamate uptake [58, 60, 62]. Phase I/II clinical trials have validated its safety and efficacy, with significant improvements in motor scores and neurological functions in cervical SCI patients [61, 62]. However, the results of the RISCIS trial, published in 2023, showed no significant difference using the upper extremity motor score as the primary endpoint [62]. Notably, this study was underpowered and failed to reach its target population after premature discontinuation amidst the COVID-19 pandemic.

In nontraumatic SCI, riluzole is associated with beneficial treatment effects as shown in the secondary analysis of the CSM-PROTECT Trial (Efficacy of Riluzole in Surgical Treatment for Cervical Spondylotic Myelopathy). Using a global statistical test that comprehensively incorporates measures of neurological, functional, quality of life, and neck/arm pain scores, the study by Fehlings et al. revealed a treatment benefit of riluzole over placebo [62]. The study provides a rationale to consider this drug for neuroprotection in patients with degenerative cervical myelopathy (DCM) undergoing surgical intervention. A similar analysis of the RISCIS trial (Safety and Efficacy of Riluzole in Acute Spinal Cord Injury Study [59]) using a more comprehensive outcome representation is currently in progress. A Phase II trial (NCT02859792) is underway to investigate optimal doses for treating chronic SCI-related spasticity, highlighting continued interest in riluzole's potential as a therapeutic agent for SCI [63–66].

10.3.6 Hepatocyte Growth Factor

Hepatocyte growth factor (HGF), produced via the c-Met pathway, is crucial for cellular regeneration in the CNS [67] (Fig. 10.2). Early studies showed that while acute-phase HGF levels rise after thoracic SCI in rats, they are not sustained into the chronic phase, leading researchers to administer exogenous HGF. This approach improved myelination, reduced neuronal apoptosis, enhanced angiogenesis, and promoted functional recovery [68]. Subsequent experiments demonstrated HGF's efficacy in reducing astrogliosis and enhancing axonal growth in cervical SCI models, improving motor skills and nerve regeneration [69, 70]. Clinical trials, including a multicenter phase I/II study, confirmed HGF's potential in improving motor function in SCI patients, indicating significant rehabilitation benefits [71]. A phase III trial (NCT04475224) is currently active to further validate these findings.

10.3.7 Minocycline

Minocycline, a synthetic tetracycline derivative, has demonstrated antioxidant, anti-apoptotic, and anti-excitotoxic neuroprotective effects in various models of SCI [38, 72, 73] (Fig. 10.2). Studies in mouse and rat models have shown that minocycline improves motor function, reduces lesion volume, and decreases axonal and oligodendrocyte death [74–76]. It also mitigates inflammation and oxidative stress [77, 78]. Clinical trials have further explored its efficacy, showing promising but variable results in improving motor recovery and reducing neuropathic pain as well as autonomic dysreflexia in SCI patients [79, 80]. Clinical studies, including a phase II trial and the Minocycline in Acute Spinal Cord Injury (MASC) phase III RCT (NCT01828203), aimed to confirm these findings and optimize therapeutic strategies for use of minocycline in acute SCI. However, the MASC trial was discontinued due to concerns regarding off-target effects and toxicity as well as poor enrollment.

10.3.8 Ba-210 and Rho Inhibition

Rho GTPase is a critical component in inhibiting axonal regrowth after SCI by mediating the neuronal apoptotic cascade [81] (Fig. 10.2). C3 transferase has been shown to effectively inhibit Rho by keeping it in an inactive state, promoting axonal regeneration and neurite growth in various studies [82]. To overcome the delivery challenges of C3 for clinical use, the C3 fusion protein Ba-210 was developed, which enhanced tissue penetration and functional recovery when applied topically to the spinal dura mater [83].

Clinical trials, including a phase I/IIa study, tested the safety and tolerability of Ba-210, showing low systemic exposure and no serious adverse effects across different doses. The most effective outcomes were observed in cervical SCI patients treated with 3 mg of Ba-210, though less effect was noted in thoracic SCI cases [84]. However, a subsequent phase III trial was terminated early due to a lack of significant motor improvements in patients, highlighting the challenges in translating promising preclinical results into effective clinical treatments [85].

10.3.9 Erythropoietin

Human recombinant erythropoietin (hR-EPO) has demonstrated potential neuroprotective effects in various models of SCI, including SCI ischemia (SCIsc), with doses ranging from 350 to 1000 units/kg, leading to improved neurological scores and reduced motoneuron apoptosis [86, 87] (Fig. 10.2). EPO's anti-apoptotic and motor function enhancement capabilities were observed across thoracic SCI, cervical SCI, and lumbar spinal cord ischemia models, suggesting it mitigates inflammation and oxidative stress, contributing to its therapeutic effects [88, 89]. Studies also indicate EPO may promote neurological recovery by reducing levels of harmful proteins and increasing beneficial growth factors [90, 91]. Despite these promising preclinical outcomes, clinical trials—including one comparing EPO with methylprednisolone—have not yet confirmed significant functional improvements in patients with acute cervical SCI, indicating a need for further research to fully understand and harness EPO's potential in SCI treatment [92, 93].

10.3.10 Lithium

Lithium, known for inhibiting glycogen synthase kinase 3-beta (GSK-3beta), promotes neurogenesis and motor recovery after SCI [94] (Fig. 10.2). Research has shown that lithium enhances the survival, proliferation, and differentiation of neural progenitor cells (NPCs) in various SCI models, leading to improved locomotion and reduced scar formation [95]. It also fosters axonal sprouting and enhances motor function recovery [96, 97]. Lithium's potential benefits include anti-apoptotic, anti-inflammatory, antioxidative, and pro-autophagic effects, contributing to its therapeutic potential in SCI [98]. Clinical trials have further explored lithium's efficacy, noting improvements in pain management but not in functional recovery [99, 100].

10.3.11 Granulocyte Colony-Stimulating Factor

Granulocyte colony-stimulating factor (G-CSF) is recognized for its role in promoting myeloid cell growth and has demonstrated significant therapeutic effects in SCI recovery, including anti-apoptotic, anti-inflammatory, antioxidative, and anti-excitotoxic properties [101, 102] (Fig. 10.2). Studies have shown that G-CSF enhances hindlimb recovery, improves myelin integrity, and stimulates axonal regeneration in various SCI models [103, 104]. Clinical trials have further highlighted its potential for improving motor function and sensory scores in patients with cervical and thoracic SCI. Specifically, trials have documented improvements in ASIA Impairment Scale (AIS) and motor scores at varying doses of G-CSF, suggesting its efficacy in enhancing neurologic recovery [105, 106].

But despite promising results in phase I/II trials, a phase III randomized controlled trial did not show significant motor improvements, indicating mixed outcomes and the need for further investigation to solidify the role of G-CSF in SCI treatment [107, 108]. This ongoing research underscores the potential of G-CSF but also highlights the complexity of translating preclinical success into clinical therapies for SCI patients.

10.3.12 Methylprednisolone

Methylprednisolone, a synthetic glucocorticoid, is known for its anti-inflammatory properties and has been a focus of research for its potential to treat SCI (Fig. 10.2). This drug works by reducing lipid peroxidation, stabilizing cell membranes, improving blood flow, decreasing inflammatory cytokines, and preventing the formation of free radicals, thereby impacting multiple mechanisms that contribute to secondary injury after SCI [109, 110]. Several animal studies have demonstrated that steroids improve neurological outcomes in animals with SCI. However, the evidence supporting the use of steroids in clinical practice is still limited and controversial [111].

Three randomized trials (NASCIS I, NASCIS II, and NASCIS III) have evaluated the potential effects and safety of methylprednisolone in the treatment of SCI. In these trials, patients were treated with either high-dose methylprednisolone, low-dose methylprednisolone, or other medications. The inclusion criteria and the doses of methylprednisolone were different in each study, and the results were heterogeneous [112–114].

A systematic review was conducted to assess the effectiveness of high-dose methylprednisolone versus no pharmacological treatment in patients with SCI. In total, 13 studies were included. The authors suggested that when commenced within 8 hours of injury, a high-dose 24-hour regimen of methylprednisolone confers a small positive benefit on long-term motor recovery and should be considered a treatment option for patients with traumatic SCI [115, 116].

Despite its potential, the use of methylprednisolone in SCI treatment remains controversial due to inconsistent evidence and possible severe side effects [117, 118]. Current guidelines suggest that while a 24-hour high-dose infusion of methylprednisolone may be considered within 8 hours of SCI, extending the treatment to 48 hours post-injury is not recommended due to the limited evidence of efficacy [115, 116]. The decision to use high-dose corticosteroids should be left to the discretion of the physician and patient.

10.3.13 Nimodipine

Nimodipine, an L-type Ca2+ channel antagonist, has been explored as a potential treatment for SCI due to its role in regulating pathological intraneuronal calcium shifts [119–121] (Fig. 10.2). However, preclinical results have been mixed. While some studies reported no improvement in histological, motor, and sensory recovery, and noted possible adverse effects like hypotension [122, 123], others observed enhancements in spinal cord blood flow, reduced lesion size, and improvement in locomotion and tissue preservation when combined with pressor agents or in stand-alone treatments [124–127].

Recent studies have also indicated potential reductions in spasticity and pain-related behaviors with nimodipine use after SCI [128]. Despite these promising observations, randomized clinical trials have yet to demonstrate significant neurological improvement with nimodipine compared to other treatments like methylprednisolone, with one notable study being underpowered [129, 130]. Thus, while nimodipine shows some therapeutic potential, more robust clinical trials are required to conclusively determine its efficacy and safety in treating SCI.

10.3.14 Magnesium and Polyethylene Glycol

Magnesium (Mg2+), known for its neuroprotective properties, prevents calcium-induced cellular injuries and has shown promise in reducing apoptosis as well as preserving axons, nuclear membranes, and myelin after thoracic SCI [131, 132] (Fig. 10.2). However, the clinical application of Mg2+ has been challenging due to the high doses required for effectiveness.

To enhance its therapeutic potential and reduce dosage issues, Mg2+ has been combined with polyethylene glycol (PEG), a hydrophilic polymer noted for inducing vascular and axonal regeneration in traumatic brain injury models [133]. This combination therapy has improved extracellular and intracellular magnesium levels, helping mitigate excitotoxic glutamate levels at injury sites [134]. In preclinical studies, Mg2+ plus PEG showed promising results in cervical SCI models, with treated animals exhibiting fewer motor errors and greater tissue preservation than controls [135]. However, the combination did not produce significant improvements in locomotion or spinal cord preservation in a minipig thoracic SCI model [136], and a phase II double-blind randomized controlled trial was terminated early due to insufficient participant enrollment (NCT01750684). These findings indicate that while Mg2+ and PEG have potential neuroprotective benefits, further research is necessary to optimize the therapy and confirm its efficacy in clinical settings.

10.4 Conclusion

Numerous novel pharmaceutical therapies are currently being explored as potential treatments for SCI (Fig. 10.3). These therapies attempt to improve outcomes by affecting a variety of physiologic processes, including axonal regeneration, neuroexcitation, inflammation, and neurotrophic-mediated effects. While further work is required on each of the candidates discussed in this review, our current state of knowledge hints that these novel therapies may enhance neural regeneration, reduce inflammation, and improve functional outcomes. Additionally, synergy with advances in other treatments like surgical procedures, cell therapies, and biomaterials may create even more options for new therapeutic interventions. These combined approaches may significantly enhance the overall treatment landscape for SCI, offering new hope for improved recovery and quality of life for these patients.

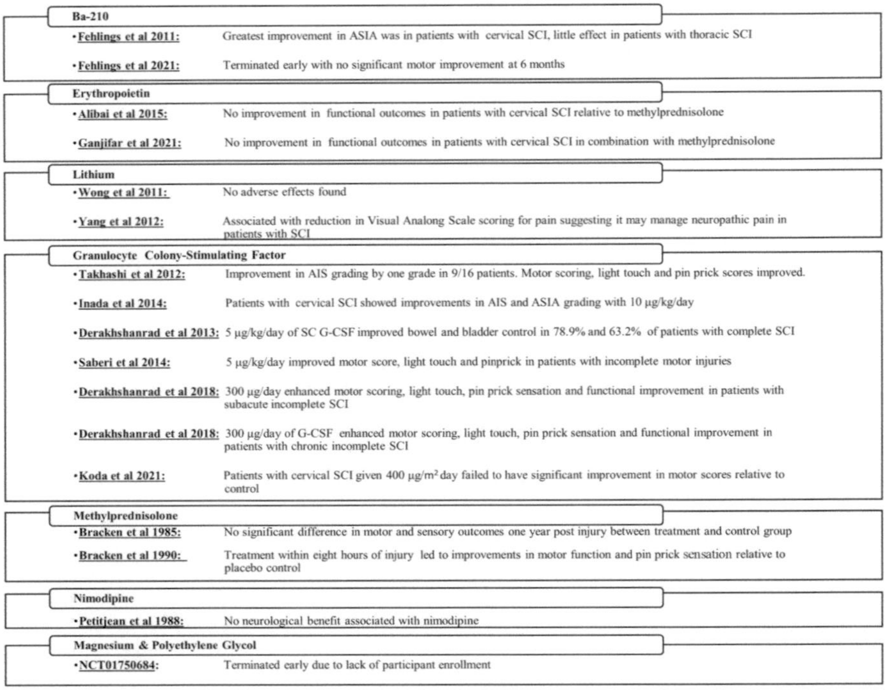

Fig. 10.3 The results of previous pharmaceutical trials for candidate medications targeting SCI

References

1. Zhu S, Chen M, Chen M, Ye J, Ying Y, Wu Q, et al. Fibroblast growth factor 22 inhibits ER stress-induced apoptosis and improves recovery of spinal cord injury. Front Pharmacol. 2020;11:18.
2. Aljović A, Jacobi A, Marcantoni M, Kagerer F, Loy K, Kendirli A, et al. Synaptogenic gene therapy with FGF22 improves circuit plasticity and functional recovery following spinal cord injury. EMBO Mol Med. 2023;15(2):e16111.
3. Rommel C, Bodine SC, Clarke BA, Rossman R, Nunez L, Stitt TN, et al. Mediation of IGF-1-induced skeletal myotube hypertrophy by PI(3)K/Akt/mTOR and PI(3)K/Akt/GSK3 pathways. Nat Cell Biol. 2001;3(11):1009–13.
4. Moghaddam A, Sperl A, Heller R, Kunzmann K, Graeser V, Akbar M, et al. Elevated serum insulin-like growth factor 1 levels in patients with neurological remission after traumatic spinal cord injury. PLoS One. 2016;11(7):e0159764.
5. Bellini MJ, Labombarda F. Brain and spinal cord trauma: what we know about the therapeutic potential of insulin growth factor 1 gene therapy. Neural Regen Res. 2022;18(2):253–7.
6. Zakharova IO, Bayunova LV, Zorina II, Sokolova TV, Shpakov AO, Avrova NF. Insulin and α-tocopherol enhance the protective effect of each other on brain cortical neurons under oxidative stress conditions and in rat two-vessel forebrain ischemia/reperfusion injury. Int J Mol Sci. 2021 Jan;22(21):11768.
7. Maugeri G, D'Agata V, Musumeci G. Role of exercise in the brain: focus on oligodendrocytes and remyelination. Neural Regen Res. 2023;18(12):2645–6.

8. Ma K, Xu H, Zhang J, Zhao F, Liang H, Sun H, et al. Insulin-like growth factor-1 enhances neuroprotective effects of neural stem cell exosomes after spinal cord injury via an miR-219a-2-3p/YY1 mechanism. Aging (Albany NY). 2019;11(24):12278–94.
9. Boulenguez P, Liabeuf S, Bos R, Bras H, Jean-Xavier C, Brocard C, et al. Down-regulation of the potassium-chloride cotransporter KCC2 contributes to spasticity after spinal cord injury. Nat Med. 2010 Mar;16(3):302–7.
10. Chen B, Li Y, Yu B, Zhang Z, Brommer B, Williams PR, et al. Reactivation of dormant relay pathways in injured spinal cord by KCC2 manipulations. Cell. 2018;174(3):521–535.e13.
11. Bilchak JN, Yeakle K, Caron G, Malloy D, Côté MP. Enhancing KCC2 activity decreases hyperreflexia and spasticity after chronic spinal cord injury. Exp Neurol. 2021 Apr;1(338):113605.
12. Sánchez-Brualla I, Boulenguez P, Brocard C, Liabeuf S, Viallat-Lieutaud A, Navarro X, et al. Activation of 5-HT2A receptors restores KCC2 function and reduces neuropathic pain after spinal cord injury. Neuroscience. 2018 Sep;1(387):48–57.
13. Watanabe K, Ishibashi M, Suzuki T, Otsuka A, Yoshimura N, Miyake H, et al. Therapeutic effects of KCC2 chloride transporter activation on detrusor overactivity in mice with spinal cord injury. American Journal of Physiology-Renal Physiology. 2023 Apr;324(4):F353–61.
14. Sabatini DM. mTOR and cancer: insights into a complex relationship. Nat Rev Cancer. 2006 Sep;6(9):729–34.
15. Ma XM, Blenis J. Molecular mechanisms of mTOR-mediated translational control. Nat Rev Mol Cell Biol. 2009 May;10(5):307–18.
16. Liu K, Lu Y, Lee JK, Samara R, Willenberg R, Sears-Kraxberger I, et al. PTEN deletion enhances the regenerative ability of adult corticospinal neurons. Nat Neurosci. 2010 Sep;13(9):1075–81.
17. Gutilla EA, Buyukozturk MM, Steward O. Long-term consequences of conditional genetic deletion of PTEN in the sensorimotor cortex of neonatal mice. Exp Neurol. 2016 May;1(279):27–39.
18. Lemons ML, Howland DR, Anderson DK. Chondroitin sulfate proteoglycan immunoreactivity increases following spinal cord injury and transplantation. Exp Neurol. 1999 Nov;160(1):51–65.
19. Zuo J, Neubauer D, Dyess K, Ferguson TA, Muir D. Degradation of chondroitin sulfate proteoglycan enhances the neurite-promoting potential of spinal cord tissue. Exp Neurol. 1998 Dec;154(2):654–62.
20. Massey JM, Hubscher CH, Wagoner MR, Decker JA, Amps J, Silver J, et al. Chondroitinase ABC digestion of the perineuronal net promotes functional collateral sprouting in the cuneate nucleus after cervical spinal cord injury. J Neurosci. 2006;26(16):4406–14.
21. Chau CH, Shum DKY, Li H, Pei J, Lui YY, Wirthlin L, et al. Chondroitinase ABC enhances axonal regrowth through Schwann cell-seeded guidance channels after spinal cord injury. FASEB J. 2004 Jan;18(1):194–6.
22. Houle JD, Tom VJ, Mayes D, Wagoner G, Phillips N, Silver J. Combining an autologous peripheral nervous system "bridge" and matrix modification by chondroitinase allows robust, functional regeneration beyond a hemisection lesion of the adult rat spinal cord. J Neurosci. 2006;26(28):7405–15.
23. Tester NJ, Plaas AH, Howland DR. Effect of body temperature on chondroitinase ABC'S ability to cleave chondroitin sulfate glycosaminoglycans. J Neurosci Res. 2007 Apr;85(5):1110–8.
24. Moradi K, Shirdel SA, Shamsi M, Jafarian V, Khalifeh K. Investigating the structural and functional features of representative recombinants of chondroitinase ABC I. Enzym Microb Technol. 2017 Dec;1(107):64–71.
25. Wollman LB, Streeter KA, Fusco AF, Gonzalez-Rothi EJ, Sandhu MS, Greer JJ, et al. Ampakines stimulate phrenic motor output after cervical spinal cord injury. Exp Neurol. 2020 Dec;1(334):113465.
26. Rana S, Sunshine MD, Greer JJ, Fuller DD. Ampakines stimulate diaphragm activity after spinal cord injury. J Neurotrauma. 2021;38(24):3467–82.

27. Hachem LD, Mothe AJ, Tator CH. Positive modulation of AMPA receptors promotes survival and proliferation of neural stem/progenitor cells from the adult rat spinal cord. Stem Cells Dev. 2017 Dec;26(23):1675–81.
28. Zhang C, Hu A, Jing Y, Yang D, Li J. Mannitol reduces spinal cord edema in rats with acute traumatic spinal cord injury. Letters in Drug Design & Discovery. 2019;17(6):676–83. https://doi.org/10.2174/1570180816666190731112158.
29. Barry KG, Berman AR. Mannitol Infusion. Part III. The acute effect of the intravenous Infusion of mannitol on blood and plasma volume. New Eng- land J Med 1961; 264:1085–1088.
30. McGraw CP, Howard G. The effect of mannitol on increased intracranial pressure. Neurosurgery. 1983;13:269–71.
31. Cruz J, Miner ME, Allen SJ, et al. Continuous monitoring of cerebral oxygenation in acute brain. J Neurosurg. 1990;73:725–30.
32. Marshall LF, Smith RW, Rauscher LA, et al. Manni- Tol dose requirements in brain-injured patients. J Neurosurg. 1978;48:169–72.
33. Schwab JM, Conrad S, Monnier PP, Julien S, Mueller BK, Schluesener HJ. Spinal cord injury-induced lesional expression of the repulsive guidance molecule (RGM). Eur J Neurosci. 2005 Mar;21(6):1569–76.
34. Hata K, Fujitani M, Yasuda Y, Doya H, Saito T, Yamagishi S, et al. RGMa inhibition promotes axonal growth and recovery after spinal cord injury. J Cell Biol. 2006;173(1):47–58.
35. Kyoto A, Hata K, Yamashita T. Synapse formation of the cortico-spinal axons is enhanced by RGMa inhibition after spinal cord injury. Brain Res. 2007 Dec;1186:74–86.
36. Kitayama M, Ueno M, Itakura T, Yamashita T. Activated microglia inhibit axonal growth through RGMa. PLoS One. 2011;6(9):e25234.
37. Mothe AJ, Tassew NG, Shabanzadeh AP, Penheiro R, Vigouroux RJ, Huang L, et al. RGMa inhibition with human monoclonal antibodies promotes regeneration, plasticity and repair, and attenuates neuropathic pain after spinal cord injury. Sci Rep. 2017;7(1):10529.
38. Chen MS, Huber AB, van der Haar ME, et al. Nogo-a is a myelin-associated neurite outgrowth inhibitor and an antigen for monoclonal antibody IN-1. Nature. 2000a;403:434–9.
39. Kempf A, Schwab ME. Nogo-a represses anatomical and synaptic plasticity in the central nervous system. Physiology (Bethesda). 2013;28:151–63.
40. Merkler D, Metz GA, Raineteau O, Dietz V, Schwab ME, Fouad K. Locomotor recovery in spinal cord-injured rats treated with an antibody neutralizing the myelin-associated neurite growth inhibitor Nogo-A. J Neurosci. 2001;21:3665–73.
41. Freund P, Schmidlin E, Wannier T, et al. Nogo-A-specific antibody treatment enhances sprouting and functional recovery after cervical lesion in adult primates. Nat Med. 2006;12:790–2.
42. Abrams MB, Nilsson I, Lewandowski SA, Kjell J, Codeluppi S, Olson L, et al. Imatinib enhances functional outcome after spinal cord injury. PLoS One. 2012;7(6):e38760.
43. Liu L, Zhou J, Wang Y, Qi T, Wang Z, Chen L, et al. Imatinib inhibits oxidative stress response in spinal cord injury rats by activating Nrf2/HO-1 signaling pathway. Exp Ther Med. 2020 Jan;19(1):597–602.
44. Yao F, Luo Y, Liu YC, Chen YH, Li YT, Hu XY, et al. Imatinib inhibits pericyte-fibroblast transition and inflammation and promotes axon regeneration by blocking the PDGF-BB/PDGFRβ pathway in spinal cord injury. Inflamm Regen. 2022;42(1):44.
45. Sharp KG, Yee KM, Steward O. A re-assessment of treatment with a tyrosine kinase inhibitor (imatinib) on tissue sparing and functional recovery after spinal cord injury. Exp Neurol. 2014 Apr;254:1–11.
46. Deng J, Zhang Y, Wang L, Zhao J, Song B, Li L. The effects of Glivec on the urinary bladder excitation of rats with suprasacral or sacral spinal cord transection. J Surg Res. 2013 Aug;183(2):598–605.
47. Kjell J, Finn A, Hao J, Wellfelt K, Josephson A, Svensson CI, et al. Delayed Imatinib treatment for acute spinal cord injury: functional recovery and serum biomarkers. J Neurotrauma. 2015;32(21):1645–57.
48. Tzekou A, Fehlings MG. Treatment of spinal cord injury with intravenous immunoglobulin G: preliminary evidence and future perspectives. J Clin Immunol. 2014;34(Suppl 1):132–8.

49. Chio JCT, Wang J, Surendran V, Li L, Zavvarian MM, Pieczonka K, et al. Delayed administration of high dose human immunoglobulin G enhances recovery after traumatic cervical spinal cord injury by modulation of neuroinflammation and protection of the blood spinal cord barrier. Neurobiol Dis. 2021 Jan;1(148):105187.
50. Brennan FH, Kurniawan ND, Vukovic J, Bartlett PF, Käsermann F, Arumugam TV, et al. IVIg attenuates complement and improves spinal cord injury outcomes in mice. Annals of Clinical and Translational Neurology. 2016;3(7):495–511.
51. Stutzmann JM, Pratt J, Boraud T, Gross C. The effect of riluzole on post-traumatic spinal cord injury in the rat. Neuroreport. 1996;7(2):387.
52. Wu Y, Satkunendrarajah K, Teng Y, Chow DSL, Buttigieg J, Fehlings MG. Delayed post-injury administration of riluzole is neuroprotective in a preclinical rodent model of cervical spinal cord injury. J Neurotrauma. 2013;30(6):441–52.
53. Schwartz G, Fehlings MG. Evaluation of the neuroprotective effects of sodium channel blockers after spinal cord injury: improved behavioral and neuroanatomical recovery with riluzole. J Neurosurg Spine. 2001;94(2):245–56.
54. Mu X, Azbill RD, Springer JE. Riluzole and methylprednisolone combined treatment improves functional recovery in traumatic spinal cord injury. J Neurotrauma. 2000 Sep;17(9):773–80.
55. Mazzone GL, Nistri A. Delayed neuroprotection by riluzole against excitotoxic damage evoked by kainate on rat organotypic spinal cord cultures. Neuroscience. 2011 Sep;5(190):318–27.
56. Wu Q, Zhang Y, Zhang Y, Zhang W, Zhang W, Liu Y, et al. Riluzole improves functional recovery after acute spinal cord injury in rats and may be associated with changes in spinal microglia/macrophages polarization. Neurosci Lett. 2020 Apr;1(723):134829.
57. Satkunendrarajah K, Nassiri F, Karadimas SK, Lip A, Yao G, Fehlings MG. Riluzole promotes motor and respiratory recovery associated with enhanced neuronal survival and function following high cervical spinal hemisection. Exp Neurol. 2016 Feb;276:59–71.
58. Miller RG, Mitchell JD, Lyon M, Moore DH. Riluzole for amyotrophic lateral sclerosis (ALS)/motor neuron disease (MND). Amyotroph Lateral Scler Other Motor Neuron Disord. 2003;4(3):191–206. https://doi.org/10.1080/14660820310002601.
59. Safety and Efficacy of Riluzole in Acute Spinal Cord Injury Study (RISCIS): A Multi-Center, Randomized, Placebo-Controlled, Double-Blinded Trial—PubMed. (n.d.). Retrieved April 28, 2024, from https://pubmed.ncbi.nlm.nih.gov/37279301/
60. Serag I, Abouzid M, Elmoghazy A, Sarhan K, Alsaad SA, Mohamed RG. An updated systematic review of neuroprotective agents in the treatment of spinal cord injury. Neurosurg Rev. 2024;47(1):132. https://doi.org/10.1007/s10143-024-02372-6.
61. Grossman RG, Fehlings MG, Frankowski RF, Burau KD, Chow DSL, Tator C, et al. A prospective, multicenter, phase I matched-comparison group trial of safety, pharmacokinetics, and preliminary efficacy of riluzole in patients with traumatic spinal cord injury. J Neurotrauma. 2014;31(3):239–55.
62. Fehlings MG, Moghaddamjou A, Harrop JS, Stanford R, Ball J, Aarabi B, et al. Safety and efficacy of Riluzole in acute spinal cord injury study (RISCIS): a multi-center, randomized, placebo-controlled. Double-Blinded Trial Journal of Neurotrauma. 2023;40(17–18):1878–88.
63. Balbinot G. Neuromodulation to guide circuit reorganization with regenerative therapies in upper extremity rehabilitation following cervical spinal cord injury. Frontiers in Rehabilitation Sciences. 2023;4 https://doi.org/10.3389/FRESC.2023.1320211.
64. Fehlings MG, Nakashima H, Nagoshi N, Chow DSL, Grossman RG, Kopjar B. Rationale, design and critical end points for the Riluzole in acute spinal cord injury study (RISCIS): a randomized, double-blinded, placebo-controlled parallel multi-center trial. Spinal Cord. 2016;54(1):8–15. https://doi.org/10.1038/sc.2015.95.
65. Fehlings MG, Pedro KM, Alvi MA, et al. Riluzole for Degenerative Cervical Myelopathy: A Secondary Analysis of the CSM-PROTECT Trial. JAMA Netw Open. 2024;7(6):e2415643. https://doi.org/10.1001/jamanetworkopen.2024.15643.
66. Fehlings MG, Pedro KM, Alvi MA, et al. The sodium-glutamate antagonist riluzole improves outcome after acute spinal cord injury: results from the RISCIS randomised controlled trial analysed using a global statistical analytic technique. EBioMedicine. 2025;118:105863. https://doi.org/10.1016/j.ebiom.2025.105863.

67. Kitamura K, Nagoshi N, Tsuji O, Matsumoto M, Okano H, Nakamura M. Application of hepatocyte growth factor for acute spinal cord injury: the road from basic studies to human treatment. Int J Mol Sci. 2019;20(5):1054.
68. Kitamura K, Iwanami A, Nakamura M, Yamane J, Watanabe K, Suzuki Y, et al. Hepatocyte growth factor promotes endogenous repair and functional recovery after spinal cord injury. J Neurosci Res. 2007;85(11):2332–42.
69. Jeong SR, Kwon MJ, Lee HG, Joe EH, Lee JH, Kim SS, et al. Hepatocyte growth factor reduces astrocytic scar formation and promotes axonal growth beyond glial scars after spinal cord injury. Exp Neurol. 2012 Jan;233(1):312–22.
70. Kitamura K, Fujiyoshi K, Yamane JI, Toyota F, Hikishima K, Nomura T, et al. Human hepatocyte growth factor promotes functional recovery in primates after spinal cord injury. PLoS One. 2011;6(11):e27706.
71. Nagoshi N, Tsuji O, Kitamura K, Suda K, Maeda T, Yato Y, et al. Phase I/II study of intrathecal Administration of Recombinant Human Hepatocyte Growth Factor in patients with acute spinal cord injury: a double-blind, randomized clinical trial of safety and efficacy. J Neurotrauma. 2020;37(15):1752–8.
72. Amin AR, Attur MG, Thakker GD, Patel PD, Vyas PR, Patel RN, et al. A novel mechanism of action of tetracyclines: effects on nitric oxide synthases. Proc Natl Acad Sci USA. 1996;93(24):14014–9.
73. Chen M, Ona VO, Li M, Ferrante RJ, Fink KB, Zhu S, et al. Minocycline inhibits caspase-1 and caspase-3 expression and delays mortality in a transgenic mouse model of Huntington disease. Nat Med. 2000b Jul;6(7):797–801.
74. Wells JEA, Hurlbert RJ, Fehlings MG, Yong VW. Neuroprotection by minocycline facilitates significant recovery from spinal cord injury in mice. Brain. 2003;126(7):1628–37.
75. Lee SM, Yune TY, Kim SJ, Park DW, Lee YK, Kim YC, et al. Minocycline reduces cell death and improves functional recovery after traumatic spinal cord injury in the rat. J Neurotrauma. 2003 Oct;20(10):1017–27.
76. Teng YD, Choi H, Onario RC, Zhu S, Desilets FC, Lan S, et al. Minocycline inhibits contusion-triggered mitochondrial cytochrome c release and mitigates functional deficits after spinal cord injury. Proc Natl Acad Sci USA. 2004;101(9):3071–6.
77. Sonmez E, Kabatas S, Ozen O, Karabay G, Turkoglu S, Ogus E, et al. Minocycline treatment inhibits lipid peroxidation, preserves spinal cord ultrastructure, and improves functional outcome after traumatic spinal cord injury in the rat. Spine (Phila Pa 1976). 2013 Jul 1;38(15):1253–9.
78. Aras M, Altas M, Motor S, Dokuyucu R, Yilmaz A, Ozgiray E, et al. Protective effects of minocycline on experimental spinal cord injury in rats. Injury. 2015 Aug;46(8):1471–4.
79. Casha S, Zygun D, McGowan MD, Bains I, Yong VW, John HR. Results of a phase II placebo-controlled randomized trial of minocycline in acute spinal cord injury. Brain. 2012;135(4):1224–36.
80. Squair JW, Ruiz I, Phillips AA, Zheng MMZ, Sarafis ZK, Sachdeva R, et al. Minocycline reduces the severity of autonomic Dysreflexia after experimental spinal cord injury. J Neurotrauma. 2018;35(24):2861–71.
81. Dergham P, Ellezam B, Essagian C, Avedissian H, Lubell WD, McKerracher L. Rho signaling pathway targeted to promote spinal cord repair. J Neurosci. 2002;22(15):6570–7.
82. Wilde C, Aktories K. The rho-ADP-ribosylating C3 exoenzyme from clostridium botulinum and related C3-like transferases. Toxicon. 2001;39(11):1647–60.
83. Lord-Fontaine S, Yang F, Diep Q, Dergham P, Munzer S, Tremblay P, et al. Local inhibition of rho signaling by cell-permeable recombinant protein BA-210 prevents secondary damage and promotes functional recovery following acute spinal cord injury. J Neurotrauma. 2008 Nov;25(11):1309–22.
84. Fehlings MG, Theodore N, Harrop J, Maurais G, Kuntz C, Shaffrey CI, et al. A phase I/IIa clinical trial of a recombinant rho protein antagonist in acute spinal cord injury. J Neurotrauma. 2011 May;28(5):787–96.

85. Fehlings MG, Chen Y, Aarabi B, Ahmad F, Anderson KD, Dumont T, et al. A randomized controlled trial of local delivery of a rho inhibitor (VX-210) in patients with acute traumatic cervical spinal cord injury. J Neurotrauma. 2021 Aug;38(15):2065–72.
86. Celik M, Gökmen N, Erbayraktar S, Akhisaroglu M, Konakç S, Ulukus C, et al. Erythropoietin prevents motor neuron apoptosis and neurologic disability in experimental spinal cord ischemic injury. Proc Natl Acad Sci USA. 2002;99(4):2258–63.
87. Arishima Y, Setoguchi T, Yamaura I, Yone K, Komiya S. Preventive effect of erythropoietin on spinal cord cell apoptosis following acute traumatic injury in rats. Spine. 2006;31(21):2432.
88. Ning B, Zhang A, Song H, Gong W, Ding Y, Guo S, et al. Recombinant human erythropoietin prevents motor neuron apoptosis in a rat model of cervical sub-acute spinal cord compression. Neurosci Lett. 2011;490(1):57–62.
89. Wang S, Wu Z, Chiang P, Fink DJ, Mata M. Vector-mediated expression of erythropoietin improves functional outcome after cervical spinal cord contusion injury. Gene Ther. 2012 Sep;19(9):907–14.
90. Fang X, qian, Fang M, Fan S wu, Gu C long. Protection of erythropoietin on experimental spinal cord injury by reducing the expression of thrombospondin-1 and transforming growth factor-beta. Chin Med J. 2009;122(14):1631–5.
91. Hong Z, Hong H, Chen H, Wang Z, Hong D. Protective effects of erythropoietin in experimental spinal cord injury by reducing the C/EBP-homologous protein expression. Neurol Res. 2012 Jan;34(1):85–90.
92. Alibai EA, Baghban F, Farrokhi MR, Mohebali N, Ashraf MH. Effects of human erythropoietin on functional outcome of patients with traumatic cervical cord injury; a pilot randomized clinical trial. Bull Emerg Trauma. 2015 Jul;3(3):79–85.
93. Ganjeifar B, Rezaee H, Keykhosravi E, Tavallaii A, Bahadorkhan G, Nakhaei M, et al. The effect of combination therapy with erythropoietin and methylprednisolone in patients with traumatic cervical spinal cord injury: a pilot randomized controlled trial. Spinal Cord. 2021 Mar;59(3):347–53.
94. Rodriguez-Jimenez FJ, Vilches A, Perez-Arago MA, Clemente E, Roman R, Leal J, et al. Activation of neurogenesis in multipotent stem cells cultured in vitro and in the spinal cord tissue after severe injury by inhibition of glycogen synthase Kinase-3. Neurotherapeutics. 2021;18(1):515–33.
95. Su H, Chu TH, Wu W. Lithium enhances proliferation and neuronal differentiation of neural progenitor cells in vitro and after transplantation into the adult rat spinal cord. Exp Neurol. 2007 Aug;206(2):296–307.
96. Dill J, Wang H, Zhou F, Li S. Inactivation of glycogen synthase kinase 3 promotes axonal growth and recovery in the CNS. J Neurosci. 2008;28(36):8914–28.
97. Kim Y, Kim J, Ahn M, Shin T. Lithium ameliorates rat spinal cord injury by suppressing glycogen synthase kinase-3β and activating heme oxygenase-1. Anatomy & Cell Biology. 2017;50(3):207–13.
98. He Z, Zhou Y, Wang Q, Li J, Zheng Z, Chen J, et al. Inhibiting endoplasmic reticulum stress by lithium chloride contributes to the integrity of blood-spinal cord barrier and functional recovery after spinal cord injury. Am J Transl Res. 2017;9(3):1012–24.
99. Wong YW, Tam S, So KF, Chen JYH, Cheng WS, Luk KDK, et al. A three-month, open-label, single-arm trial evaluating the safety and pharmacokinetics of oral lithium in patients with chronic spinal cord injury. Spinal Cord. 2011 Jan;49(1):94–8.
100. Yang ML, Li JJ, So KF, Chen JYH, Cheng WS, Wu J, et al. Efficacy and safety of lithium carbonate treatment of chronic spinal cord injuries: a double-blind, randomized, placebo-controlled clinical trial. Spinal Cord. 2012 Feb;50(2):141–6.
101. Nishio Y, Koda M, Kamada T, Someya Y, Kadota R, Mannoji C, et al. Granulocyte colony-stimulating factor attenuates neuronal death and promotes functional recovery after spinal cord injury in mice. J Neuropathol Exp Neurol. 2007 Aug;66(8):724–31.

102. Guo Y, Liu S, Wang P, Zhang H, Wang F, Bing L, et al. Granulocyte colony-stimulating factor improves neuron survival in experimental spinal cord injury by regulating nucleophosmin-1 expression. J Neurosci Res. 2014 Jun;92(6):751–60.
103. Urdzíková L, Jendelová P, Glogarová K, Burian M, Hájek M, Syková E. Transplantation of bone marrow stem cells as well as mobilization by granulocyte-colony stimulating factor promotes recovery after spinal cord injury in rats. J Neurotrauma. 2006 Sep;23(9):1379–91.
104. Claudia, Pitzer Stefan, Klussmann Carola, Krüger Elisabeth, Letellier Christian, Plaas Tanjew, Dittgen Friederike, Kirsch Bram, Stieltjes Daniela, Weber Rico, Laage Ana, Martin-Villalba Armin, Schneider. The hematopoietic factor granulocyte-colony stimulating factor improves outcome in experimental spinal cord injury Journal of Neurochemistry 2010;113(4):930–42. https://doi.org/10.1111/jnc.2010.113.issue-4. https://doi.org/10.1111/j.1471-4159.2010.06659.x.
105. Takahashi H, Yamazaki M, Okawa A, Sakuma T, Kato K, Hashimoto M, et al. Neuroprotective therapy using granulocyte colony-stimulating factor for acute spinal cord injury: a phase I/IIa clinical trial. Eur Spine J. 2012 Dec;21(12):2580–7.
106. Inada T, Takahashi H, Yamazaki M, Okawa A, Sakuma T, Kato K, et al. Multicenter prospective nonrandomized controlled clinical trial to prove neurotherapeutic effects of granulocyte colony-stimulating factor for acute spinal cord injury: analyses of follow-up cases after at least 1 year. Spine (Phila Pa 1976). 2014 Feb 1;39(3):213–9.
107. Koda M, Hanaoka H, Fujii Y, Hanawa M, Kawasaki Y, Ozawa Y, et al. Randomized trial of granulocyte colony-stimulating factor for spinal cord injury. Brain. 2021;144(3):789–99.
108. Derakhshanrad N, Saberi H, Yekaninejad MS, Joghataei MT, Sheikhrezaei A. Granulocyte-colony stimulating factor administration for neurological improvement in patients with postrehabilitation chronic incomplete traumatic spinal cord injuries: a double-blind randomized controlled clinical trial. J Neurosurg Spine. 2018;29(1):97–107.
109. Esen E, Taşar F, Akhan O. Determination of the anti-inflammatory effects of methylprednisolone on the sequelae of third molar surgery. J Oral Maxillofac Surg. 1999;57(10):1201–6.
110. Bains M, Hall ED. Antioxidant therapies in traumatic brain and spinal cord injury Biochimica et Biophysica Acta (BBA) - Molecular Basis of Disease. 2012;1822(5):675–84.
111. Chen WT, Zhou YP, Zhang GS. The progress and controversies regarding steroid use in acute spinal cord injury. Eur Rev Med Pharmacol Sci. 2023 Jul;27(13):6101–10. https://doi.org/10.26355/eurrev_202307_32966.
112. Bracken MB, Shepard MJ, Hellenbrand KG, Collins WF, Leo LS, Freeman DF, Wagner FC, Flamm ES, Eisenberg HM, Goodman JH, et al. Methylprednisolone and neurological function 1 year after spinal cord injury. Results of the National Acute Spinal Cord Injury Study. J Neurosurg. 1985 Nov;63(5):704–13. https://doi.org/10.3171/jns.1985.63.5.0704.
113. Bracken MB, Shepard MJ, Collins WF, Holford TR, Young W, Baskin DS, Eisenberg HM, Flamm E, Leo-Summers L, Maroon J, et al. A randomized, controlled trial of methylprednisolone or naloxone in the treatment of acute spinal-cord injury. Results of the second national acute spinal cord injury study. N Engl J Med. 1990;322(20):1405–11. https://doi.org/10.1056/NEJM199005173222001.
114. Bracken MB, Shepard MJ, Holford TR, Leo-Summers L, Aldrich EF, Fazl M, Fehlings M, Herr DL, Hitchon PW, Marshall LF, Nockels RP, Pascale V, Perot PL Jr, Piepmeier J, Sonntag VK, Wagner F, Wilberger JE, Winn HR, Young W. Administration of methylprednisolone for 24 or 48 hours or tirilazad mesylate for 48 hours in the treatment of acute spinal cord injury. Results of the Third National Acute Spinal Cord Injury Randomized Controlled Trial. National Acute Spinal Cord Injury Study. JAMA 1997 277(20):1597–604.
115. Fehlings MG, Wilson JR, Harrop JS, Kwon BK, Tetreault LA, Arnold PM, Singh JM, Hawryluk G, Dettori JR. Efficacy and Safety of Methylprednisolone Sodium Succinate in Acute Spinal Cord Injury: A Systematic Review. Global Spine J. 2017a Sep;7(3 Suppl):116S–137S. https://doi.org/10.1177/2192568217706366. Epub 2017 Sep 5. PMID: 29164020; PMCID: PMC5684849.

116. Fehlings MG, Tetreault LA, Wilson JR, Kwon BK, Burns AS, Martin AR, Hawryluk G, Harrop JS. A Clinical Practice Guideline for the Management of Acute Spinal Cord Injury: Introduction, Rationale, and Scope. Global Spine J. 2017b Sep;7(3 Suppl):84S–94S. https://doi.org/10.1177/2192568217703387. Epub 2017 Sep 5. PMID: 29164036; PMCID: PMC5684846.
117. Hurlbert RJ. Methylprednisolone for acute spinal cord injury: an inappropriate standard of care. J Neurosurg Spine. 2000;93(1):1–7.
118. Sauerland S, Nagelschmidt M, Mallmann P, Neugebauer EAM. Risks and benefits of preoperative high dose methylprednisolone in surgical patients. Drug-Safety. 2000;23(5):449–61.
119. Happel RD, Smith KP, Banik NL, Powers JM, Hogan EL, Balentine JD. Ca2+-accumulation in experimental spinal cord trauma. Brain Res. 1981;211(2):476–9.
120. Stokes BT, Fox P, Hollinden G. Extracellular calcium activity in the injured spinal cord. Exp Neurol. 1983 Jun;80(3):561–72.
121. Tymianski M, Tator CH. Normal and abnormal calcium homeostasis in neurons: a basis for the pathophysiology of traumatic and ischemic central nervous system injury. Neurosurgery. 1996 Jun;38(6):1176–95.
122. Faden AI, Jacobs TP, Smith MT. Evaluation of the calcium channel antagonist nimodipine in experimental spinal cord ischemia. J Neurosurg. 1984 Apr;60(4):796–9.
123. Ford RW, Malm DN. Failure of nimodipine to reverse acute experimental spinal cord injury. Cent Nerv Syst Trauma. 1985;2(1):9–17.
124. Guha A, Tator CH, Piper I. Effect of a calcium channel blocker on posttraumatic spinal cord blood flow. J Neurosurg. 1987;66(3):423–30.
125. Guha A, Tator CH, Smith CR, Piper I. Improvement in post-traumatic spinal cord blood flow with a combination of a calcium channel blocker and a vasopressor. J Trauma. 1989 Oct;29(10):1440–7.
126. Fehlings MG, Tator CH, Linden RD. The effect of nimodipine and dextran on axonal function and blood flow following experimental spinal cord injury. J Neurosurg. 1989;71(3):403–16.
127. Marcantoni M, Fuchs A, Löw P, Bartsch D, Kiehn O, Bellardita C. Early delivery and prolonged treatment with nimodipine prevents the development of spasticity after spinal cord injury in mice. Science Translational Medicine. 2020;12(539):eaay0167.
128. Guo F, Zheng X, He Z, Zhang R, Zhang S, Wang M, et al. Nimodipine promotes functional recovery after spinal cord injury in rats. Front Pharmacol. 2021 Sep;13(12):733420.
129. Petitjean M, Pointillart V, Dixmerias F, Wiart L, Sztark F, Lassié P, et al. Traitement médicamenteux de la lésion médullaire traumatique au stade aigu. Annales Françaises d'Anesthésie et de Réanimation. 1998;17(2):114–22.
130. Hawryluk GWJ, Rowland J, Kwon BK, Fehlings MG. Protection and repair of the injured spinal cord: a review of completed, ongoing, and planned clinical trials for acute spinal cord injury. Neurosurg Focus. 2008;25(5):E14.
131. Muir KW, Lees KR. A randomized, double-blind, placebo-controlled pilot trial of intravenous magnesium sulfate in acute stroke. Stroke. 1995 Jul;26(7):1183–8.
132. Kirkland AE, Sarlo GL, Holton KF. The role of magnesium in neurological disorders. Nutrients. 2018;10(6):730.
133. Carballo-Molina OA, Velasco I. Hydrogels as scaffolds and delivery systems to enhance axonal regeneration after injuries. Front Cell Neurosci. 2015 Feb;17(9):13.
134. Huang Z, Filipovic Z, Mp N, Ung C, Troy EL, Colburn RW, et al. AC105 increases extracellular magnesium delivery and reduces Excitotoxic glutamate exposure within injured spinal cords in rats. J Neurotrauma. 2017 Feb;34(3):685–94.
135. Lee JHT, Roy J, Moon Sohn H, Cheong M, Liu J, Stammers AT, et al. Magnesium in a polyethylene glycol formulation provides neuroprotection after unilateral cervical spinal cord injury. Spine. 2010;35(23):2041.
136. Streijger F, Lee JHT, Manouchehri N, Okon EB, Tigchelaar S, Anderson LM, et al. The evaluation of magnesium chloride within a polyethylene glycol formulation in a porcine model of acute spinal cord injury. J Neurotrauma. 2016;33(24):2202–16.

Special Populations: Older Adults, Pregnant, Pediatric, and Polytrauma Patients

11

Navpreet K. Dhillon and Mira H. Ghneim

11.1 SCI in Older Adults

SCI is occurring increasingly in older adults, particularly older men. Part of this rise is attributed to an aging population due to increasing life expectancies. These injuries often occur after ground-level falls, comprising up to 60% of cases [1]. In fact, SCI rates have been rising over the last several decades, specifically due to the climbing incidence of falls in the geriatric population. Other leading causes of SCI include motor vehicle collisions and sports and/or recreational injuries.

Pre-existing musculoskeletal abnormalities contribute to spinal cord vulnerability after injury. Factors that increase the risk of SCI include underlying hyperostotic spinal conditions, such as ankylosing spondylitis, as well as disc space collapse and osteophyte development. These anatomic changes contribute to spinal stenosis, narrowing the area available for the spinal cord, and may subsequently result in spinal cord compression and injury [2]. A significant proportion of males over 50 years and females over 60 years have radiographic evidence of degenerative changes on imaging [3]. Additionally, one in four asymptomatic patients over 65 years will have some degree of spinal stenosis on magnetic resonance imaging [4].

The C4 to C7 segment is particularly prone to injury due to the relative immobility in older patients, especially in the presence of external forces [5]. Some patients may instead have clinical manifestations of myelopathy from chronic spinal cord

N. K. Dhillon (✉)
Division of Trauma and Acute Care Surgery, Riverside University Health System Medical Center, Moreno Valley, CA, USA

Department of Surgery, Loma Linda University School of Medicine, Loma Linda, CA, USA
e-mail: n.dhillon@ruhealth.org

M. H. Ghneim
Program in Trauma, R Adams Cowley Shock Trauma Center, University of Maryland, Baltimore, MD, USA
e-mail: mira.ghneim@som.umaryland.edu

E. Brogi et al. (eds.), *Traumatic Spinal Cord Injury*, Hot Topics in Acute Care Surgery and Trauma, https://doi.org/10.1007/978-3-031-99890-4_11

compression; symptoms include disturbances in gait and coordination, along with motor and sensory deficits, which can contribute to falls and further injury [2].

SCI in older adults often presents within three contexts: (1) central cord syndrome, (2) cervical extension/distraction injuries, and (3) odontoid fractures [2]. Central cord syndrome is often seen in older patients with pre-existing cervical spondylosis and is characterized by disproportionate weakness of the upper extremities compared to the lower extremities. These are frequently seen after a hyperextension injury without an associated fracture; because there is often no associated fracture, delays in diagnosis may occur. Surgical decompression should be considered, but must be weighed against the risks. Decompression allows for potential improvement in neurologic function and recovery. Earlier decompression is associated with decreased lengths of stay and better motor recovery, specifically in patients who have central cord syndrome due to an acute disc herniation or an associated fracture [6]. However, patients who have developed central cord syndrome from spinal stenosis or spondylosis are unlikely to have improved motor function after early decompression. Decompression may be coupled with spinal fusion to prevent further traumatic injury.

Extension/distraction injuries occur due to a fracture that opens or lengthens the anterior column of the spine and can result in a SCI if severe [7]. These often happen in older patients with ankylosing spondylitis and stabilization is the mainstay of therapy. Stabilization may prevent further translation of the fracture and subsequent SCI in those who do not have cord injury at the time of presentation.

Odontoid fractures often result from cranial impact wherein the odontoid process is displaced either anteriorly or posteriorly [2]. The classification schema is based on the location of the fracture: type I odontoid fractures are an avulsion fracture of the apex, type II involves the base of the dens, and type III fractures extend into the body of the axis. Among these, type II fractures are most likely to be unstable. Type II fractures have the potential to migrate, resulting in spinal cord compression, neurologic deficits, and even death. Of note, few patients will initially present with neurologic deficits because of the large cervical column canal size in this area. Patients may be placed in a halo; however, this often is associated with airway issues and swallowing dysfunction, particularly in older patients. In fact, halos are associated with higher rates of pneumonia, pin site complications, and impairments in mobility in older patients [8]. Injuries that are unstable or do not improve with mobilization should be considered for internal fixation.

As the cervical spinal cord is disproportionately injured in older patients who sustain SCI, the topic of tracheostomies becomes increasingly relevant. Cervical SCI can result in impairment of respiratory muscles, inability to clear secretions, and prolonged ventilator dependence. Patients with cervical SCI who had an early tracheostomy, as defined as a tracheostomy performed within four days of initial intubation, had fewer respiratory complications regardless of the level of cervical SCI, more ventilator-free and intensive care unit-free days, and shorter hospital length of stays compared to patients who had a tracheostomy done at least five days from intubation [9]. Of note, in-hospital mortality was similar between cohorts.

Although early tracheostomy may appear advantageous, it becomes imperative for the care team to understand the goals of care and to understand if tracheostomy and/or feeding tube placement would be consistent with the patient's wishes. It is also important for the team to set realistic expectations. Survival rates decrease significantly after injury. In one investigation by DeVivo et al., seven-year survival rates among patients 50 years and older with SCI decreased from 86.7% to 22.7% [10]. While older patients are more likely to benefit from rehabilitation compared to their younger counterparts, older patients are less likely to achieve independence and are more likely to remain immobile. This immobility is associated with higher rates of decubitus ulcers, venous thromboembolism, and infectious complications.

11.2 SCI in Pregnancy

Traumatic SCI during pregnancy is a rare occurrence. The most commonly impacted region is the thoracic spine, and among pregnant patients with some degree of SCI in the thoracic spine, nearly 40% patients will have a complete SCI [11]. As emphasized in the Advanced Trauma Life Support course, the life of the mother takes priority over the life of the fetus, and thus, all resuscitative efforts should focus on stabilizing the mother. This strategy also helps to optimize the chances of fetal survival.

One common maneuver often discussed in the acute resuscitation of the pregnant patient is to place the patient in a left lateral tilt position. This allows for the uterus to displace from the inferior vena cava, resulting in increased preload and increased cardiac output. The left lateral tilt position must be done while maintaining full spine precautions in a patient whose spinal injury is suspected. Spinal precautions can be accomplished by keeping the patient on a spinal board and placing towels or blankets underneath the spinal board such that there is a 15-degree tilt.

While attempts are often made to minimize radiation exposure in pregnant patients, computed tomography should be obtained liberally to better identify injuries if there is a high suspicion of SCI. While magnetic resonance imaging can be used, it may not identify significant injuries to the spine in a timely fashion.

Literature on pregnancy outcomes in patients with SCI is generally lacking. If SCI occurs within the first trimester, there is an approximately 10% risk of fetal loss and malformations due to fetal hypoxia and hypotension secondary to spinal shock [12]. The risk of fetal loss is lower if SCI occurs either in the second or third trimester [13].

It becomes important to counsel pregnant patients about what to expect during their pregnancy when they have a traumatic SCI. Patients with a SCI above T4 may develop significant respiratory issues due to impaired ventilation, particularly as the pregnancy progresses. These patients may develop nocturnal hypercapnia and may need either continuous positive airway pressure or even mechanical ventilation, depending on the severity [14]. Spasticity, which often develops in patients with SCI, is typically managed with medications such as baclofen and tizanidine; however, these medications are not recommended during pregnancy. Due to this, physical therapy and routine stretching are the main form of therapy during pregnancy. It is not uncommon for patients to require a chronic indwelling Foley catheter because of reduced mobility and incontinence. Regional anesthesia with epidurals is safe in patients with SCI. Insertion may be difficult in patients with prior instrumentation or surgery. Patients should be counseled that future fertility is not affected by traumatic SCI, nor does pregnancy impact neurologic function after a SCI. Few patients will experience an obstetric complication [11]. Pregnant patients with SCI, in particular, are at a high risk for venous thromboembolism, and some have advocated for extended venous thromboembolism chemoprophylaxis after discharge [15].

11.3 SCI in Pediatric Patients

The cervical spine in younger patients is characterized by incomplete ossification and ligamentous laxity, which is why there are lower rates of injury in pediatric patients compared to their adult counterparts [16]. The pediatric cervical spine is more likely to resemble the adult cervical spine once a child is approximately eight years old which corresponds to when skeletal maturation occurs. The literature reports a low incidence of spine injuries and SCI among pediatric patients, although it most commonly occurs in the cervical region if it does occur. In a retrospective study of pediatric patients admitted to a Level 1 trauma center over a 25-year study period, 1.3% of the patients had a cervical spine injury. As expected, the rate of cervical SCI was substantially lower at 0.1%. Although SCI is rare, the injuries can be devastating due to a multitude of anatomic issues such as a large head-to-trunk ratio and weak nuchal musculature. This is another reason why SCI is more likely to occur in the upper spine compared to the lower spine [17].

Imaging is critical in diagnosing and managing SCI as a general principle. There is an overall reluctance to image pediatric patients due to the risk of exposure from ionizing radiation. And there is substantial variation among trauma centers with respect to which imaging modality is used to work up pediatric patients, if any [18]. Due to this reluctance, there may be delays in diagnosing spinal injuries, and some may be missed altogether. The Pediatric Emergency Care Applied Research Network (PECARN) has recently provided guidance on which patients should undergo cervical spine imaging after blunt trauma [19]. A computed tomography should be obtained in patients with a Glasgow Coma Scale between three and eight, those who are unresponsive on the Alert, Verbal, Pain, Unresponsive (AVPU) scale, any patient with an abnormal airway, breathing, or circulation status, or if focal neurologic deficits are present. Plain films should be considered in patients with a Glasgow Coma Scale between nine and fourteen, those who are able to verbalize or demonstrate pain according to the AVPU scale, patients who report neck pain or tenderness on exam, and/or in patients with substantial head or torso injuries. Such substantial injuries include skull fractures, pneumothoraces, solid organ injury, additional spine fractures, and pelvic fractures. The cervical spine can otherwise be clinically cleared if the aforementioned risk factors are absent.

One phenomenon that is often discussed within the context of pediatric trauma is Spinal Cord Injury Without Any Radiographic Abnormality, otherwise known as SCIWORA [20]. This has been classically defined as damage to the spinal cord with no corresponding abnormality identified on x-ray or computed tomography. With more ubiquitous use of magnetic resonance imaging (MRI), injuries that were previously classified as SCIWORA are now detected on advanced imaging. Patients with SCIWORA most commonly present after high-energy mechanisms such as motor vehicle accidents [21]. A subanalysis of a multicenter study in pediatric trauma patients compared patients with SCIWORA who had normal MRI imaging to patients with abnormal imaging findings [21]. One in five patients with SCIWORA had abnormal cord signaling on MRI. Patients with abnormal MRI findings were more likely to require an intervention and more likely to have persistent deficits when compared to their counterparts with normal imaging. Further classification of SCIWORA patients based on MRI findings may allow for early prognostication, as MRI findings often correlate well with American Spinal Injury Association scores [21]. Operative intervention is often recommended in cases with cord compression; however, there are no comparative analyses that demonstrate a strong benefit in pediatric patients [22].

Children who sustain a SCI before their growth spurt can develop scoliosis as they grow. Neurological outcomes in pediatric patients are generally better compared to adults with similar injuries.

11.4 SCI in Patients with Polytrauma

Spinal injuries can occur in up to a third of patients with polytrauma [23]. Patients presenting with polytrauma can be particularly challenging. There may be multiple injuries that require urgent stabilization, and setting priorities becomes imperative. Maintaining circulation and adequate oxygenation, and ventilation are the highest priorities in any trauma patient. Consequently, spinal injuries are often not immediately addressed in polytrauma scenarios. While it is ideal to stabilize unstable fractures immediately to either prevent or exacerbate SCI, these operations are often prolonged, require special positioning, are invasive, and are associated with increased bleeding, making these interventions particularly unsuitable in critically ill patients.

Regardless of the presence or absence of a neurologic deficit, the literature recommends early fixation of unstable spinal fractures. In a randomized controlled trial of 35 patients with SCI from a thoracolumbar injury, patients underwent either early surgical decompression, defined as decompression within 24 hours of injury, or late decompression, defined as decompression within 24–72 hours of injury [24]. Neurologic function did not differ in patients with timing of decompression among the subset of patients with a complete SCI. Patients with an incomplete injury had greater improvements in motor function if decompression was completed early. Many studies advocate for early stabilization in patients with neurologic deficits [23, 25]. Earlier surgery is associated with decreased hospital lengths of stay, shorter stays in the intensive care unit, fewer days of mechanical ventilation, and fewer pulmonary complications [26]. However, these studies, along with others, do not contextualize the injury within the polytrauma setting.

Most of the literature that accounts for polytrauma does not accurately characterize the overall injury burden or the corresponding physiologic state. A recently published retrospective review attempted to address both and demonstrated that patients who underwent early total care for both spinal and non-spinal injuries were more likely to have non-lethal abdominal injuries [27]. Patients with severe traumatic brain injury often had definitive care after 48 hours, regardless of the presence of other severe injuries. Those patients who had early definitive surgery had a higher survival rate; however, this is more likely to reflect the injury burden that these patients sustained.

The World Society of Emergency Surgery and the European Association of Neurosurgical Societies collaborated to create recommendations about the management of spinal cord injury in polytrauma patients [28]. Given the nature of polytrauma, patients will often undergo multiple interventions prior to spine stabilization. As they undergo these interventions, close attention to positioning should be given to avoid secondary injuries to the spine. The authors recommend maintaining a mean arterial pressure above 85 mmHg while other interventions are being delivered. This threshold may need to be lowered in the setting of ongoing bleeding. There are also strong recommendations for maintaining the PaO2 between 60 and 100 mmHg, PaCO2 between 35 and 40 mmHg, a platelet count of at least 50,000 per microliter, and the use of adjunctive testing to restore normal coagulation profiles. Additionally, early administration of reversal agents should be considered in any patient on a prehospital anticoagulant or antiplatelet agent. Importantly, the authors strongly recommend against high-dose corticosteroid therapy.

The management of SCI in polytrauma patients is incredibly complex and requires strong multidisciplinary collaboration, clear communication, and coordination.

11.5 Conclusions

Managing spinal cord injuries is inherently complex, and it becomes even more challenging when considering specific subpopulations of trauma patients whose unique anatomical and physiological characteristics may influence both diagnosis and treatment. Each subpopulation requires its own set of considerations to be effectively addressed. Understanding these intricacies is crucial for optimizing outcomes in patients with SCI.

References

1. Jeanmonod R, Varacallo M. Geriatric cervical spine injury. In: StatPearls. StatPearls Publishing; 2024. Accessed 20 Sept 2024. http://www.ncbi.nlm.nih.gov/books/NBK470375/.
2. Jabbour P, Fehlings M, Vaccaro AR, Harrop JS. Traumatic spine injuries in the geriatric population. Neurosurg Focus. 2008;25(5):E16.
3. Young WF. Cervical spondylotic myelopathy: a common cause of spinal cord dysfunction in older persons. Am Fam Physician. 2000;62(5):1064–73.
4. Teresi LM, Lufkin RB, Reicher MA, et al. Asymptomatic degenerative disk disease and spondylosis of the cervical spine: MR imaging. Radiology. 1987;164(1):83–8.
5. Dvorak J, Froehlich D, Penning L, Baumgartner H, Panjabi MM. Functional radiographic diagnosis of the cervical spine: flexion/extension. Spine (Phila Pa 1976). 1988;13(7):748–55.
6. Hagen EM, Aarli JA, Gronning M. The clinical significance of spinal cord injuries in patients older than 60 years of age. Acta Neurol Scand. 2005;112(1):42–7.
7. Magee DJ, Zachazewski JE, Quillen WS, Manske RC. Pathology and intervention in musculoskeletal rehabilitation—E-book. Elsevier Health Sciences; 2015.
8. van Middendorp JJ, Slooff WBM, Nellestein WR, Öner FC. Incidence of and risk factors for complications associated with halo-vest immobilization: a prospective, descriptive cohort study of 239 patients. JBJS. 2009;91(1):71.
9. Anand T, Hanna K, Kulvatunyou N, et al. Time to tracheostomy impacts overall outcomes in patients with cervical spinal cord injury. J Trauma Acute Care Surg. 2020;89(2):358–64.
10. DeVivo MJ, Kartus PL, Stover SL, Rutt RD, Fine PR. Seven-year survival following spinal cord injury. Arch Neurol. 1987;44(8):872–5.
11. Rajkovic C, Kiss A, Lee A, et al. Management of spinal trauma in pregnant patients: a systematic review of the literature. J Trauma Acute Care Surg Published online August 30; 2024. p. 969.
12. Baranović S, Maldini B, Cengić T, Kolundzić R. Anesthetic management of acute cervical spinal cord injury in pregnancy. Acta Clin Croat. 2014;53(1):98–101.
13. Engel S, Ferrara G. Obstetric outcomes in women who sustained a spinal cord injury during pregnancy. Spinal Cord. 2013;51(2):170–1.
14. Robertson K, Ashworth F. Spinal cord injury and pregnancy. Obstet Med. 2022;15(2):99–103.
15. Eichinger S, Eischer L, Sinkovec H, et al. Risk of venous thromboembolism during rehabilitation of patients with spinal cord injury. PLoS One. 2018;13(3):e0193735.
16. Platzer P, Jaindl M, Thalhammer G, et al. Cervical spine injuries in pediatric patients. J Trauma. 2007;62(2):389–96. discussion 394–396
17. Hofbauer M, Jaindl M, Höchtl LL, Ostermann RC, Kdolsky R, Aldrian S. Spine injuries in polytraumatized pediatric patients: characteristics and experience from a Level I trauma center over two decades. J Trauma Acute Care Surg. 2012;73(1):156–61.
18. Massoumi R, Wertz J, Duong T, Tseng CH, Jen HCH. Variation in pediatric cervical spine imaging across trauma centers—a cause for concern? J Trauma Acute Care Surg. 2021;91(4):641–8.
19. Leonard JC, Harding M, Cook LJ, et al. PECARN prediction rule for cervical spine imaging of children presenting to the emergency department with blunt trauma: a multicentre prospective observational study. Lancet Child Adolesc Health. 2024;8(7):482–90.
20. Dickman CA, Zabramski JM, Rekate HL, Sonntag VK. Spinal cord injuries in children without radiographic abnormalities. West J Med. 1993;158(1):67–8.
21. Boese CK, Oppermann J, Siewe J, Eysel P, Scheyerer MJ, Lechler P. Spinal cord injury without radiologic abnormality in children: a systematic review and meta-analysis. J Trauma Acute Care Surg. 2015;78(4):874–82.

22. Muzumdar D, Ventureyra ECG. Spinal cord injuries in children. J Pediatr Neurosci. 2006;1(2):43.
23. Mugesh Kanna R, Prasad Shetty A, Rajasekaran S. Timing of intervention for spinal injury in patients with polytrauma. J Clin Orthop Trauma. 2021;12(1):96–100.
24. Rahimi-Movaghar V, Niakan A, Haghnegahdar A, Shahlaee A, Saadat S, Barzideh E. Early versus late surgical decompression for traumatic thoracic/thoracolumbar (T1-L1) spinal cord injured patients. Primary results of a randomized controlled trial at one year follow-up. Neurosciences (Riyadh). 2014;19(3):183–91.
25. Chipman JG, Deuser WE, Beilman GJ. Early surgery for thoracolumbar spine injuries decreases complications. J Trauma. 2004;56(1):52–7.
26. Dimar JR, Carreon LY, Riina J, Schwartz DG, Harris MB. Early versus late stabilization of the spine in the polytrauma patient. Spine (Phila Pa 1976). 2010;35(21 Suppl):S187–92.
27. Halvachizadeh S, Pfeifer R, Duncan J, et al. Does the injury pattern drive the surgical treatment strategy in multiply injured patients with major fractures? J Trauma Acute Care Surg. 2024;96(6):931–7.
28. Picetti E, Demetriades AK, Catena F, et al. Early management of adult traumatic spinal cord injury in patients with polytrauma: a consensus and clinical recommendations jointly developed by the World Society of Emergency Surgery (WSES) & the European Association of Neurosurgical Societies (EANS). World J Emerg Surg. 2024;19(1):4.

Part III

Neurological Injury and Its Sequelae

Hemodynamic Monitoring and Cardiovascular Complications in Traumatic Spinal Cord Injury

12

Saad L. Sahi and Ali Salim

12.1 Hemodynamic Changes After SCI

12.1.1 Neurogenic Shock and Spinal Shock Syndrome

The hemodynamic changes following SCI can present significant challenges to the care team. Understanding the pathophysiology behind these changes is necessary to provide appropriate care to the patient. Therefore, it is important to first differentiate between neurogenic shock and spinal shock syndrome, both of which are critical complications of SCI and distinct in how they manifest.

Sympathetic and parasympathetic divisions of the autonomic nervous system innervate the heart and blood vessels and, in turn, regulate cardiovascular responses to stimuli [2, 4, 7–9]. Neurogenic shock refers to the loss of sympathetic tone below the level of injury, often resulting in unopposed parasympathetic activity, which can lead to hypotension, bradycardia, and hypothermia [10, 11]. Cervical and high thoracic SCI above the level of the T6 vertebra results in greater loss of sympathetic tone, especially to the heart, and thus the body's control over autonomic functions such as blood pressure, heart rate, and temperature control [2, 12]. Lower thoracic SCI below T6 preserves greater sympathetic outflow, allowing for better regulation of autonomic functions, but can still result in hypotension due to relative hypovolemia secondary to vasodilation and venous pooling [8, 12]. Regardless of the level of injury, neurogenic shock refers specifically to the hemodynamic consequences of

S. L. Sahi · A. Salim (✉)
Division of Trauma and Acute Care Surgery, Mass General Brigham, Boston, MA, USA
e-mail: ssahi@mgb.org; asalim1@bwh.harvard.edu

E. Brogi et al. (eds.), *Traumatic Spinal Cord Injury*, Hot Topics in Acute Care Surgery and Trauma, https://doi.org/10.1007/978-3-031-99890-4_12

impaired autonomic function in SCI, which can manifest as severe hypotension and bradycardia [4].

Spinal shock syndrome, on the other hand, refers to the transient reduction or absence of somatic functions, including reflexes distal to the level of injury, which resolve temporally [8, 11]. Symptoms progress through phases from areflexia to hyperreflexia and can last from days to weeks, sometimes months. The severity and location of injury can affect the overall duration of symptoms, with the resolution of spinal shock being marked by the gradual return of reflex activity below the level of injury [2, 6, 9, 11, 12]. Spinal shock thus refers specifically to impaired somatic function in SCI, which can manifest as a loss of sensory, motor, and reflex functions [4, 6]. Importantly, spinal shock syndrome is a transient physiologic response to injury, whereas paralysis results from irreversible damage to the spinal cord itself [13].

The clinical presentation of neurogenic shock includes persistent hypotension (defined as a systolic blood pressure of less than 90 mmHg) and bradycardia (defined as a heart rate of less than 60 bpm) without hypovolemia [14, 15]. The impact of neurogenic shock on systemic circulation includes vasodilation, venous pooling, and reduced cardiac output, resulting in inadequate tissue perfusion [8, 12, 16]. Therefore, maintaining hemodynamic stability is essential for reducing the risk of secondary ischemic injury and improving outcomes in SCI patients [2, 6, 17]. Diagnosis involves continuous monitoring of blood pressure and heart rate to identify hemodynamic instability. Neurogenic shock usually resolves within 4–6 weeks post-injury but can persist longer in severe cases, necessitating ongoing hemodynamic support [2, 8].

12.2 Hemodynamic Management

12.2.1 Hemodynamic Monitoring

Close hemodynamic monitoring of patients with acute SCI in an intensive care unit (ICU) or similar setting is critical for early detection and treatment of cardiovascular dysfunction and hemodynamic instability [14, 15]. In the laboratory setting, hypotension exacerbated secondary injury by reducing spinal cord blood flow and perfusion, making continuous monitoring a crucial prerequisite for prompt intervention [13]. Key hemodynamic parameters to monitor include blood pressure, heart rate, cardiac output, and central venous pressure [6, 10, 17]. And while hypotension is typically defined using a systolic blood pressure threshold, hemodynamic monitoring in SCI patients generally focuses on mean arterial pressure (MAP) as it better correlates with spinal cord perfusion [18].

Hemodynamic monitoring in SCI patients is best achieved using invasive techniques, including arterial lines, central venous catheters, and, less frequently, pulmonary artery catheters, all of which provide a detailed hemodynamic assessment [6, 10, 17]. Non-invasive methods can serve as useful adjuncts for supplemental information, such as echocardiography, and are increasingly used for their safety and efficacy [6, 10]. Advanced hemodynamic monitoring systems, such as the Pulse Contour Cardiac Output (PiCCO) system and the FloTrac system, which utilizes a Vigileo monitor, provide detailed insights into cardiac function and fluid status, thus enhancing the ability to detect and respond to hemodynamic changes in real time [19].

12.2.2 Volume Resuscitation and Vasoactive Medications

Volume resuscitation is a fundamental aspect of hemodynamic management in SCI, as ensuring adequate tissue perfusion and maintaining blood pressure are critical to prevent further spinal cord damage and improve overall outcomes [4, 8, 10, 11]. Initially, crystalloids such as normal saline or lactated Ringer's solution are commonly administered to quickly expand intravascular volume. This is often necessary after SCI given the effects of vasodilation on hemodynamic stability [8, 10, 11]. The choice of fluid may then shift to blood products or colloids based on the specific clinical scenario and patient response, such as in polytrauma patients presenting with hemorrhagic shock or cirrhotic patients presenting with chronic hypoalbuminemia.

However, clinicians must be cautious to avoid excessive volume administration, as volume overload can result in significant complications. Overloading the patient with fluids can lead to pulmonary edema, impairing gas exchange and causing respiratory distress, or congestive heart failure, potentially exacerbating cardiac dysfunction and leading to further hemodynamic instability [6, 8]. Therefore, careful monitoring of fluid balance, regular assessment of the patient's clinical status, and judicious use of fluids are essential to optimize outcomes and minimize the risk of adverse effects. When euvolemia has been achieved and volume resuscitation is insufficient to maintain target MAP goals, vasoactive medications are indicated [2, 8, 12]. The selection and dosage of vasoactive agents should consider patient-specific factors, including the level of injury and be guided by continuous hemodynamic monitoring to achieve optimal outcomes [12].

In the acute phase of SCI, intravenous vasoactive agents, including norepinephrine, phenylephrine, and dopamine, can be used to maintain hemodynamic stability (Table 12.1) [12]. Norepinephrine is a potent vasopressor with strong alpha-adrenergic agonist properties, leading to vasoconstriction, and some beta-adrenergic effects that increase heart rate and contractility. It is often considered the first-line agent for managing hypotension in SCI, particularly for high thoracic and cervical injuries, providing a balanced approach to increasing blood pressure and cardiac output. Phenylephrine, a pure alpha-1 agonist, is recommended for injuries below T6 or in patients who cannot tolerate increased heart rate, as it effectively increases vascular tone and blood pressure without significant cardiac stimulation. Dopamine acts on dopaminergic, beta, and alpha receptors depending on the dose, making it more complex to manage and achieve the desired effect. It is typically used as a last resort given its association with increased cardiovascular complications. Contrastingly, epinephrine is rarely used in clinical practice, with experimental

Table 12.1 Comparison of vasoactive medications

Intravenous agents			
	Receptors	Effect	Use case
Norepinephrine	Alpha, beta	↑ BP and ↑ HR	First-line; high thoracic and cervical injuries
Phenylephrine	Alpha-1	↑ BP	Injuries below T6; patients with tachycardia
Dopamine	Dopaminergic, beta, alpha	Dose-dependent	Last resort due to cardiovascular complications
Enteral agents			
	Receptors	Effect	Use case
Midodrine	Alpha-1	↑ BP	Persistent hypotension without bradycardia
Pseudoephedrine	Alpha and beta	↑ BP and ↑ HR	Persistent hypotension with bradycardia

studies in animals suggesting that it does not significantly increase spinal cord blood flow and may cause arrhythmias [20, 21].

In the chronic phase of SCI, enteral vasoactive agents, including midodrine and pseudoephedrine, can be used to wean off intravenous agents and support long-term hemodynamic stability (Table 12.1) [12]. As an alpha-1 agonist, midodrine is used for persistent hypotension without concomitant bradycardia, whereas pseudoephedrine is used to manage persistent hypotension and bradycardia by increasing venous return through both alpha and beta agonism. These enteral vasoactive agents can especially help progress care as patients transition out of the ICU setting and into rehabilitation facilities.

12.2.3 Guidelines and Recommendations

In 2013, the American Association of Neurological Surgeons (AANS) and the Congress of Neurological Surgeons (CNS) jointly published guidelines for the management of acute SCI (Table 12.2) [15]. They recommended continuous monitoring in an ICU setting with the immediate correction of hypotension, defined as a systolic blood pressure of less than 90 mmHg, while maintaining a MAP between 85 and 90 mmHg for the first seven days post-injury to reduce overall morbidity and improve neurological outcomes in SCI patients. They also recommended volume resuscitation with crystalloids and blood products to correct hypovolemia, with escalation to the use of norepinephrine as the preferred vasopressor for maintaining MAP when volume resuscitation is insufficient.

While these recommendations have been widely adopted in clinical practice and routinely referenced in the literature, they remain difficult to implement on a practical level given the tight range of target MAP goals over a fixed duration of therapy. Given these challenges, along with new research that acknowledges the limitations of current evidence on the relationship between MAP and neurologic recovery, a multidisciplinary guideline development group was formed to review

Table 12.2 Comparison of consensus guidelines

Recommendation	2013 AANS/CNS guidelines	2024 AO spine and praxis guidelines
Monitoring	Continuous in ICU	Continuous in ICU
Target MAP goals	85–90 mmHg	75–80 mmHg (lower limit) 90–95 mmHg (upper limit)
Duration of MAP goals	First 7 days post-injury	First 3–7 days based on injury severity
Preferred vasopressor	Norepinephrine	Clinical discretion advised
Implementation	Widely adopted but challenging	More personalized approach to treatment

and update the 2013 AANS/CNS guidelines. In 2024, the AO Spine and Praxis Spinal Cord Institute published their own recommendations on the hemodynamic management of acute traumatic SCI (Table 12.2) [14]. Recognizing that hemodynamic management is one of the only available treatment options that likely improves neurologic outcomes in patients with acute traumatic SCI, the group sought to make recommendations on the range of target MAP goals, the duration of therapy for MAP augmentation, and the choice of vasopressor to achieve the desired MAP. They also sought to make a recommendation on spinal cord perfusion pressure (SCPP) targets.

The updated guidelines continue to emphasize the need for continuous monitoring in an ICU setting along with the avoidance of systemic hypotension. They were not able to make any specific recommendations on the choice of vasopressors or SCPP targets due to insufficient evidence, instead advising clinical discretion. They do, however, recommend a broader range for both target MAP goals and duration of therapy post-injury. Specifically, they set a lower limit MAP target of 75–80 mmHg and an upper limit MAP target of 90–95 mmHg, effectively liberalizing the target MAP goals in acute traumatic SCI patients, allowing for greater clinical compliance. They also recommend a duration of therapy of 3–7 days, allowing for a more personalized approach to treatment based on injury severity and a patient's need for aggressive and prolonged MAP augmentation. Importantly, the upper limit MAP target is intended for patients requiring active MAP augmentation with medical intervention, and not for those patients who achieve a MAP at or above 95 mmHg without medical intervention. In other words, MAP augmentation achieved with vasopressor support should not exceed the upper limit MAP target as the cardiovascular risks likely outweigh the neurologic benefits.

12.2.4 Additional Considerations

In addition to volume resuscitation and vasoactive medications, which form the cornerstone of hemodynamic management in SCI, several factors can affect hemodynamic stability. One important factor is thermoregulation, which is impaired in SCI [9, 22]. Fluctuations in body temperature can significantly affect cardiovascular function and overall stability, making careful temperature management a critical component of care [23]. Pain management and sedation also play a significant role in hemodynamic stability. Effective pain control and appropriate sedation are necessary as poorly managed pain can lead to increased stress responses, while inadequate sedation can cause agitation, both of which can destabilize hemodynamics [24]. Additionally, the management of electrolyte imbalances is critical. Regular monitoring and timely correction of electrolyte levels are necessary to maintain hemodynamic stability. Electrolyte disturbances can adversely affect cardiac function and blood pressure, leading to further complications if not properly addressed [25].

12.3 Cardiovascular Complications

12.3.1 Arrhythmias

Arrhythmias are a prevalent complication in SCI, particularly in those with high thoracic and cervical injuries [7]. The incidence of bradycardia is notably high in this population, ranging from 14–77% when defined as a heart rate of less than 60 bpm, due to autonomic dysregulation and the disruption of cardiac innervation pathways that result from the injury [26]. Autonomic dysregulation impairs the normal balance between sympathetic and parasympathetic control of the heart, leading to various cardiac rhythm disturbances [4]. While bradycardia is the most commonly observed arrhythmia, supraventricular and ventricular tachycardia, including atrial fibrillation, have also been reported with an incidence of 18–27% [26].

Continuous cardiac monitoring and regular electrocardiograms (ECGs) are essential for the early detection and timely management of arrhythmias in SCI patients. Continuous cardiac monitoring allows for the immediate identification of bradycardia, tachycardia, and other rhythm abnormalities, facilitating prompt intervention. Routine ECGs provide valuable diagnostic information, helping to monitor the progression of arrhythmias and assess the effectiveness of treatment interventions [27].

Treatment strategies for arrhythmias in SCI patients are tailored to the specific type and severity of the arrhythmia. For symptomatic bradycardia resulting in hemodynamic instability, the administration of atropine is a common and effective intervention [15]. While there is no reported threshold of heart rate below which atropine should be administered, many clinicians will keep the medication at the bedside during the acute phase of injury and choose a minimum acceptable heart rate at which it should be administered, regardless of symptoms. Atropine works by blocking the vagus nerve's influence on the heart, thereby increasing the heart rate [9, 28]. In cases where bradycardia is refractory to atropine or when it is severe, temporary or permanent pacing may be necessary to maintain an adequate heart rate and ensure sufficient cardiac output [7, 15].

For tachyarrhythmias, including atrial fibrillation, the use of antiarrhythmic drugs is a primary treatment strategy. Amiodarone is the most frequently used antiarrhythmic drug in the ICU setting, while beta-blockers, calcium channel blockers, digoxin, and magnesium are also commonly used in practice [29]. These medications help control the heart rate and rhythm, reducing the risk of complications such as stroke and heart failure. The choice of antiarrhythmic drug is guided by the specific arrhythmia, underlying health conditions, and potential drug interactions. In some cases, electrical cardioversion may be required to restore normal sinus rhythm, especially if pharmacological interventions are ineffective [29].

In addition to pharmacological and electrical interventions, managing underlying factors that contribute to arrhythmias is crucial. This includes optimizing electrolyte balance, ensuring adequate oxygenation, and addressing any other instigating factors that might increase parasympathetic tone, such as suctioning and turning, all of which may exacerbate cardiac rhythm disturbances [7]. Multidisciplinary care involving cardiologists, neurologists, and rehabilitation specialists is often necessary to provide comprehensive management of arrhythmias in SCI patients, aiming to improve their overall cardiovascular stability and quality of life.

12.3.2 Secondary Ischemic Injury

Hemodynamic instability can significantly exacerbate ischemic injury to the spinal cord, thereby leading to secondary damage [2, 15]. This secondary damage can result in further deterioration of neurological function and worsen the overall prognosis. Ensuring adequate perfusion pressure through aggressive hemodynamic management is crucial for preventing secondary ischemic injury and optimizing patient outcomes [6]. Strategies include maintaining target MAP goals, early volume resuscitation, and the use of vasoactive medications as discussed in the previous section of this chapter.

12.3.3 Autonomic Dysreflexia

Autonomic dysreflexia (AD) is a serious and potentially life-threatening condition characterized by a severe hypertensive response to stimuli below the level of SCI [2, 6, 9, 27]. It is most observed in individuals with high thoracic and cervical injuries [11, 13]. This condition arises due to disrupted communication between the brain and the sympathetic nervous system, resulting in unregulated sympathetic outflow and subsequent vasoconstriction below the level of injury [11].

In individuals with injury above the T6 level, the ability of the central nervous system to modulate autonomic responses is impaired. Normally, afferent stimuli from the body are processed in the brain, which then modulates the autonomic response appropriately. However, in SCI this regulatory pathway is disrupted [9]. Consequently, stimuli such as bladder distension, bowel impaction, or skin sores can trigger an exaggerated sympathetic response, leading to widespread vasoconstriction and severe hypertension [4].

Autonomic dysreflexia is a complex and critical condition requiring prompt recognition and management. By understanding the underlying pathophysiology, identifying common triggers, and implementing both immediate and long-term management strategies as discussed in a later chapter, clinicians can significantly reduce the morbidity associated with this condition and improve the quality of life for individuals with spinal cord injuries.

12.4 Other Complications

12.4.1 DVT and Prophylaxis

Deep vein thrombosis (DVT) and pulmonary embolism (PE) pose a significant risk to SCI patients, with a recent meta-analysis reporting a 10.9% incidence of DVT along with a 4.5% incidence of PE in the acute phase of injury even with prophylaxis [30, 31]. Moreover, the mortality rate for PE has been reported as 3.5% in this patient population compared to 0.46% in the general population [31, 32]. The combination of venous stasis from prolonged immobility, endothelial damage, and a hypercoagulable state significantly elevates the risk [8, 10]. Prophylactic measures are crucial and include the use of anticoagulants such as low molecular weight heparins (LMWH) and mechanical devices like compression stockings [11]. Early mobilization and physical therapy also play a vital role in preventing DVT by promoting circulation [7].

In cases of confirmed DVT, immediate treatment is essential to prevent complications like PE [10]. Initial anticoagulation with heparin, either unfractionated or LMWH, is followed by long-term oral anticoagulation using agents such as warfarin or direct oral anticoagulants (DOACs) [10, 11, 27]. Suspected PE requires prompt diagnostic imaging, typically spiral CT, and may necessitate thrombolytic therapy in severe cases [10].

Long-term management of DVT in SCI patients often involves extended anticoagulation therapy, potentially up to six months or longer, depending on individual risk factors [7, 33]. Regular monitoring and follow-up are essential to ensure the effectiveness and safety of the treatment. Patient education about recognizing symptoms and adhering to preventive measures is critical for reducing the risk of recurrence and improving overall outcomes.

12.5 Future Developments

Advances in hemodynamic monitoring technologies, such as intrathecal pressure monitors and epidural near-infrared spectroscopy (NIRS) sensors, offer significant promise for improving the accuracy and efficiency of hemodynamic assessment in SCI patients [14, 22, 34]. These tools provide real-time data on spinal cord blood flow and oxygenation, crucial for optimizing perfusion pressure and minimizing secondary ischemic injury.

Temperature management, particularly therapeutic hypothermia, is being investigated for its potential neuroprotective benefits in SCI patients [3]. Hypothermia may reduce secondary injury by decreasing metabolic demand and limiting inflammatory responses. Studies have shown that controlled hypothermia may be beneficial in the acute phase of SCI, theoretically leading to better long-term neurological outcomes. However, precise protocols for its application, including timing, duration, and degree of cooling, require further research and clinical validation.

Evidence suggests that a cardio-centric hemodynamic management strategy using dobutamine may be more effective than norepinephrine in augmenting spinal cord blood flow and oxygenation while reducing the risk of hemorrhagic complications [17]. Dobutamine, a positive inotrope, enhances cardiac output and improves perfusion to the spinal cord without significantly increasing systemic vascular resistance. This property makes it particularly useful in managing hemodynamic instability in SCI patients, where maintaining optimal perfusion is critical for preventing secondary ischemic damage.

The management principles used in traumatic brain injury (TBI), such as monitoring intracranial pressure (ICP) and cerebral perfusion pressure (CPP), are being adapted for traumatic SCI with a focus on intraspinal pressure (ISP) and spinal cord perfusion pressure (SCPP) [22]. Monitoring ISP and SCPP can provide valuable insights into the hemodynamic status of the spinal cord, guiding interventions to maintain adequate perfusion and oxygenation. Multi-center validation of ISP monitoring findings and the development of probes for non-surgical insertion are necessary to advance this approach. Improved multimodality monitoring tools, integrating various physiological parameters, will further enhance the management of traumatic SCI.

Ultimately, future research should focus on refining hemodynamic management strategies, exploring new therapeutic options, and developing advanced monitoring systems to address the complex challenges of managing cardiovascular complications in SCI patients. Continued investigation into temperature management, neuroprotective and regenerative treatments, and innovative monitoring technologies will help improve the prognosis and quality of life for SCI patients.

12.6 Summary and Recommendations

The hemodynamic changes following SCI present significant challenges, requiring a deep understanding of the pathophysiology for appropriate patient care. It is crucial to distinguish between neurogenic shock and spinal shock syndrome, both critical complications of SCI. Neurogenic shock results from the loss of sympathetic tone below the injury, leading to unopposed parasympathetic activity and symptoms such as hypotension, bradycardia, and hypothermia. The severity of these symptoms varies depending on the injury level, with cervical and high thoracic injuries causing more significant autonomic dysfunction. Spinal shock syndrome, conversely, involves a transient loss of somatic functions below the injury level, progressing through phases from areflexia to hyperreflexia over days to weeks.

Hemodynamic management is vital for patients with acute SCI, emphasizing continuous monitoring in intensive care settings. Key parameters include blood pressure, heart rate, cardiac output, and central venous pressure, with mean arterial pressure (MAP) being particularly important for spinal cord perfusion. Invasive techniques such as arterial lines and central venous catheters provide detailed assessments, while non-invasive methods like echocardiography offer additional insights. Updated guidelines recommend maintaining a MAP of 75–95 mmHg for the first 3–7 days post-injury, with volume resuscitation using crystalloids and blood products and norepinephrine as the preferred vasopressor, promoting a personalized approach to treatment based on injury severity and patient needs.

Cardiovascular complications such as arrhythmias are common in SCI, particularly with high thoracic and cervical injuries. Continuous cardiac monitoring and regular electrocardiograms are essential for early detection and management. Bradycardia may require atropine or pacing, while tachyarrhythmias might need antiarrhythmic drugs or electrical cardioversion. Preventing secondary ischemic injury involves aggressive hemodynamic management to ensure adequate perfusion pressure. Autonomic dysreflexia, a severe hypertensive response, requires prompt recognition and management. DVT prophylaxis includes anticoagulants, mechanical devices, early mobilization, and physical therapy. Long-term management may involve extended anticoagulation therapy and regular monitoring to prevent complications such as pulmonary embolism.

Key Recommendations

1. Differentiate neurogenic shock and spinal shock:
   - Neurogenic shock: Loss of sympathetic tone leading to hypotension, bradycardia, and hypothermia.
   - Spinal shock: Transient loss of reflexes and somatic functions below the injury level.
2. Hemodynamic monitoring and management:
   - Use invasive techniques (arterial lines, central venous catheters) for detailed assessment.
   - Employ volume resuscitation and vasoactive medications as needed, with norepinephrine as the preferred vasopressor.
   - Maintain MAP of 75–95 mmHg for the first 3–7 days post-injury.
3. Cardiovascular complications:
   - Continuous cardiac monitoring and regular ECGs for early arrhythmia detection.
   - Use atropine or pacing for bradycardia; antiarrhythmic drugs or cardioversion for tachyarrhythmias.
4. Prevent secondary ischemic injury:
   - Ensure adequate perfusion pressure through aggressive hemodynamic management.
5. Manage autonomic dysreflexia:
   - Recognize and promptly manage this hypertensive response in high thoracic and cervical injuries.

6. DVT prophylaxis:
   - Use anticoagulants and mechanical devices.
   - Promote early mobilization and physical therapy.
   - Long-term management may require extended anticoagulation therapy and regular monitoring.

References

1. National Spinal Cord Injury Statistical Center. Facts and figures at a glance. Birmingham, AL: University of Alabama at Birmingham; 2017.
2. Stein DM, Sheth KN. Management of acute spinal cord injury. Contin: Lifelong Learn Neurol. 2015;21:159–87. https://doi.org/10.1212/01.con.0000461091.09736.0c.
3. Ahmad FU, Wang MY, Levi AD. Hypothermia for acute spinal cord injury—a review. World Neurosurg. 2014;82:207–14. https://doi.org/10.1016/j.wneu.2013.01.008.
4. Phillips AA, Krassioukov AV. Contemporary cardiovascular concerns after spinal cord injury: mechanisms, Maladaptations, and management. J Neurotrauma. 2015;32:1927–42. https://doi.org/10.1089/neu.2015.3903.
5. Ropper AE, Neal MT, Theodore N. Acute management of traumatic cervical spinal cord injury. Pr Neurol. 2015;15:266. https://doi.org/10.1136/practneurol-2015-001094.
6. Stevens RD, Bhardwaj A, Kirsch JR, Mirski MA. Critical care and perioperative management in traumatic spinal cord injury. J Neurosurg Anesthesiol. 2003;15:215–29. https://doi.org/10.1097/00008506-200307000-00009.
7. Calvo-Infante R, Narvaez-Rojas A, Padilla-Zambrano H, et al. Cardiovascular complications associated with spinal cord injury. J Acute Dis. 2018;7:139. https://doi.org/10.4103/2221-6189.241006.
8. Furlan JC, Fehlings MG. Cardiovascular complications after acute spinal cord injury: pathophysiology, diagnosis, and management. Neurosurg Focus. 2008;25:E13. https://doi.org/10.3171/foc.2008.25.11.e13.
9. Partida E, Mironets E, Hou S, Tom VJ. Cardiovascular dysfunction following spinal cord injury. Neural Regen Res. 2016;11:189–94. https://doi.org/10.4103/1673-5374.177707.
10. Ball PA. Critical Care of Spinal Cord Injury. Spine. 2001;26:S27–30. https://doi.org/10.1097/00007632-200112151-00006.
11. Grigorean VT, Sandu AM, Popescu M, et al. Cardiac dysfunctions following spinal cord injury. J Med Life. 2009;2:133–45.
12. Iovine JA, Villanueva RD, Werth CM, et al. Contemporary hemodynamic management of acute spinal cord injuries with intravenous and enteral vasoactive agents: a narrative review. Am J Heal-Syst Pharm. 2022;79:1521–30. https://doi.org/10.1093/ajhp/zxac164.
13. Wang TY, Park C, Zhang H, et al. Management of acute traumatic spinal cord injury: a review of the literature. Front Surg. 2021;8:698736. https://doi.org/10.3389/fsurg.2021.698736.
14. Kwon BK, Tetreault LA, Martin AR, et al. A clinical practice guideline for the management of patients with acute spinal cord injury: recommendations on hemodynamic management. Glob Spine J. 2024;14:187S–211S. https://doi.org/10.1177/21925682231202348.
15. Ryken TC, Hurlbert RJ, Hadley MN, et al. Chapter 7: the acute cardiopulmonary management of patients with cervical spinal cord injuries. Neurosurgery. 2013;72:84–92. https://doi.org/10.1227/neu.0b013e318276ee16.
16. Wecht J, Harel N, Guest J, et al. Cardiovascular autonomic dysfunction in spinal cord injury: epidemiology, diagnosis, and management. Semin Neurol. 2020;40:550–9. https://doi.org/10.1055/s-0040-1713885.

17. Williams AM, Manouchehri N, Erskine E, et al. Cardio-centric hemodynamic management improves spinal cord oxygenation and mitigates hemorrhage in acute spinal cord injury. Nat Commun. 2020;11:5209. https://doi.org/10.1038/s41467-020-18905-8.
18. Hawryluk G, Whetstone W, Saigal R, et al. Mean arterial blood pressure correlates with neurological recovery after human spinal cord injury: analysis of high frequency physiologic data. J Neurotrauma. 2015;32:1958–67. https://doi.org/10.1089/neu.2014.3778.
19. Sangkum L, Liu GL, Yu L, et al. Minimally invasive or noninvasive cardiac output measurement: an update. J Anesthesia. 2016;30:461–80. https://doi.org/10.1007/s00540-016-2154-9.
20. Lee Y-S, Kim K-T, Kwon BK. Hemodynamic management of acute spinal cord injury: a literature review. Neurospine. 2020;18:7–14. https://doi.org/10.14245/ns.2040144.072.
21. Ploumis A, Yadlapalli N, Fehlings MG, et al. A systematic review of the evidence supporting a role for vasopressor support in acute SCI. Spinal Cord. 2010;48:356–62. https://doi.org/10.1038/sc.2009.150.
22. Saadoun S, Papadopoulos MC. Targeted perfusion therapy in spinal cord trauma. Neurotherapeutics. 2020;17:511–21. https://doi.org/10.1007/s13311-019-00820-6.
23. Liu C, Yavar Z, Sun Q. Cardiovascular response to thermoregulatory challenges. Am J Physiol-Hear Circ Physiol. 2015;309:H1793–812. https://doi.org/10.1152/ajpheart.00199.2015.
24. Kong CY, Hosseini AM, Belanger LM, et al. A prospective evaluation of hemodynamic management in acute spinal cord injury patients. Spinal Cord. 2013;51:466–71. https://doi.org/10.1038/sc.2013.32.
25. Salazar LM, Agrawal A, Satyarthee G, et al. Hyponatremia in the acute phase of spinal cord trauma: review. J Acute Dis. 2018;7:103. https://doi.org/10.4103/2221-6189.236823.
26. Hector SM, Biering-Sørensen T, Krassioukov A, Biering-Sørensen F. Cardiac arrhythmias associated with spinal cord injury. J Spinal Cord Med. 2013;36:591–9. https://doi.org/10.1179/2045772313y.0000000114.
27. Furlan JC, Verocai F, Palmares X, Fehlings MG. Electrocardiographic abnormalities in the early stage following traumatic spinal cord injury. Spinal Cord. 2016;54:872–7. https://doi.org/10.1038/sc.2016.11.
28. Part 7.3: Management of Symptomatic Bradycardia and Tachycardia. Circulation 2005; 112:IV-67–IV-77. https://doi.org/10.1161/circulationaha.105.166558.
29. Wetterslev M, Pirracchio R, Jung C. Management of supraventricular arrhythmias in the intensive care unit: a step in the right direction. Intensiv Care Med. 2023;49:1383–5. https://doi.org/10.1007/s00134-023-07236-z.
30. Shang Z, Wanyan P, Zhang B, et al. Incidence and risk factors of deep vein thrombosis in patients with spinal cord injury: a systematic review with meta-analysis. Front Cardiovasc Med. 2023;10:1153432. https://doi.org/10.3389/fcvm.2023.1153432.
31. Alabed S, de Heredia LL, Naidoo A, et al. Incidence of pulmonary embolism after the first 3 months of spinal cord injury. Spinal Cord. 2015;53:835–7. https://doi.org/10.1038/sc.2015.105.
32. Barco S, Valerio L, Gallo A, et al. Global reporting of pulmonary embolism–related deaths in the World Health Organization mortality database: vital registration data from 123 countries. Res Pr Thromb Haemost. 2021;5:e12520. https://doi.org/10.1002/rth2.12520.
33. Yue JK, Winkler EA, Rick JW, et al. Update on critical care for acute spinal cord injury in the setting of polytrauma. Neurosurg Focus. 2017;43:E19. https://doi.org/10.3171/2017.7.focus17396.
34. Hejrati N, Fehlings MG. Commentary on "hemodynamic management of acute spinal cord injury". Neurospine. 2021;18:15–6. https://doi.org/10.14245/ns.2121077.075.

13 Respiratory Complications and the Role of the Respiratory Therapist: Noninvasive and Invasive Ventilation

Giuliana Stagni, Federico Pozzi, Stefano Marelli, and Arturo Chieregato

13.1 Introduction

Respiratory complications represent some of the most significant challenges faced by individuals with spinal cord injury (SCI), particularly those with injuries at the cervical spine level. These injuries often result in profound impairments in respiratory function due to paralysis or weakness of the diaphragm, intercostal muscles, and abdominal muscles, all of which are essential for effective ventilation and airway clearance [1].

In the acute phase following SCI, respiratory failure is a leading cause of mortality. This is primarily attributed to the inability to maintain adequate ventilation, which can rapidly result in hypoxemia and hypercapnia. Additional acute challenges include atelectasis, caused by reduced lung expansion; aspiration pneumonia, stemming from impaired swallowing and cough reflexes; and ventilator-associated pneumonia (VAP), which is a common complication in mechanically ventilated patients.

In the post-acute phase, respiratory complications remain a dominant cause of morbidity and mortality, accounting for approximately 20% of deaths in the SCI population, as reported by the 2023 National Spinal Cord Injury Statistical Center. Long-term risks include chronic respiratory insufficiency, recurrent pneumonia, and complications from reduced airway clearance. Impaired secretion management, coupled with weakened cough strength, predisposes patients to mucus plugging and recurrent lower respiratory tract infections. Over time, these issues can lead to progressive lung damage and chronic respiratory failure.

The role of the respiratory therapist (RT) is critical in mitigating these complications. Early interventions, such as the use of cough assistance techniques and noninvasive ventilation, play a pivotal role, particularly immediately after extubation. Cough assistance devices, such as mechanical insufflation-exsufflation systems,

G. Stagni (✉) · F. Pozzi · S. Marelli · A. Chieregato
Neurointensive Care Unit, ASST Grande Ospedale Metropolitano Niguarda, Milan, Italy

E. Brogi et al. (eds.), *Traumatic Spinal Cord Injury*, Hot Topics in Acute Care Surgery and Trauma, https://doi.org/10.1007/978-3-031-99890-4_13

help compensate for the reduced expiratory force, facilitating effective secretion clearance. Similarly, NIV can provide respiratory support without the need for re-intubation, reducing the risk of complications associated with invasive mechanical ventilation. By implementing these strategies promptly, respiratory therapists can significantly improve respiratory outcomes and reduce both acute and long-term morbidity and mortality in patients with cervical SCI [2].

The respiratory system relies on the coordinated action of several muscle groups, primarily the diaphragm, intercostal muscles, and accessory muscles. Spinal cord injury disrupts this coordination, leading to respiratory dysfunction characterized by reduced lung volumes, impaired cough, and, as a consequence, an increased risk of respiratory infections and atelectasis. Effective management of respiratory complications in SCI patients involves thorough assessment, targeted interventions, and continuous monitoring.

Non-invasive ventilation has become a cornerstone in the management of respiratory failure in SCI, providing support without the need for intubation. It offers numerous benefits, including reduced risk of ventilator-associated pneumonia, preservation of speech and swallowing, and enhanced patient comfort. However, the success of NIV depends on early identification of respiratory compromise and timely intervention.

For injuries at or below C4, the decision to keep the patient intubated or to perform a tracheotomy is related to the extent of the injury and, in some cases, to the patient's age, which can result in greater management difficulties due to pre-existing conditions and reduced chances of returning home. The choice of ventilatory mode and settings is tailored to the individual's needs, considering factors such as lung mechanics, the risk of ventilator-induced lung injury (VILI), and the presence of concomitant medical conditions [3].

The RT plays a pivotal role in both noninvasive and invasive ventilation. This includes conducting ventilatory assessments, managing mechanical ventilation, providing respiratory muscle training, and implementing secretion management techniques. The expertise of the RT is essential in optimizing respiratory care, enhancing patient outcomes, and improving quality of life for individuals with SCI.

13.2 Ventilatory Assessment

13.2.1 Monitoring Diaphragmatic Function: Ultrasound

Assessing diaphragmatic function is a useful evaluation in patients with SCI to determine the need for ventilatory support and to guide therapeutic interventions. This assessment can be performed daily using various techniques, including fluoroscopy, ultrasonography, and transdiaphragmatic pressure measurements. A particularly useful tool could be diaphragmatic ultrasound, which is a noninvasive and reliable method for evaluating diaphragmatic movement and thickness, providing real-time information about muscle function and fatigue [4].

By placing an ultrasound probe on the patient's abdomen or lower chest, clinicians can visualize the diaphragm in real-time, measuring its thickness and evaluating its excursion during respiration. This method is particularly valuable in diagnosing diaphragmatic dysfunction, monitoring respiratory muscle strength, and assessing patients with conditions such as chronic obstructive pulmonary disease (COPD), neuromuscular disorders, or post-surgical complications. It can also provide information for determining the need for interventions like respiratory support or rehabilitation.

Particularly in patients with SCI is useful to evaluate the ability of the diaphragmatic muscle to support respiratory movement. Ultrasound assessment of the diaphragm can comprehend:

1. Diaphragmatic thickness (Tdi): it requires measurement of diaphragm thickness at end-expiration (Tdi,ee). It is useful to assess the development of atrophy over time, but it is not a measure of effort per se.
2. Diaphragmatic thickening fraction (TFdi): it requires absolute measurement of diaphragm thickness (Tdi), diaphragm thickness at end-expiration (Tdi,ee), and diaphragm thickness at end-inspiration (Tdi,ei). It is better to perform this measurement when the patient has low or no pressure support, to assess the diaphragm's true contractile capacity.
3. Diaphragmatic excursion: It assesses diaphragm movements during tidal breathing. In contrast to the TFdi, assessment of diaphragm movement should only be conducted in patients disconnected from the ventilator, as ventilator assistance will result in caudal movement of the diaphragm.

Reference values are still a matter of debate; most validated normal ranges are listed below (Table 13.1) and refer to assessment of patients in semi-recumbent position.

Ultrasound offers several advantages, including its non-invasive nature, low cost, quick learning curve, and straightforward calculations, making it suitable for bedside assessment of breathing effort. However, there are certain technical and methodological limitations to using ultrasound for this purpose. Due to the diaphragm's thin structure, even minor measurement errors can lead to significant overestimation or underestimation of its thickness and thickening fraction (this is the reason why the reference ranges are broad). Moreover, visualizing the left hemidiaphragm is more challenging compared to the right side due to the different ultrasound window determined by the liver and the spleen. Additionally, TFdi does not account for the duration and frequency of contractions, nor does it consider the involvement of accessory and expiratory muscles. In fact, when the load on the diaphragm increases relative to its capacity, the accessory inspiratory muscles (such as the parasternal, external intercostal, scalene, and sternocleidomastoid muscles) are recruited. With further loading, the expiratory muscles (like the transversus abdominis and the internal and external oblique muscles) are activated to assist. For this reason, recent literature suggests new ultrasound techniques to assess the accessory muscles and their recruitment, although these methods are still under investigation.

Table 13.1 Main information about the execusion of diaphragmatic ultrasound measurements, together with actual reference values

Technique	Utility	Probe placement	Measurement	Reference values
Tdi	Assess the development of atrophy over time	Linear array; mid-axillary line (zone of apposition)	Tdi,ee	1.5–2.4 mm at end-expiration
TFdi	Measure of contractile activity	Linear array; mid-axillary line (zone of apposition)	TFdi = (Tdi,ei – Tdi,ee)/ Tdi,ee*100%	24–53% during quiet breathing, up to 157% during vigorous effort
Diaphragmatic excursion	See the diaphragm displacement during tidal breathing	Phased or curved array, below the subcostal arch at the midclavicular line	Using M-mode to measure excursion	1.6–1.8 cm during quiet breathing, up to 7.5 cm during deep breathing

. Despite these drawbacks, ultrasound remains a promising technique in clinical care, particularly for bedside evaluations. The ultrasound evaluation of the diaphragm should not be the sole tool for assessing the need and duration of NIV trials; it must be correlated with the person's ability to perform rehabilitation and daily activities without relying on accessory muscles.

13.2.2 Spirometry

Spirometry is a fundamental tool in the ventilatory assessment of SCI patients. For each patient, preliminary normal values have to be predicted based on age, sex, height, and ethnicity (REF). Spirometry measures key pulmonary function parameters such as forced vital capacity (FVC), forced expiratory volume in one second (FEV1), peak expiratory flow rate (PEFR), and peak expiratory flow during cough (PCEF). These parameters help quantify the degree of restrictive lung disease and monitor changes over time, detecting early signs of respiratory compromise and assessing the effectiveness of therapeutic interventions. Signs of respiratory compromise could be:

- Reduced FVC: suggests weakened respiratory muscles and reduced lung compliance, indicating restrictive lung disease.
- Decrease FEV1: can indicate muscle weakness, leading to inadequate airway clearance and increased risk of respiratory infections and atelectasis.

- Decreased FEV1/FVC ratio: in the context of SCI, if FEV1 and FVC are both reduced the ratio is normal or high, but monitoring this ratio helps identify any superimposed obstructive processes.
- Reduced PEFR/PCEF: indicates weakened expiratory muscles and compromised airway clearance, increasing the risk of mucus plugging and respiratory infections.
- Lower inspiratory capacity (IC): suggests impaired diaphragmatic function and reduced lung volumes, contributing to restrictive lung patterns.
- Reduced maximal voluntary ventilation (MVV) in SCI patients indicates significant respiratory muscle weakness and potential for ventilatory failure.

Cut-offs (Table 13.2):

- FVC: less than 80% of the predicted value is generally considered indicative of restrictive lung disease.
- FEV1: less than 80% of the predicted value is considered abnormal.
- FEV1/FVC: a ratio below 0.70 suggests obstructive lung disease.
- PEFR: values less than 80% of the predicted value indicate compromised airway clearance.

  PCEF: values above 160 L/min are requtired for effective cough and less than 270 L/min is associated with increased secretion retention and risk of infection.
- IC: less than 80% of the predicted value suggests restrictive lung disease.
- MVV: less than 70% of the predicted value indicates significant respiratory muscle weakness.

Table 13.2 Summary of the main spirometry parameters and the cut-offs associated with different degrees of impairment

Parameter	Normal value	Mild impairment	Severe impairment
FVC	≥ 80% of predicted[a]	< 80% of predicted	< 50% of predicted
FEV1	≥ 80% of predicted	< 80% of predicted	< 50% of predicted
FEV1/FVC ratio	> 0.70 (or 70%)	< 0.70 suggests obstruction	Not applicable for restriction
PEFR	≥ 80% of predicted	< 80% of predicted	< 50% of predicted
PCEF	≥ 270 L/min	≥ 160 L/min but <270 L/min	< 160 L/min
IC	≥ 80% of predicted	< 80% of predicted	< 50% of predicted
MVV	≥ 70% of predicted	< 70% of predicted	< 50% of predicted

[a]Normal values are usually predicted based on age, sex, height, and ethnicity

13.2.3 Maximal Inspiratory Pressure (MIP) and Sniff Nasal Inspiratory Pressure

Maximal inspiratory pressure (MIP) is a measure of the strength of the inspiratory muscles, primarily the diaphragm. It is assessed by having the patient inhale forcefully against an occluded airway. Sniff nasal inspiratory pressure (SNIP) is an alternative measure that evaluates inspiratory muscle strength during a maximal sniff through the nose. Both MIP and SNIP are valuable in assessing respiratory muscle function and predicting the need for ventilatory support. These measures must also be correlated with a comprehensive evaluation, as MIP (measured non-invasively) could be affected by compensatory muscle activity above the level of the injury.

13.2.3.1 Cut-offs

- MIP: less than 60 cmH2O for males and less than 40 cmH2O for females are indicative of significant respiratory muscle weakness and may suggest the need for further evaluation and potential ventilatory support.
- SNIP: less than 40 cmH2O is often used as a threshold to identify significant inspiratory muscle weakness.

13.2.4 Ability to Cough

The ability to cough effectively is important for clearing secretions and preventing respiratory infections in SCI patients. Cough strength can be assessed by measuring peak cough flow (PCF) using a peak flow meter. A PCF below 270 L/min indicates an impaired cough, necessitating interventions with mechanical and manual cough assistance. Assessing cough ability is essential for developing appropriate secretion management strategies.

13.2.5 The Role of the Respiratory Therapist in SCI Patients

The fundamental role of the RT is to integrate seamlessly with the care team. From the team, the RT gathers critical information about the extent and completeness of the spinal cord injury, as well as any associated organ dysfunctions and scheduled interventions or procedures in the coming days. Based on this comprehensive data and their understanding of the typical trajectory of recovery in spinal cord injury patients—which involves both neuronal and muscular reorganization—the RT assumes responsibility for implementing a ventilatory strategy that initially replaces and subsequently supports the patient's recovering respiratory functions [5, 6].

The ability to map out this recovery trajectory without suppressing the patient's intrinsic capacity for recovery, while simultaneously preventing complications associated with premature withdrawal from mechanical ventilation, is a delicate and essential process. This iterative approach, balancing support and autonomy, allows the RT to play a pivotal role in guiding the patient through this critical phase of respiratory rehabilitation.

13.2.6 Ventilator Management and Coughing Assistance

The RT, in collaboration with the intensivist, plays a crucial role in managing mechanical ventilation for SCI patients, as with other ICU patients, ensuring that ventilator settings are tailored to meet the patient's needs while minimizing the risk of lung injury. This includes fine-tuning tidal volumes, respiratory rates, and oxygen levels based on continuous monitoring of blood gases and respiratory mechanics. The approach to mechanical ventilation in SCI patients is distinct, as the goal is not merely to remove mechanical support but to transition to 24-hour NIV, recognizing the need to prevent respiratory fatigue and muscle exhaustion, even when initial endurance appears sufficient.

In addition to ventilator management, the unique challenges of SCI include impaired synchrony and effort of the respiratory muscles, which significantly diminish the effectiveness of the cough reflex. As NIV temporarily substitutes for weakened ventilatory muscle function, the RT assumes a pivotal role in cough assistance. Techniques such as manually assisted cough and mechanical insufflation-exsufflation are employed to enhance secretion clearance and maintain airway patency, addressing a critical aspect of care that differs from other forms of acute respiratory failure [7].

13.2.7 Cough Assist Device: Mechanical Insufflator-Exsufflator

The mechanical insufflator–exsufflator, also known as a cough assist device, is a critical tool for managing respiratory secretions in SCI patients. It simulates a natural cough by delivering pre-cough volume by means of an insufflation in simultaneous combination with external manual compression, which mimics the function of ineffective abdominal muscles and prevents early closure of distal airways, should be considered. The settings of the cough assist device must be personalized based on needs (e.g., more recruitment function versus expectoration function or vice versa). However, it should be noted that inspiratory and expiratory pressures below +/− 40 cmH2O are not sufficient to achieve adequate pre-cough volumes and resulting cough peaks. The RT is responsible for training patients and caregivers in the use of this device and integrating it into the overall respiratory care plan.

13.2.8 Effects of Elastic Abdominal Binders

Elastic abdominal binders are commonly used in SCI patients to support the abdominal contents and improve diaphragmatic function. By increasing intra-abdominal pressure, these binders enhance the efficiency of the diaphragm, leading to improved ventilation and reduced respiratory fatigue. The RT evaluates the appropriate use of abdominal binders and monitors their effects on respiratory mechanics and overall function.

13.3 Ventilation Strategy in SCI (TSCI): Non-invasive Ventilation

Non-invasive ventilation is relevant in the management of respiratory failure in most SCI patients. Non-invasive ventilation involves the delivery of positive pressure ventilation through a mask or nasal interface, avoiding the need for invasive procedures like intubation. This approach offers several benefits, including reduced risk of ventilator-associated pneumonia, preservation of upper airway function, and greater patient comfort. In more severe patients or in those with multiple injuries, NIV can be applied after lifesaving mechanical ventilation. In other less compromised patients, NIV could also be considered in the early stages of respiratory compromise or during periods of increased respiratory demand, such as during infections or following surgical procedures [8].

For the success of NIV, even apparently minor details have to be considered. The RT is fundamental in initiating NIV, selecting appropriate interfaces, and titrating ventilator settings to achieve optimal support. Continuous monitoring of blood gases, respiratory rate, and patient comfort is essential to ensure the effectiveness of NIV. Moreover, NIV settings cannot disregard the assessment and identification of any pre-existing issues, which are increasingly common with the rise of SCI in adulthood/senescence, such as COPD or OSAS [9].

Proper ventilation settings provide the patient with the necessary resources to start the rehabilitation process and transition back to their home and pre-injury life. In many cases, NIV will continue to be used at home, and in higher-level injuries, it may be utilized at work or school (e.g., mouthpiece, nasal mask). For this reason, selecting one or more interfaces to alternate during therapy can help minimize the risk of pressure sores, reducing the likelihood of NIV failure and the need for reintubation.

Successful implementation of NIV requires thorough patient education and training. The RT teaches patients and caregivers how to properly use and maintain NIV equipment, recognize signs of NIV failure, and troubleshoot common issues. Patient adherence and comfort are key factors in the long-term success of NIV, together with regular follow-ups that can identify early potential respiratory issues, such as the development of an obstructive sleep disorder absent during the acute phase and related to anatomical changes induced by the injury (e.g., overdevelopment of supra-lesional neck muscles) [10].

13.4 Timing of Tracheal Intubation

Determining the appropriate timing for tracheal intubation in SCI patients is important for optimizing outcomes. Early intubation may be necessary in cases of severe respiratory compromise, while avoided intubation can be beneficial in less severe cases. The decision to intubate is based on a combination of clinical assessment and ventilatory parameters.

In the specific setting of NIV failure, the key ventilatory parameters that predict the need for intubation include worsening hypoxemia ($PaO2/FiO2$ ratio < 200), hypercapnia ($PaCO2 > 50$ mmHg), and signs of respiratory muscle fatigue (increased respiratory rate, use of accessory muscles). Additionally, a decline in mental status or inability to protect the airway necessitates prompt intubation [11].

The RT plays a role in monitoring these parameters and providing timely feedback to the medical team. Early recognition of NIV failure allows for timely intubation, preventing further deterioration and potential complications such as respiratory arrest or aspiration.

13.5 Ventilation Strategy in SCI (TSCI): Invasive Ventilation

When non-invasive ventilation is insufficient, invasive ventilation becomes necessary to support respiratory function in SCI patients. Invasive ventilation typically involves endotracheal intubation or tracheostomy; the latter should be performed in selected cases where it is proven that extubation combined with immediate NIV use is not feasible.

The primary objectives of invasive ventilation in patients with SCI are to ensure adequate oxygenation and carbon dioxide elimination, prevent ventilator-induced lung injury, and reduce respiratory fatigue. Unlike other forms of ventilatory failure, extubation in SCI does not signify complete weaning from mechanical ventilation but rather a transition from invasive to non-invasive interfaces. In the early phases of SCI, diffusion-limited oxygenation is rarely an issue. Instead, positive pressure ventilation compensates for the inadequate negative pressure generated by weakened respiratory muscles, ensuring effective gas exchange. Unlike comatose patients, individuals with SCI retain upper airway defense reflexes, meaning intubation is not inherently necessary for airway protection. However, the combination of inspiratory muscle weakness and reduced expiratory effort, such as during coughing, complicates the transition from invasive ventilation [12].

In cases of incomplete injuries at lower levels, respiratory mechanics are generally preserved but remain fragile, requiring careful management. The weaning process in SCI cannot follow a "trial-and-error" strategy, as these patients are rarely capable of being fully and immediately weaned from ventilation. During the acute phase, continuous NIV is typically required, and as recovery progresses, ventilation may only be needed during the night, particularly in cervical-level injuries or in cases with sleep-disordered breathing.

The RT plays a pivotal role in the management of invasive ventilation, from the initial setup to continuous monitoring and adjustment. Selecting the appropriate ventilatory mode and settings is essential for ensuring optimal outcomes. In the acute phase, patients with SCI demonstrate unique predictors of ventilatory failure that differ from other conditions, such as ARDS or COPD exacerbations. While intubated but no longer sedated, ventilator settings should prioritize the elimination of respiratory fatigue and lung recruitment rather than a stepwise reduction of pressure support and PEEP to achieve full extubation. The goal is to transition smoothly to non-invasive ventilation while maintaining a comparable ventilatory regimen, avoiding complications related to sedation and the obstruction caused by the tube cuff.

Fraction of inspired oxygen (FiO_2) should be titrated to the lowest level necessary to ensure adequate gas exchange, with prompt action taken to address lung recruitment or airway clearance when needed. Continuous monitoring of blood gases, lung volumes, and respiratory pressures guides adjustments to maintain ventilation that is both effective and safe. Preventing complications such as ventilator-induced lung injury, barotrauma, and ventilator-associated pneumonia is a priority. Additionally, early mobilization and lung-protective ventilation strategies are integral to care [13].

Weaning from invasive ventilation in SCI is a gradual and complex process that demands careful planning and collaboration among the RT, intensivists, and nursing staff. Readiness for weaning is assessed through spontaneous breathing trials and other evaluations, aiming for a smooth transition to non-invasive ventilation. The process balances maintaining effective respiratory support with allowing the patient's respiratory muscles to recover, ensuring both safety and a successful outcome [14].

13.6 Conclusions

Respiratory complications are a major concern for patients with spinal cord injury, significantly impacting morbidity and mortality. The role of the RT is pivotal in managing these complications through both noninvasive and invasive ventilation strategies. Effective respiratory care involves comprehensive assessment, targeted interventions, and continuous monitoring to optimize respiratory function and improve patient outcomes [15].

Noninvasive ventilation offers numerous benefits, including reduced infection risk and improved patient comfort, but requires timely initiation and diligent monitoring [16].

The RT's expertise extends beyond ventilation management: mechanical/manual cough assistance, lung recruitment maneuvers, choice of the best NIV interface, and the identification of sentinel events such as predictive indicators of exacerbation and muscle fatigue (e.g., increased secretions, loss of volume, use of accessory muscles during ventilation or respiratory support).

Ultimately, the goal of respiratory therapy in SCI patients is to support respiratory function, promote independence, and enhance quality of life. The RT's comprehensive approach, combining clinical expertise with patient-centered care, is essential for achieving these outcomes. As advancements in respiratory care continue, the role of the RT will remain integral to the multidisciplinary management of SCI patients, ensuring they receive the best possible care throughout their recovery journey.

References

1. Brown R, DiMarco AF, Hoit JD, Garshick E. Respiratory dysfunction and management in spinal cord injury. Respir Care. 2006;51(8):853–68.
2. Bach JR, Burke L, Chiou M. Noninvasive respiratory management of spinal cord injury. Phys Med Rehabil Clin N Am. 2020;31(3):397–413. https://doi.org/10.1016/j.pmr.2020.03.006.
3. Kumar A, Khandelwal A, Jamil S. Ventilatory strategies in traumatic cervical spinal cord injury: controversies and current updates. Asian Spine J. 2023;17(4):615–9. https://doi.org/10.31616/asj.2023.0094. Epub 2023 Aug 21. PMID: 37614075; PMCID: PMC10460671
4. Laveneziana P, Albuquerque A, Aliverti A, Babb T, Barreiro E, Dres M, Dubé BP, Fauroux B, Gea J, Guenette JA, Hudson AL, Kabitz HJ, Laghi F, Langer D, Luo YM, Neder JA, O'Donnell D, Polkey MI, Rabinovich RA, Rossi A, Series F, Similowski T, Spengler CM, Vogiatzis I, Verges S. ERS statement on respiratory muscle testing at rest and during exercise. Eur Respir J. 2019;53(6):1801214. https://doi.org/10.1183/13993003.01214-2018. PMID: 30956204
5. Toki A, Nakamura T, Nishimura Y, Sumida M, Tajima F. Clinical introduction and benefits of non-invasive ventilation for above C3 cervical spinal cord injury. J Spinal Cord Med. 2021;44(1):70–6. https://doi.org/10.1080/10790268.2019.1644474. Epub 2019 Aug 12. PMID: 31403375; PMCID: PMC7919887
6. Krause JS, Cao Y, DeVivo MJ, DiPiro ND. Risk and protective factors for cause-specific mortality after spinal cord injury. Arch Phys Med Rehabil. 2016;97(10):1669–78. https://doi.org/10.1016/j.apmr.2016.07.001. Epub 2016 Jul 20. PMID: 27449321
7. Berlowitz DJ, Tamplin J. Respiratory muscle training for cervical spinal cord injury. Cochrane Database Syst Rev. 2013;2013(7):CD008507. https://doi.org/10.1002/14651858.CD008507.pub2. PMID: 23881660; PMCID: PMC11089516
8. Berlowitz DJ, Wadsworth B, Ross J. Respiratory problems and management in people with spinal cord injury. Breathe (Sheff). 2016;12(4):328–40. https://doi.org/10.1183/20734735.012616. PMID: 28270863; PMCID: PMC5335574
9. Bach JR, Saporito LR. Criteria for extubation and tracheostomy tube removal for patients with ventilatory failure. A different approach to weaning. Chest. 1996;110(6):1566–71. https://doi.org/10.1378/chest.110.6.1566. PMID: 8989078
10. McMichan JC, Michel L, Westbrook PR. Pulmonary dysfunction following traumatic quadriplegia. Recognition, prevention, and treatment. JAMA. 1980;243(6):528–31. PMID: 7351783
11. de Vries H, Jonkman A, Shi ZH, Spoelstra-de Man A, Heunks L. Assessing breathing effort in mechanical ventilation: physiology and clinical implications. Ann Transl Med. 2018;6(19):387. https://doi.org/10.21037/atm.2018.05.53. PMID: 30460261; PMCID: PMC6212364
12. Chatwin M, Simonds AK. The addition of mechanical insufflation/exsufflation shortens airway-clearance sessions in neuromuscular patients with chest infection. Respir Care. 2009;54(11):1473–9. PMID: 19863831

13. Tzeng AC, Bach JR. Prevention of pulmonary morbidity for patients with neuromuscular disease. Chest. 2000;118(5):1390–6. https://doi.org/10.1378/chest.118.5.1390. PMID: 11083691
14. Chatwin M, Toussaint M, Gonçalves MR, Sheers N, Mellies U, Gonzales-Bermejo J, Sancho J, Fauroux B, Andersen T, Hov B, Nygren-Bonnier M, Lacombe M, Pernet K, Kampelmacher M, Devaux C, Kinnett K, Sheehan D, Rao F, Villanova M, Berlowitz D, Morrow BM. Airway clearance techniques in neuromuscular disorders: a state of the art review. Respir Med. 2018;136:98–110. https://doi.org/10.1016/j.rmed.2018.01.012. Epub 2018 Feb 6. PMID: 29501255
15. Berlly M, Shem K. Respiratory management during the first five days after spinal cord injury. J Spinal Cord Med. 2007;30(4):309–18. https://doi.org/10.1080/10790268.2007.11753946. PMID: 17853652; PMCID: PMC2031940
16. Zimmer MB, Nantwi K, Goshgarian HG. Effect of spinal cord injury on the respiratory system: basic research and current clinical treatment options. J Spinal Cord Med. 2007;30(4):319–30. https://doi.org/10.1080/10790268.2007.11753947. PMID: 17853653; PMCID: PMC2031930

Mechanical Ventilation Management, Indications and Timing of Tracheotomy and the Role of Diaphragmatic Pacing Stimulation in Spinal Cord Injury

14

Federico Pozzi, Giuliana Stagni, Stefano Marelli, and Arturo Chieregato

14.1 Introduction

Transitioning from mechanical ventilation is often an unavoidable step in the management of patients with TSCI, who are usually intubated at admission to intensive care unit (ICU). This necessity arises not only due to acute respiratory distress but also in response to other clinical challenges such as agitation, the requirement for surgical intervention, or the need for advanced diagnostic procedures at admission.

The management of mechanical ventilation in TSCI patients is inherently complex, as it requires a nuanced understanding of the pathophysiological alterations caused by the injury. Depending on the level and severity of the trauma, different physiological impairments occur, such as reduced or absent diaphragmatic function, compromised chest wall mechanics, and impaired cough and secretion clearance. Each of these factors necessitates an individualized approach to ventilation and subsequent care planning [1–3].

An essential consideration in this context is recognizing that TSCI patients often follow diverse clinical trajectories. While some may achieve early weaning and transition to NIV, others may require prolonged invasive mechanical ventilation (IMV) and, potentially, tracheostomy [4–6]. The chosen ventilatory approach and its adjustments over time depend on the patient's evolving physiological status, the presence of comorbidities, and their response to initial interventions. The trajectory of care must therefore be meticulously tailored to optimize outcomes and address both immediate and long-term respiratory needs.

F. Pozzi (✉) · G. Stagni · S. Marelli · A. Chieregato
Neurointensive Care Unit, ASST Grande Ospedale Metropolitano Niguarda, Milan, Italy
e-mail: federico.pozzi@ospedaleniguarda.it

E. Brogi et al. (eds.), *Traumatic Spinal Cord Injury*, Hot Topics in Acute Care Surgery and Trauma, https://doi.org/10.1007/978-3-031-99890-4_14

Early-phase management should include a thorough assessment of the patient's ventilatory needs, with consideration of key factors such as the extent of neurological impairment, respiratory muscle strength, and the presence of complications like atelectasis or pneumonia [2]. This underscores the importance of a multidisciplinary approach that incorporates critical care physicians and nurses, respiratory therapists, and rehabilitation specialists to establish a trajectory that promotes stabilization, reduces complications, and aligns with the patient's potential for recovery.

By understanding the variability in these clinical pathways and the specific needs of each patient, clinicians can better anticipate the challenges of mechanical ventilation and proactively adapt strategies. These efforts not only improve respiratory outcomes but also lay the groundwork for potential tracheostomy decannulation, NIV trials, and, in some cases, the implementation of advanced techniques like Diaphragmatic Pacing Stimulation (DPS).

This chapter will begin by examining the initial ventilatory management of TSCI patients, highlighting the importance of delineating a potential care trajectory (Fig. 14.1). It will then explore the broader processes of weaning from mechanical ventilation, tracheostomy timing, and long-term respiratory care strategies, providing a comprehensive framework for optimizing outcomes in this vulnerable population.

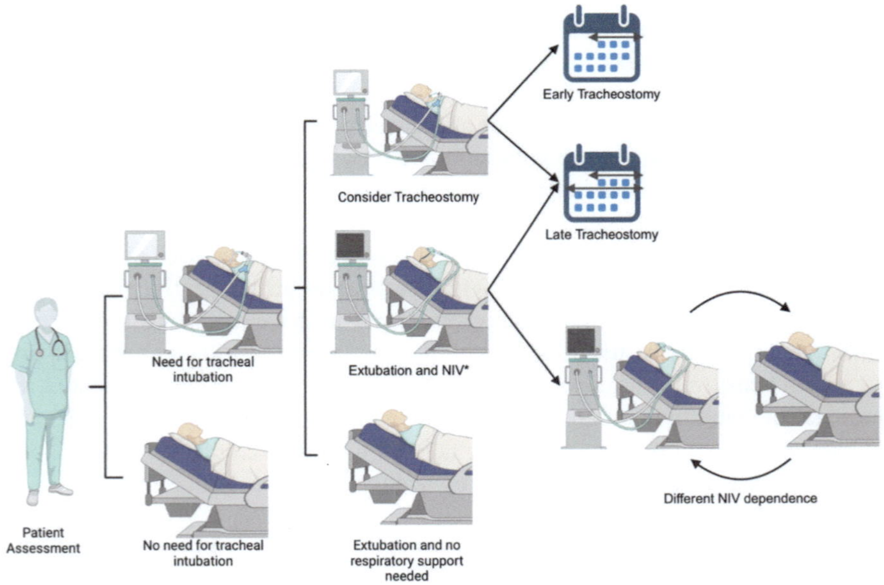

Fig. 14.1 Illustrating potential care trajectories for ventilatory support in patients with TSCI from admission throughout the entire hospitalization, ranging from intubation and tracheostomy to the need for non-invasive ventilation (NIV*). (Created in BioRender. Marelli, S. (2025) BioRender.com/w91u714)

14.2 Respiratory Dysfunction After Traumatic Spinal Cord Injury (TSCI)

14.2.1 Respiratory Pathophysiology

Traumatic Spinal cord injury results in significant alterations in respiratory physiology, primarily due to the interruption of neural pathways that control respiratory muscles. The severity and nature of respiratory dysfunction are closely related to the level and completeness of the TSCI. High cervical injuries (C1-C4) often result in near-complete paralysis of the respiratory muscles, including the diaphragm, necessitating mechanical ventilation. Injuries at the lower cervical level (C5-C8) may allow some degrees of diaphragm function but can severely compromise intercostal and accessory muscle activity, leading to restrictive lung disease and ineffective cough.

14.2.2 Changes in Respiratory Mechanics

Respiratory mechanics are profoundly affected by TSCI. The diaphragm, innervated by the phrenic nerve originating from C3-C5, is the primary muscle of inspiration. High cervical injuries usually lead to diaphragmatic paralysis and reliance on accessory muscles. These are at least initially mechanically inadequate to support the ventilatory workload, frequently leading to rapid muscle fatigue, reduction in lung volumes, and deterioration in gas exchange [1]. Additionally, the loss of intercostal muscle function further compromises chest wall stability and lung expansion, contributing to atelectasis and ventilation-perfusion mismatch. However, it is important to consider that the initial respiratory system alterations due to spinal shock tend to partially resolve over time, and the trajectory of ventilator failure is expected to improve.

14.2.3 Relationship Between Injury Level and Respiratory Compromise

The level of injury is a critical determinant of respiratory compromise following TSCI (Fig. 14.2). High cervical injuries typically necessitate immediate and conventional long-term ventilatory support or Diaphragmatic stimulation due to the loss of phrenic nerve function. These patients, observing their evolution, can be reevaluated over the days to consider the indication of NIV. A considerable ratio of lower cervical and thoracic injuries could avoid invasive ventilation, and require longer or shorter trials of NIV and mechanical cough assistance to provide the necessary respiratory reserve. The degree of respiratory impairment is also influenced by the completeness of the injury, with complete injuries leading to more

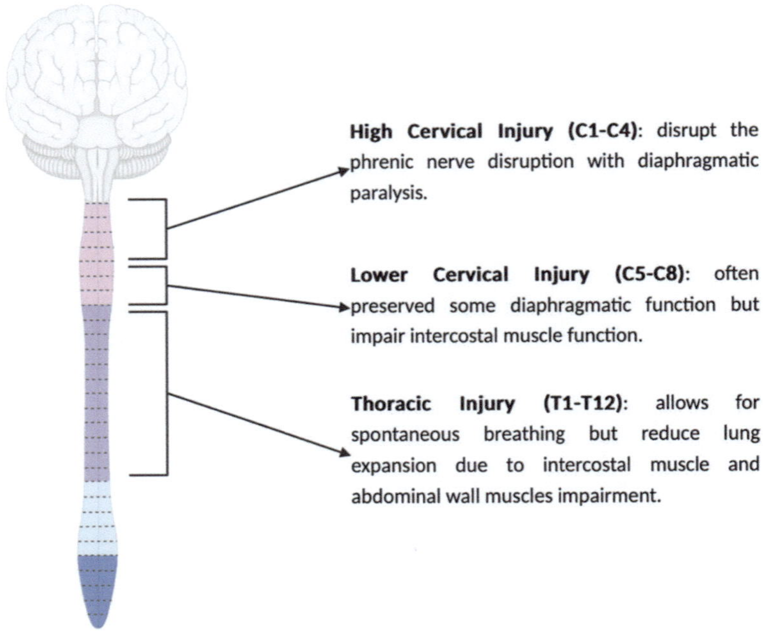

Fig. 14.2 Possible level of injury and associated respiratory compromise, divided by high cervical injury, lower cervical injury, and thoracic injury. (Created in BioRender. Marelli, S. (2024) BioRender.com/l27j988)

pronounced deficits; nevertheless, incomplete injury is associated with early development of hypertonia, and automatisms can cause greater difficulty in respiratory management.

14.3 Weaning from Mechanical Ventilation and Predicting Extubation Failure

Considering the potential pathophysiological challenges associated with alterations in respiratory mechanics, weaning from mechanical ventilation in TSCI patients is a complex process that demands meticulous planning and execution to achieve successful extubation and prevent respiratory failure. The process involves several stages, including clinical stability assessment, optimization of IIMV, patient education, extubation, and the use of NIV and mechanical/manual cough assistance post-extubation.

14.3.1 Evaluation of Injury Level and Respiratory Capacity

The evaluation of the level and completeness of a TSCI is a fundamental aspect in assessing respiratory mechanics and determining the potential for extubation or the necessity for progressing to tracheostomy. This assessment should be conducted through a meticulous clinical examination, complemented by respiratory function tests as outlined in the following chapter. Understanding the extent and nature of the injury allows clinicians to anticipate potential challenges in respiratory management and guide the weaning process from mechanical ventilation. In cases where a patient presents with an injury level that may permit extubation, the possibility of compensating for mechanical deficiencies caused by muscle weakness must be assessed. This can be achieved through techniques such as assisted coughing and NIV [7]. These interventions aim to support the patient's respiratory function and facilitate the removal of secretions, thus preventing complications such as atelectasis and respiratory infections.

However, the decision-making process regarding extubation should not rely solely on respiratory parameters. A holistic assessment of the patient is essential, taking into consideration the overall clinical picture, the patient's general health status, and the compliance of both the patient and their family members. While family support is more immediately relevant at the time of discharge, it can also play a role during extubation, albeit less directly. Additionally, the patient's personality traits, particularly their ability to cope with stress or uncertainty, may influence the extubation outcome. This is especially important for patients who, unlike those with traumatic brain injuries, remain fully conscious and aware throughout the process. A comprehensive evaluation that includes psychological, social, and emotional factors is key in predicting extubation success and identifying those at risk for extubation failure.

14.3.2 Clinical Stability

Before initiating the weaning process, clinically stable must be assessed. This includes adequate oxygenation ($PaO2 > 60$ mmHg on $FiO2 \leq 0.4$), stable hemodynamics without significant vasopressor support, the absence of acute infection or metabolic disturbances, and a recovered gastrointestinal function with a non-tender abdomen. Given the limited respiratory muscle reserve, the team must carefully assess the significance of these conditions and optimize them before initiating the extubation pathway.

14.3.3 Optimization of Invasive MV

Optimizing IMV involves adjusting ventilator settings to ensure patient comfort and readiness for weaning. This involves ensuring adequate humidification and addressing any issues related to airway clearance. Support should be set to eliminate respiratory fatigue to prevent muscle exhaustion, and an appropriate PEEP should be used to counteract the absence of abdominal muscles, which, especially in a seated posture, place the diaphragm in a disadvantageous length/tension situation. For these reasons, it is important to fine-tune IMV settings and ensure the patient receives appropriate ventilatory support.

Optimizing IMV involves adjusting ventilator settings to ensure patient comfort and readiness for weaning. This may include reducing ventilator support gradually, ensuring adequate humidification, and addressing any issues related to airway clearance. Technical parameters such as P0.1 (airway occlusion pressure at 100 ms), Pmusc (muscle pressure), and ultrasound assessment offer valuable insights into a patient's respiratory drive and effort. These parameters are integral to the comprehensive respiratory evaluation of the patient, aiding in the optimization of ventilatory support, ensuring appropriate assistance, and facilitating the weaning process [8].

14.3.4 Patient Education and Compliance

Educating the patient and their family about the weaning process is essential. This includes explaining the steps involved, setting realistic expectations, and addressing any concerns or fears. The RT provides education regarding mechanical and manual cough assistance techniques and all aspects necessary to achieve the maximum possible respiratory autonomy based on the injury and the individual's resources is essential. It is important to obtain full collaboration from both the patient and their family throughout the entire process, whether it involves extubation, decannulation, or adaptation to invasive ventilation.

14.3.5 Postures and Recruitment Maneuvers

Positioning the patient in different postures, such as supine and lateral decubitus positions, facilitates lung recruitment maneuvers and clearance of bronchial obstruction, reducing the risk of new atelectasis and enhancing lung recruitment. Different postures are connected to different lung movements and different respiratory physiology (Fig. 14.3). The RT encourages frequent changes in posture to prevent complications such as pressure ulcers and pneumonia.

Usually, respiratory volumes should increase with sitting upright, but in this case, the gravitational displacement of the abdominal contents plays a detrimental role. Moreover, the paralysis and atony of the abdominal wall muscles make it impossible to maintain the position of the abdominal organs. The downward stretch exerted by the displaced abdominal contents may also expand the total intrathoracic volume, but this action places the diaphragm into a position of disadvantage—in this position, it is already halfway descended. Thus, the diaphragm has little further travel available, and its contraction only expands the intrathoracic volume by a small proportion. (Created in BioRender. Marelli, S. (2024) BioRender.com/j17o820).

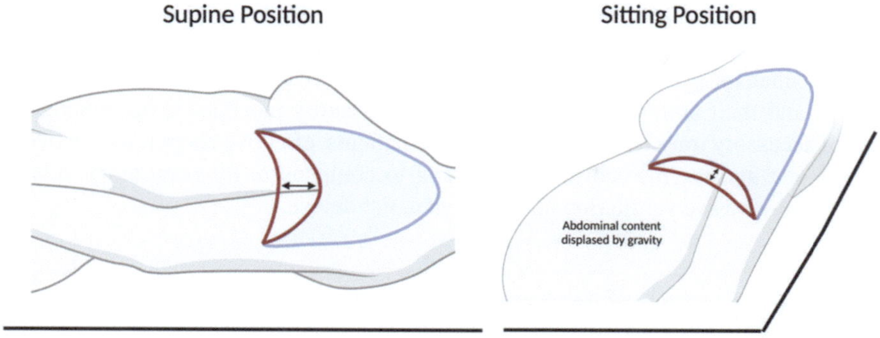

Fig. 14.3 The patients seem to breathe easier when supine, particularly if the diaphragm is alone in the generation of respiratory effort. The reason for this is thought to be greater stretch of the diaphragm, which places it into a position of increased mechanical advantage

14.3.6 Extubation

Successful extubation is based on three main aspects: overall clinical stability, the ability to compensate for the existing spinal cord injury using NIV (e.g., assisted coughing), adequate patient education of the extubation process, and good NIV interface choice to enhance patient cooperation. The team ensures the patient is prepared for extubation by clearing secretions, optimizing ventilator settings, and providing psychological support. Immediate post-extubation care is pivotal and includes monitoring for signs of respiratory distress, early use of NIV, and mechanical and manual cough assistance maneuvers.

14.3.7 Immediate NIV and Mechanical/Manual Cough Assistance

Post-extubation, NIV supports the patient's respiratory function and prevents re-intubation. Mechanical/manual cough assistance techniques, such as the use of a cough assist device or manually assisted cough, are essential for maintaining airway patency and preventing atelectasis. The RT is skilled in these techniques and ensures their appropriate use.

In conclusion, for TSCI patients, we can consider a new paradigm in the extubation pathway, which is based on three key principles:

- Adequate clinical reserve
- Patient education and cooperation
- Ability to compensate for deficits using a cough assist device and NIV

In fact, the extubation process for TSCI patients varies primarily based on the injury level and the respiratory mechanics impairment due to muscle deficit. Unlike the typical extubation protocol for critically ill patients (connected to Spontaneous Breathing Trial), these patients must be extubated under optimal clinical conditions, ensuring they have adequate respiratory and hemodynamic reserves to tolerate the process. In addition, TSCI patients are expected to show improvements in respiratory mechanics for two main reasons: the progressive reduction of perilesional edema and their ability to adapt to the new respiratory mechanics, optimizing the use of accessory muscles. Moreover, in these patients, effective cooperation between the patient and the medical team is crucial to compensate for respiratory deficits using non-invasive ventilation and a cough assist device.

14.4 Evaluation of Performing Tracheostomy and Timing of Tracheostomy

14.4.1 Guidelines About Tracheostomy in TSCI Patients

As highlighted at the beginning of the chapter (Fig. 14.1), tracheostomy is a cornerstone intervention in managing respiratory complications associated with TSCI, particularly in patients with cervical injuries. High-level cervical injuries (C1-C4) often cause complete paralysis of the diaphragm, necessitating long-term IMV. Early tracheostomy (ET), defined as within 7 days of intubation, has shown significant benefits in reducing ventilator-associated complications such as pneumonia (VAP), decreasing ICU and hospital length of stay, and shortening the duration of IMV. Late tracheostomy (LT), on the other hand, may lead to prolonged intubation-related complications like subglottic stenosis and mucosal damage.

Despite evidence supporting early intervention [9–11], standardized guidelines for tracheostomy timing in TSCI are lacking. Current practices often depend on individual assessments based on neurological level of injury (NLI), severity as measured by the ASIA Impairment Scale (AIS), and overall patient prognosis. Clinical protocols integrating these parameters are critical to ensure timely and effective decision-making.

14.4.2 Timing: Early vs. Late Tracheostomy

Meta-analyses comparing ET and LT underscore the clinical benefits of early intervention in these patients [11]. ET has been associated with:

- Reduced ICU and Hospital Stay: By minimizing complications such as VAP and airway trauma, ET shortens recovery times.
- Decreased Complication Rates: Patients undergoing ET have a lower incidence of tracheostomy-related complications, including airway stenosis and granulation tissue formation.
- Enhanced Weaning Success: Early tracheostomy facilitates ventilator weaning by improving airway resistance and reducing sedation requirements.

LT may be considered in patients with improving respiratory function to try avoiding unnecessary surgical interventions. As previously mentioned, TSCI patients often experience progressive improvements in respiratory competence. This unique characteristic allows for an individualized approach to decision-making regarding the patient's potential respiratory trajectory, as illustrated in Fig. 14.1.

Predictive models incorporating factors such as AIS grade, neurological level of injury (NLI) [10, 12], age, and Injury Severity Score (ISS) have been proposed to guide clinical decisions and optimize outcomes. A multidisciplinary evaluation is essential to better assess the patient's prognosis, starting from the pathophysiological characteristics associated with the level of injury.

14.4.3 Indications and Non-indications of Tracheostomy in Different TSCI Categories

High Cervical Injuries (C1-C4) are associated with complete loss of diaphragmatic function, resulting in immediate respiratory failure. In such patients:

- Indications: Long-term IMV requirement, ineffective airway clearance, and persistent hypoxemia despite non-invasive support.
- Contraindications: Patients with severe multi-system injuries or comorbidities where the risks of tracheostomy outweigh potential benefits.
- Physiological challenges: Complete respiratory muscle paralysis and inability to clear secretions effectively increase the risk of complications like aspiration pneumonia.

Low Cervical Lesions (C5-C8) result in partial diaphragmatic function with varying degrees of accessory muscle impairment. In this category:

- Indications: Failure to wean from IMV within a reasonable time frame, recurrent respiratory infections, or severe secretion retention.
- Contraindications: Patients with incomplete lesions (AIS B-D) showing early signs of respiratory recovery and effective weaning potential.
- Physiological challenges: Reduced inspiratory reserve capacity and fatigue of accessory muscles.

Thoracic Lesions rarely impair respiratory function unless accompanied by chest trauma. In such cases:

- Indications: Severe pulmonary contusions, flail chest, or the need for prolonged IMV due to associated injuries.
- Contraindications: Stable patients with isolated thoracic injury and preserved lung mechanics.
- Physiological challenges: Impaired expiratory function leading to secretion retention and a higher risk of atelectasis.

14.4.4 Preventive Perspectives: Non-tracheostomy Approaches

A growing body of evidence supports non-invasive respiratory management strategies to minimize or avoid the need for tracheostomy in TSCI patients [9]. Bach et al. [7] emphasize that many ventilator-dependent SCI patients, even those categorized as "unweanable," can be successfully transitioned to non-invasive ventilatory support and managed without invasive tracheostomy tubes. Different techniques are suggested to achieve this result:

1. Lung volume recruitment (LVR): it is critical for maintaining pulmonary compliance and improving vital capacity. Active air stacking through mouthpiece or nasal interfaces helps SCI patients maintain effective cough flows, prevent atelectasis, and reduce the risk of pneumonia. Passive LVR techniques can support patients who cannot perform air stacking due to glottic dysfunction.
2. Mechanical insufflation-exsufflation (MIE): it is a cornerstone of secretion management in non-invasive care. It effectively clears secretions without the discomfort or complications of suctioning, reducing the risk of respiratory infections and acute respiratory failure (ARF). Regular use of MIE helps maintain normal oxygen saturation levels and facilitates extubation or decannulation for patients transitioning from invasive ventilation.
3. Continuous non-invasive ventilatory support (CNVS): this can completely replace invasive mechanical ventilation in most cases. Daytime support with mouthpiece ventilation and sleep support with nasal NIV provide adequate ventilation while preserving natural airway integrity. Patients using CNVS show improved quality of life and autonomy compared to those reliant on tracheostomy.
4. Glossopharyngeal breathing (GPB): also called "frog breathing," allows patients with intact bulbar innervation to independently breathe without ventilators for short periods. This technique empowers patients to manage emergencies, such as ventilator disconnections, and fosters greater self-reliance.
5. Phrenic nerve and diaphragm pacing: while not strictly non-invasive, phrenic nerve and diaphragm pacing can reduce ventilator dependency in select cases. However, these methods should be considered complementary to non-invasive strategies and not a replacement for them, especially given their limitations in managing secretions and sleep-disordered breathing.

These approaches emphasize the importance of early, individualized assessments to identify patients who could benefit from non-invasive strategies. Adopting protocols such as the oximetry-driven CNVS/MIE regimen significantly reduces respiratory complications, hospitalization rates, and the need for tracheostomy. Non-invasive techniques are associated with longer survival, fewer complications, and improved patient satisfaction compared to traditional invasive methods.

14.4.5 Polytrauma Patients with TSCI: Specific Considerations for Tracheostomy Management

A special mention should be made of polytrauma patients with TSCI, who represent a distinct and particularly challenging subgroup due to their complex medical needs. These individuals often present with additional injuries, such as chest trauma, traumatic brain injury (TBI), or abdominal injuries, which significantly influence the decision to perform tracheostomy. The interplay between TSCI, systemic injuries, and pre-existing comorbidities makes them less likely to follow a "non-indication" pathway and often necessitates aggressive respiratory support strategies.

Key Characteristics of Polytrauma Patients with TSCI:

1. High Risk of Respiratory Complications:
   - Chest Trauma: Rib fractures, flail chest, pulmonary contusions, or hemothorax exacerbate respiratory insufficiency caused by TSCI.
   - Secretion Clearance Issues: These patients may have compromised cough mechanisms due to TSCI, compounded by pulmonary injuries.
   - VAP: Prolonged intubation increases the risk of infections in this subgroup.
2. Systemic Instability:
   - Hemodynamic instability, often seen in polytrauma, complicates the timing and safety of surgical procedures like tracheostomy.
   - Coagulopathies, frequent in polytrauma, elevate the risk of bleeding during and after tracheostomy.
3. Prevalence of Comorbidities:
   - Pre-existing pulmonary diseases: COPD or interstitial lung disease limits respiratory reserve.
   - Cardiac comorbidities: Congestive heart failure or coronary artery disease increases perioperative risks.
   - Neurological complications: TBI may impair consciousness and airway protection, mandating tracheostomy.

In this population, the threshold for considering tracheostomy is lower due to:

- Prolonged ventilatory support: Patients with both TSCI and significant thoracic injuries often fail extubation trials, making early tracheostomy ($\leq$7 days) advantageous to reduce complications like ventilator-associated pneumonia (VAP).
- Critical illness-associated comorbidities: Conditions like sepsis, ARDS (acute respiratory distress syndrome), or multi-organ dysfunction syndrome (MODS) increase the risk of prolonged intubation, necessitating tracheostomy.
- Weaning Cchallenges: Patients with systemic injuries or significant comorbidities (e.g., cardiovascular or renal disease) have a higher incidence of delayed ventilatory weaning due to compromised physiology.

The "non-indication" pathway, such as avoiding tracheostomy through neuromodulation or early weaning protocols, may not be feasible in polytrauma patients with TSCI due to:

- Comorbidities: Cardiac instability, hemodynamic compromise, or chronic conditions like diabetes reduce the likelihood of successful weaning or tolerance of non-invasive alternatives (e.g., phrenic nerve pacing).
- Multi-system Injuries: Associated injuries (e.g., traumatic brain injury, abdominal trauma) often delay recovery and necessitate prolonged IMV, favoring tracheostomy over less invasive approaches.
- Surgical and procedural risks: While neuromodulation (e.g., phrenic or diaphragm pacing) has promise in select patients, its invasiveness and the need for stable physiologic conditions make it less suitable for polytrauma cases.

In conclusion, polytrauma patients with TSCI require a tailored approach to tracheostomy, with an emphasis on early intervention in stable cases. However, systemic instability and comorbidities often necessitate a more cautious pathway, potentially prolonging IMV dependency. Their management highlights the importance of interdisciplinary care, involving trauma surgeons, pulmonologists, and rehabilitation specialists, to optimize outcomes.

Therefore, in all these patients decision-making framework has to include

- Early risk stratification: Use predictive tools based on ASIA Impairment Scale (AIS), ISS, neurological level of injury (NLI), and comorbid conditions to anticipate prolonged IMV needs.
- Early tracheostomy preference: Early tracheostomy is often preferred in this subgroup to reduce ICU stay, complications, and patient discomfort from prolonged intubation.
- Multidisciplinary Involvement: Decision-making should involve trauma surgeons, pulmonologists, intensivists, and rehabilitation specialists to balance risks and benefits.

14.4.6 Exemplification of a Tracheostomy Management and Care Protocol

Tracheostomy management and care protocol is an example of a standardized approach to tracheostomy care, emphasizing early intervention, multidisciplinary collaboration, and comprehensive patient assessment (Fig. 14.4). All the team members play a key role in implementing this protocol, ensuring that tracheostomy care is consistent and tailored to the patient's needs.

1. Prerequisite: ICU with in-depth and high capacity for NIV management, cough assistance manoeuvres, and management of spinal patient complexity. Homogeneous *multidisciplinary team* for training.

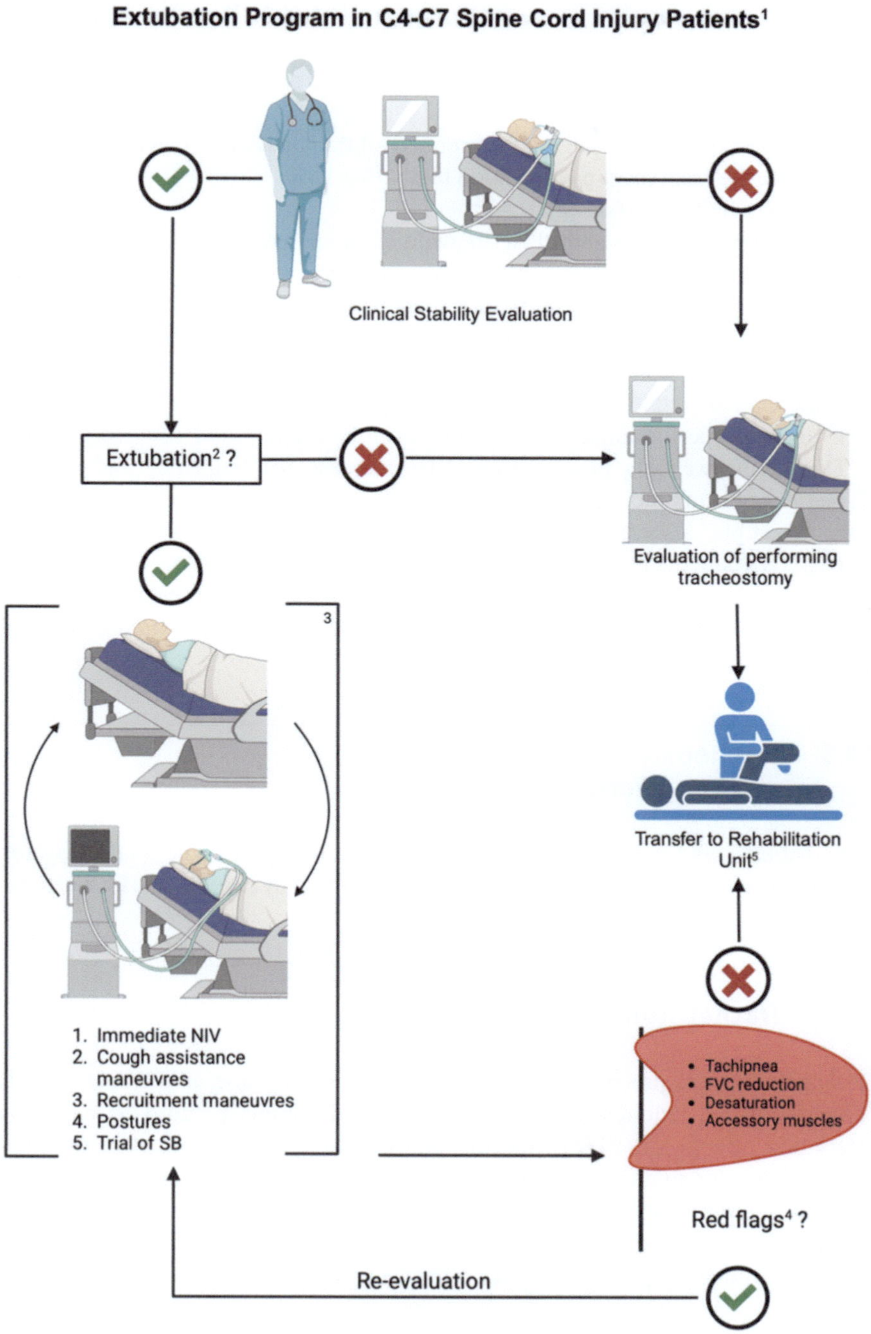

Fig. 14.4 Tracheostomy Management and Care protocol proposal used in the NeuroIntensive Care Unit in Niguarda Hospital (Milan). Here is the extubation pathway step-by-step (Created in BioRender. Marelli, S. (2025) BioRender.com/b20u478)

2. Prior to extubation is important to assess FVC and MIP and to explain post-extubation maneuvers to the patient (NIV, cough machine, postures). The team must agree on timing. It is important to verify the presence of different models of NIV masks.
3. After the extubation process, comprehend all the maneuvers listed. During this process, the team must pay attention to:
   - Lower FiO_2 to ensure $SpO_2 > 95\%$.
   - Set appropriate PS and PEEP to avoid inducing paradoxical thoracoabdominal movement and use appropriate accessories.
   - Perform clearance of secretions if there is obstruction.
   - Spontaneous Breathing (SB) trials with different timing based on the patient and duration correlated to the ventilatory pattern and desaturation.
4. If there are no red flags: perform spirometry as soon as possible and repeat daily to evaluate performance in different positions (supine and semi-recumbent). During the weaning process from NIV, increase SB frequency and increase degrees of trunk inclination until reaching the wheelchair posture.

   Chest physiotherapy maneuvers with cough assist machine pre- and post-SB trial. Evaluate the use of an abdominal binder in the wheelchair.
5. In the early post-ICU phase, a tetraplegic patient may require readmission to the ICU due to respiratory or infectious issues. Evaluate discharge timing based on rehabilitation unit characteristics.

14.5 Tracheostomy Decannulation and Long-Term Ventilation

TSCI patients who have undergone tracheostomy during the acute phase may follow one of two potential pathways in the post-acute and chronic phase: tracheostomy decannulation or long-term ventilation.

14.5.1 Tracheostomy Decannulation

Decannulation, the process of removing a tracheostomy tube, is a critical step in patient care that requires a structured and multidisciplinary approach to ensure safety and effectiveness [13]. Specific protocols may vary between institutions; therefore, is important to consult local guidelines and healthcare professionals before proceeding with a patient's decannulation.

Regardless of the specific protocol employed, it is essential to evaluate key factors to determine the patient's readiness for decannulation, including:

- Clinical stability: the patient should be free from signs of respiratory distress, exhibit stable vital signs, and show no evidence of active infection or sepsis.
- Respiratory Function: adequate oxygenation ($SpO_2 \geq 90\%$) should be maintained on low levels of supplemental oxygen (e.g., $FiO_2 \leq 0.35$ or 4 L/min via

nasal cannula). The patient should also have a $PaCO_2 \leq 60$ mmHg and demonstrate effective spontaneous breathing without mechanical ventilation support for at least 48 h.
- Airway patency: evaluate the upper airway to rule out obstructions such as tracheal stenosis or tracheomalacia. This can be achieved through flexible laryngoscopy or bronchoscopy.
- Cough strength and secretion management: assess the patient's ability to clear secretions effectively.
- Swallowing function: conduct a swallowing assessment to ensure the patient can manage oral secretions and has a low risk of aspiration. This may involve a blue dye test or a Fiberoptic Endoscopic Evaluation of Swallowing (FEES).

There are also some trials which can help evaluate patient's readiness. If the patient meets the above-mentioned criteria, proceed with the following steps:

- Speaking valve trial: Introduce a speaking valve to evaluate the patient's tolerance and upper airway patency. Begin with short periods of use, monitoring for signs of respiratory distress, desaturation, or discomfort. If tolerated, gradually increase the duration.
- Capping trial: Once the speaking valve is well-tolerated for extended periods (e.g., up to 16 h), proceed to cap the tracheostomy tube, requiring the patient to breathe entirely through the upper airway. Monitor closely for signs of respiratory distress, changes in vital signs, or difficulties in managing secretions. If the patient tolerates capping for 24–48 h without issues, they may be considered suitable for decannulation.

Once the patient's suitability for decannulation has been established, the procedure can proceed. In summary, it consists of the following steps:

- Suction the tracheostomy tube and oropharynx to remove secretions.
- Deflate the cuff of the tracheostomy tube, if present.
- Remove any securing ties or devices.
- Instruct the patient to take a deep breath and gently remove the tracheostomy tube during exhalation.
- Cover the stoma with a sterile dressing, applying light pressure to promote closure.
- Instruct the patient to apply gentle pressure over the stoma when speaking or coughing to prevent air leakage.

By following a structured and individualized approach, decannulation can be safely performed, facilitating the patient's recovery and transition to natural breathing.

14.5.2 Transtracheal Open Ventilation (TTOV)

Transtracheal open ventilation is a method of ventilatory support where oxygen is delivered directly into the trachea through tracheostomy. This tube bypasses the upper airway and delivers oxygen directly to the lungs. The "open" aspect refers to the fact that the system is not closed, meaning that exhaled gases can escape either through the upper airway, typically via the mouth or nose, or through the inserted tube.

TTOV is essential for individuals with spinal cord injury requiring mechanical invasive ventilation as life support. It allows excellent phonation and reduces not only the risk of pneumonia related to the accumulation of secretions above the cuff, with slow migration of often infected material into the lungs, but also significantly improves swallowing, reducing the risk of aspiration. Ventilator settings should be adjusted to ensure the best possible phonation without causing hypoventilation, atelectasis, or derecruitment. In some cases, it may even be maintained during the night, provided clinical stability has been achieved, thus preventing damage related to cuff pressure on the tracheal mucosa. It should be considered that TTOV is fundamental for allowing the individual to reintegrate into their social, family, and work/school environment.

14.5.3 Speech Options with Tracheostomy

In addition to tracheal open ventilation, the use of speaking valves or temporary closure of the tracheostomy tube can also be considered. A prerequisite is that the tracheostomy tube has a shape and outer diameter that do not cause an excessive increase in tracheal pressures during expiration and inspiration. A speaking valve, such as the Passy-Muir valve, allows patients to speak by redirecting airflow through the vocal cords during exhalation. It is important to note that the speaking valve excludes the normal humidification provided by airflow through the upper airways, which may lead to thicker secretions, making them more difficult to remove and increasing the risk of atelectasis. Therefore, usage should be limited or accompanied by additional active humidification.

During trials with a plug or speaking valve, respiratory mechanics should be closely monitored, paying particular attention to the use of accessory muscles, vital signs, and post-trial pulmonary recruitment. The placement of a plug or speaking valve should be considered both as a step towards decannulation and to maintain respiratory support for varying lengths of time. The use of fenestrated cannulas is less recommended as they can lead to pressure sores, granulation tissue, or may not sufficiently reduce respiratory effort due to improper alignment of the fenestration within the trachea.

Patients with tracheostomy tubes often face challenges with speech. The RT helps evaluate the patient's suitability for these options and provides training on their use, enhancing the patient's ability to communicate effectively.

14.5.4 Upper Airway Bronchoscopy

Bronchoscopy is an important tool for assessing upper airway patency and identifying potential flow obstructions such as edema or granulation tissue. Bronchoscopy is also a very important tool to assess a patient's readiness for decannulation.

Ensuring airway patency and evaluating the adequacy of the swallow are two important elements for safe decannulation. The RT also assesses the patient's ability to maintain a patent airway and perform effective swallowing, which is essential for preventing aspiration and maintaining nutritional intake.

If a patient presents with swallowing deficits, the possibility of removing the tracheostomy tube should be considered while ensuring adequate nutritional support through the placement of a PEG (percutaneous endoscopic gastrostomy). In this case, it is essential to evaluate the risk of micro aspiration of saliva, particularly during nighttime hours or when in a supine position, before decannulation. This could lead to recurrent pneumonia or atelectasis.

14.5.5 Strength of Cough

Effective cough strength is necessary for clearing secretions and maintaining airway patency. The RT evaluates the patient's cough strength using techniques such as peak cough flow measurements and provides both training and help in cough augmentation techniques if needed. The ineffectiveness of spontaneous coughing does not preclude decannulation or the use of NIV. Assisted cough, whether manual or mechanical, should be effective and could be reliably provided even in non-hospital settings.

14.5.6 Oral Feeding/Tube Feeding

The RT should collaborate with speech and language therapists to evaluate swallowing function and determine the appropriate timing for transitioning from tube feeding to oral feeding.

14.6 The Role of Diaphragmatic Pacing Stimulation in Spinal Cord Injury

In TSCI patients with high cervical injuries (C0-C4) requiring long-term ventilatory support, a diaphragmatic pacing stimulator may serve as a valuable option to reduce dependence on prolonged respiratory assistance [14].

14.6.1 Pre-operative Assessment

The success of DPS (Fig. 14.5) relies on careful patient selection and thorough pre-operative assessment. This includes evaluating the level and completeness of the spinal cord injury, the presence of intact phrenic nerve function, and the overall respiratory muscle strength [15]. A multidisciplinary equipe detailed assessments, including the integrity of the phrenic nerves, exclusion of overlapping progressive diseases, bulbar competence, absence of tracheal stenosis/malacia, and a comprehensive evaluation of the patient and family in terms of adherence to the proposed plan and the practical ability to carry out the rehabilitation program. Each candidate should be evaluated holistically by the entire team, including a psychologist.

14.6.2 Patients Suitability for Stimulation

Patients with high cervical TSCI, particularly those with injuries at C3-C5, are considered suitable candidates for DPS [14]. These patients often retain some degree of diaphragmatic function, which can be enhanced through electrical stimulation. The RT collaborates with the multidisciplinary team to identify eligible patients and develop individualized care plans.

14.6.3 Indication

DPS is indicated for patients with high cervical TSCI (C0-C4) who require long-term ventilatory support but have preserved phrenic nerve function. The goal of

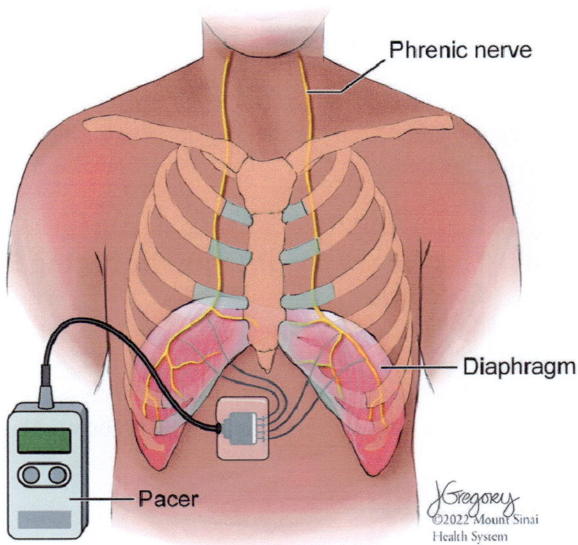

Fig. 14.5 Illustration showing the setup of a bilateral diaphragmatic pacing stimulator, where electrodes are placed in contact with the diaphragm along the course of both phrenic nerves. This system is controlled by an external pacemaker device. Diaphragmatic pacing can be a useful treatment option for central hypoventilation syndrome (CHS). (Used with permission from ©Mount Sinai Health System)

DPS is to reduce or eliminate the need for mechanical ventilation, improve respiratory muscle endurance, and enhance the patient's quality of life [16, 17].

14.6.4 Surgical Technique and Anesthesiologic Consideration

The surgical implantation of DPS involves the placement of electrodes on the diaphragm via minimally invasive techniques. Anesthesiologic considerations include ensuring adequate ventilation during the procedure and minimizing respiratory complications. Providing adequate perioperative respiratory support and closely monitoring the patient throughout the surgical process are key measures to help prevent respiratory and infectious complications.

14.6.5 Post-operative Training to Increase Diaphragmatic Endurance

Following the implantation of DPS, extensive post-operative training is essential to increase diaphragmatic endurance and optimize respiratory function [18–21]. The RT develops and implements a comprehensive training program, including regular stimulation sessions to progressively achieve weaning from mechanical ventilation.

14.7 The Role of Diaphragmatic Pacing Stimulation in Spinal Cord Injury: Living at Home with Spinal Cord Injury

Living at home with a diaphragmatic pacing stimulator offers numerous benefits for patients with cervical TSCI. Diaphragmatic Pacing Stimulator can significantly reduce the dependency on mechanical ventilation, allowing for greater mobility and participation in daily activities. The RT provides ongoing support and education to ensure patients and their families are comfortable with the use of DPS at home, to help them navigate through challenges to maintain optimal respiratory health.

The use of DPS can enhance the quality of life for patients with cervical TSCI by improving respiratory function, reducing the burden of ventilatory support, and promoting independence [4, 6]. Patients often report improved sleep, greater ease in communication, and enhanced overall well-being. In fact, DPS offers the advantage of ambulatory control, allowing patients to manage their respiratory function while engaging in daily activities. For these reasons, the RT has to provide training on the use of portable control units and ensure that patients can safely and effectively operate the DPS system at home and in the community.

14.7.1 Challenges

Despite the benefits, living with DPS also presents challenges, including the need for regular device maintenance, potential complications such as infections or electrode displacement, and the psychological impact of managing a chronic condition.

The Italian experience with 13 implanted patients has highlighted the importance of family support and the determination to maintain independent breathing despite the initial effort and fatigue required during diaphragmatic conditioning. The DPS is not a perfect system, but it can provide better life quality and independence. While it does not eliminate disability or the lack of autonomous breathing, it allows patients to regain a sense of bodily integrity without the constant presence of the ventilator circuit.

14.7.2 Family Support and Care

Family members must be involved in the long-term management of DPS. Family support can significantly impact the patient's adherence to the DPS regimen and overall quality of life. During this process the RT provides training and resources to family members, ensuring they are equipped to assist with device management and respiratory care.

14.7.3 The Necessity to Continue Ventilation/Tracheostomy

While DPS can reduce the need for mechanical ventilation, some patients may still require intermittent ventilatory support or maintain a tracheostomy for airway management. The RT assesses the patient's respiratory needs on an ongoing basis and adjusts the care plan accordingly, ensuring that all interventions are aligned with the patient's goals and preferences.

14.8 Conclusions

This chapter highlights the complexities of managing ventilatory support in patients with TSCI underscoring the need for an individualized, multidisciplinary approach. The variability in injury levels, respiratory mechanics, and patient responses demands anatomical and physiological knowledge to build tailored strategies to optimize outcomes.

Respiratory dysfunction caused by TSCI results from disruptions in neural pathways. Higher cervical injuries often lead to severe diaphragmatic paralysis, necessitating mechanical ventilation. In contrast, lower cervical injuries require a tailored approach to assess the extent of damage and customize respiratory support strategies accordingly. Successful management requires balancing the immediate need for mechanical ventilation with long-term goals such as weaning, transitioning to non-invasive ventilation, or implementing advanced interventions like diaphragmatic pacing stimulation.

Tracheostomy plays a pivotal role in TSCI care, particularly for high cervical injuries. Early tracheostomy is often favored for its benefits in reducing ventilator-associated complications and facilitating weaning. However, its timing and necessity should be carefully evaluated based on injury severity, comorbidities, and evolving patient needs. Advanced non-invasive strategies, such as mechanical insufflation-exsufflation and continuous non-invasive ventilation, offer potential alternatives for selected patients, reducing tracheostomy dependency while improving quality of life.

Decannulation represents a critical milestone, requiring comprehensive assessments of clinical stability, airway patency, and secretion management. Trials with speaking valves and capping are crucial steps in ensuring a safe transition to natural breathing. For patients unable to achieve full independence, DPS offers a transformative solution, enhancing respiratory autonomy and overall well-being.

Ultimately, effective ventilatory management in TSCI hinges on multidisciplinary collaboration. Respiratory therapists, critical care physicians and nurses, and rehabilitation specialists must integrate clinical expertise with innovative approaches to address immediate needs and support long-term recovery. By combining evidence-based protocols with patient-centered care, clinicians can improve respiratory outcomes, reduce complications, and enhance the quality of life for individuals with TSCI.

References

1. Brown R, DiMarco AF, Hoit JD, Garshick E. Respiratory dysfunction and management in spinal cord injury. Respir Care. 2006;51(8):853–68.
2. Michael B Kazuko S. Respiratory management during the first five days after spinal cord injury. J Spinal Cord Med. 2007;30(4):309–18. https://doi.org/10.1080/10790268.2007.11753946.
3. David J, Berlowitz B, Wadsworth JR. Respiratory problems and management in people with spinal cord injury Breathe. 2016;12(4):328–40. https://doi.org/10.1183/20734735.012616.
4. Krause JS, Cao Y, DeVivo MJ, DiPiro ND. Risk and protective factors for cause-specific mortality after spinal cord injury. Arch Phys Med Rehabil. 2016;97(10):1669–78. https://doi.org/10.1016/j.apmr.2016.07.001. Epub 2016 Jul 20. PMID: 27449321
5. National Spinal Cord Injury Statistical Center. Spinal cord injury facts and figures at a glance: 2020 SCI data sheet. [https://sites.uab.edu/nscisc/] 2020.
6. Shavelle RM, DeVivo MJ, Strauss DJ, Paculdo DR, Lammertse DP, Day SM. Long-term survival of persons ventilator dependent after spinal cord injury. J Spinal Cord Med. 2006;29(5):511–9. https://doi.org/10.1080/10790268.2006.11753901. PMID: 17274490; PMCID: PMC1949034
7. Bach JR, Burke L, Chiou M. Noninvasive respiratory management of spinal cord injury. Phys Med Rehabil Clin N Am. 2020;31(3):397–413. https://doi.org/10.1016/j.pmr.2020.03.006. Epub 2020 May 6. PMID: 32624102
8. Burns KEA, Soliman I, Adhikari NKJ, Zwein A, Wong JTY, Gomez-Builes C, Pellegrini JA, Chen L, Rittayamai N, Sklar M, Brochard LJ, Friedrich JO. Trials directly comparing alternative spontaneous breathing trial techniques: a systematic review and meta-analysis. Crit Care.

2017;21(1):127. https://doi.org/10.1186/s13054-017-1698-x. PMID: 28576127; PMCID: PMC5455092
9. Pozzi F, Palazzo N, Veronese G, Stagni G, Sattin L, Bastia L, Curto F, Chieregato A. Tracheostomy in patients with acute traumatic spinal cord injury: is it really a matter of timing? Anesth Analg. 2021;133(4):e49–50. https://doi.org/10.1213/ANE.0000000000005669. PMID: 34524994
10. Sun D, Liu K, Jian Y, Zhang Z, Zhao H. Tracheostomy in traumatic cervical spinal cord injury: early versus late tracheostomy. Clin Neurol Neurosurg. 2023;224:107577. https://doi.org/10.1016/j.clineuro.2022.107577. Epub 2022 Dec 26. PMID: 36580737
11. Foran SJ, Taran S, Singh JM, Kutsogiannis DJ, McCredie V. Timing of tracheostomy in acute traumatic spinal cord injury: a systematic review and meta-analysis. J Trauma Acute Care Surg. 2022;92(1):223–31. https://doi.org/10.1097/TA.0000000000003394. PMID: 34508010; PMCID: PMC8677619
12. Yan WZ, Guo D, Fan H, Lu D, Xie D, Zhang Y, Jiang P, Li HT. A meta-analysis of the influencing factors for tracheostomy after. Cervical spinal cord injury. BioMed Research International. 2018;1–10. https://doi.org/10.1155/2018/5895830.
13. Singh RK, Saran S, Baronia AK. The practice of tracheostomy decannulation-a systematic review. J Intensive Care. 2017;20(5):38. https://doi.org/10.1186/s40560-017-0234-z. PMID: 28649385; PMCID: PMC5477679
14. Gonzalez-Bermejo J, LLontop C, Similowski T, Morélot-Panzini C. Respiratory neuromodulation in patients with neurological pathologies: for whom and how? Ann Phys Rehabil Med. 2015;58(4):238–44. https://doi.org/10.1016/j.rehab.2015.07.001. Epub 2015 Aug 8. PMID: 26260006
15. Moxham J, Shneerson JM. Diaphragmatic pacing. Am Rev Respir Dis. 1993;148(2):533–6. https://doi.org/10.1164/ajrccm/148.2.533. PMID: 8342921
16. DiMarco AF, Onders RP, Kowalski KE, Miller ME, Ferek S, Mortimer JT. Phrenic nerve pacing in a tetraplegic patient via intramuscular diaphragm electrodes. Am J Respir Crit Care Med. 2002;166(12 Pt 1):1604–6. https://doi.org/10.1164/rccm.200203-175CR. PMID: 12471076
17. DiMarco AF, Onders RP, Ignagni A, Kowalski KE. Inspiratory muscle pacing in spinal cord injury: case report and clinical commentary. J Spinal Cord Med. 2006;29(2):95–108. https://doi.org/10.1080/10790268.2006.11753863. PMID: 16739553; PMCID: PMC1864798
18. Onders RP, Khansarinia S, Ingvarsson PE, Road J, Yee J, Dunkin B, Ignagni AR. Diaphragm pacing in spinal cord injury can significantly decrease mechanical ventilation in multicenter prospective evaluation. Artif Organs. 2022;46(10):1980–7. https://doi.org/10.1111/aor.14221. Epub 2022 Mar 8. PMID: 35226374
19. Onders RP, Elmo M, Kaplan C, Schilz R, Katirji B, Tinkoff G. Long-term experience with diaphragm pacing for traumatic spinal cord injury: early implantation should be considered. Surgery. 2018;164(4):705–11. https://doi.org/10.1016/j.surg.2018.06.050. Epub 2018 Sep 6. PMID: 30195400
20. Wijkstra PJ, van der Aa H, Hofker HS, Curto F, Giacomini M, Stagni G, Dura Agullo MA, Curià Casanoves FX, Benito-Penalva J, Martinez-Barenys C, Vidal J. Diaphragm pacing in patients with spinal cord injury: a European experience. Respiration. 2022;101(1):18–24. https://doi.org/10.1159/000517401. Epub 2021 Jul 16. PMID: 34274930; PMCID: PMC8820415
21. Monden KR, Coker J, Charlifue S, Bennett SJ, Draganich C, Coons D, Marino RJ, Berliner J. Long-term follow-up of patients with ventilator-dependent high tetraplegia managed with diaphragmatic pacing systems. Arch Phys Med Rehabil. 2022;103(4):773–8. https://doi.org/10.1016/j.apmr.2021.03.005. Epub 2021 Mar 22. PMID: 33766556

Hematological and Endocrinological Complications After Traumatic Spinal Cord Injury

15

Eloy Rusafa Neto, Ludhmila Abrahão Hajjar, and Wellingson Silva Paiva

15.1 Introduction

Spinal cord injury (SCI) is a catastrophic condition that leads to dysfunction in multiple systems of the human body. The systemic inflammatory immune response is responsible for various endocrinological and hematological complications that are not always detectable by standard blood tests. Nevertheless, this response is the underlying cause of infections, impaired healing, an increased risk of thrombotic events, and osteoporosis. Additionally, the hypothalamic-pituitary-gonadal and thyroid axes may be compromised, leading to hormonal alterations that can exacerbate obesity and osteoporosis, contributing to muscle mass loss, and cause fertility problems. In this chapter, we clarify the mechanisms behind the hematological and endocrinological issues associated with SCI and provide evidence-based approaches for the treatment and prevention of these complications.

15.2 Hematological Dysfunctions After SCI

The disruption of sympathetic system control caused by spinal cord injury (SCI) triggers hematopoietic dysfunction, resulting in a decentralized autonomic network and abnormal sympathetic and neuroendocrine responses. This leads to alterations in bone marrow and cellular function, including an increase in the total number of hematopoietic stem and progenitor cells (HSPCs), despite these cells being nonfunctional and unable to be adequately mobilized from the bone marrow [1].

E. R. Neto · W. S. Paiva (✉)
Division of Neurosurgery, Hospital das Clínicas da FMUSP, Sao Paulo, Brazil

L. A. Hajjar
Department of Neurology, University of Sao Paulo Medical School, Sao Paulo, Brazil

E. Brogi et al. (eds.), *Traumatic Spinal Cord Injury*, Hot Topics in Acute Care Surgery and Trauma, https://doi.org/10.1007/978-3-031-99890-4_15

The first evidence of alterations in hematopoiesis without the influence of the sympathetic system came from studies that detected anemia in the acute phase of spinal cord injury, comparing patients with and without SCI [2, 3]. However, experimental studies have sought to explain the underlying causes of these findings, as other factors such as acute blood loss, surgery, and hemodilution could also contribute to hematological changes during the acute phase of trauma.

Obayashi et al. induced sympathectomy in rats using 6-hydroxydopamine and found that anemia was induced after sympathetic blockade [4]. Additionally, Carpenter et al. published a molecular study that further elucidated the mechanisms by which SCI influences the hematopoietic system.

First, SCI leads to an increase in the proliferation of hematopoietic stem and progenitor cells (HSPCs) in the bone marrow during the acute phase, a condition that persists even one month after SCI when compared with post-laminectomy, non-SCI control mice. Second, there is a chronic expansion of bone marrow HSPCs across all types of progenitor precursors, including long-term repopulating stem cells, short-term progenitors, and myeloid, lymphoid, and granulocyte–monocyte progenitors. This expansion induces long-term replication stress. Third, the HSPCs produced are not mobilized from the bone marrow. Although stress still induces hematopoiesis in extramedullary tissues like lymphoid tissues, the progenitors do not leave the bone marrow, meaning HSPCs are not found in the spleen, and extramedullary-induced hematopoiesis does not occur in SCI. Finally, B cells are sequestered in the bone marrow, leading to a decrease in circulating leukocytes [5].

To determine the molecular mechanisms underlying these phenomena, the same authors found that the expression of all cytokines and chemokines affecting the development and function of HSPCs increased, except for Ccl2. The most important chemokine identified was CXCL12, which binds to CXCR4 and influences the retention of HSPCs in the bone marrow, a process dependent on the sympathetic branch of the autonomic nervous system. Plerixafor, a CXCR4 antagonist, facilitated the release of these cells from the bone marrow, leading to an increase in circulating leukocytes and confirming these findings. Additionally, the authors observed that SCI results in chronic impairment of bone marrow function and diminished responses to inflammatory stimuli, persisting even 24 weeks after the injury [1, 6].

The factors mentioned above contribute to the increased risk of pulmonary and urinary infections in these patients. However, other factors, such as long-term mechanical ventilation and repeated urinary catheterization, also play a role.

15.3 Blood Dyscrasias

SCI increases immobility, putting these patients at a higher risk of deep venous thrombosis (DVT) and pulmonary embolism (PE), as the skeletal muscle pump, which aids in venous return, is no longer functional. Paralysis also leads to metabolic changes in blood vessels, affecting distensibility and flow resistance [7]. In addition to immobility and stasis, two other components of the Virchow triad are present in these patients: hypercoagulability and venous intimal injury [8]. General factors that contribute to this increased risk include middle and old age, personal or family history of DVT, history of smoking, male sex, lack of compression therapy, severity of injury, diabetes, and the presence of lower limb or pelvic fractures [9, 10]. The risk of DVT is lower in patients under 14 years of age and higher in those over 45 [11, 12]. Hormonal factors and height may also be linked to the higher incidence of DVT in males.

The mechanisms behind the relationship between smoking and thrombosis include the effects of nicotine and benzopyrene, which increase platelet activation, aggregation, and blood viscosity, as well as induce endothelial injury through oxidative stress and inflammation [13]. Diabetes is another condition that leads to damage of endothelial cells and alters their function, promoting hypercoagulability with chronic inflammation. Other studies have linked protein N-linked homocysteinemia and Leiden factor V to higher risks of DVT in SCI, as these proteins are associated with higher levels of inflammation [14]. Some authors advocate that a family history of thrombosis should prompt further investigation.

The diagnosis of PE and DVT is most often made with multislice thoracic CT angiogram and deep venous color Doppler ultrasonography of the lower limbs and pelvis, as these methods are highly sensitive and specific [15]. Ventilation-perfusion scintigraphy is an alternative to CT angiogram with similar sensitivity and specificity [16]. Differential diagnosis with pneumonia is crucial since this complication is common in SCI, and symptoms can be very similar.

The incidence of DVT in SCI patients ranges from 9% to 90%, with high mortality rates of approximately 5% related to PE [17]. Early prophylaxis, combining pharmacological and mechanical treatments within the first three months, is crucial for preventing DVT and reducing morbidity and mortality [18], as the majority of cases (88%) occur within this period [19, 20]. Tissue Factor (TF) is part of the extrinsic coagulation cascade, forming a complex with Factor VIIa to initiate the extrinsic coagulation pathway. The tissue factor pathway inhibitor (TFPI) inhibits this complex and helps control thrombosis. D-dimer is another component of the coagulation cascade that reflects activation of the fibrinolytic system, and its elevation is a key parameter for detecting thrombotic events. Some studies have revealed higher levels of D-dimer in the chronic phase of SCI compared with control groups, though these levels are lower than those in the acute phase.

After 3 months of SCI, the necessity for continued anticoagulation is questioned based on autopsy studies that suggest a rare incidence of this complication [21–24]. Some studies have concluded that high levels of Tissue Factor (TF) are present up to 3 months after injury, while Tissue Factor Protein Inhibitor (TFPI) levels significantly elevate between 3 and 12 months post-SCI [25–27]. Alabed et al. found a 1.25% incidence of PE more than 90 days after SCI, which is lower than the 5–12% incidence observed in the acute phase but higher than the 0.06% per year incidence in the general population [28, 29]. Other studies have reported high incidences of DVT in chronic SCI, with rates varying from 1.25% to 12%, leading to recommendations for anticoagulation up to 6 months after SCI.

PE in the chronic phase of SCI continues to occur but seems to be less prevalent and often clinically silent. Dyspnea may be overlooked as a common symptom in SCI, hypotension may be dismissed as a typical manifestation in patients with labile blood pressure, and tetraplegic subjects may not feel chest pain. Factors such as venous stasis, decreased cardiac output, and higher risks of septicemia contribute to PE in the chronic phase. Repeated PE events can lead to chronic increases in pulmonary resistance and right-sided cardiac hypertrophy and dilatation, which may be detected by ECG as right bundle branch block (RBBB) or by transthoracic echocardiogram. The factors explained above should raise the level of suspicion in this group of patients [30–34].

Prevention of thromboembolic events in SCI involves multiple strategies. In the acute phase, anticoagulation, mechanical therapy, physical therapy, and the use of vena cava filters can reduce the risk of thromboembolic events by up to four times [37]. However, these measures may be associated with complications, including the expansion of spinal contusions, hematomas, bleeding (especially in polytrauma patients), and worsening of neurological deficits [35].

In the chronic phase (after 3 months), prevention focuses on mechanical pumps promoted by physical therapy and electrical stimulation, applied up to three times a day, along with potential anticoagulation [30]. Although the risk of PE and DVT is lower in the chronic phase of SCI, the optimal method for preventing these complications remains unclear, as the incidence is still higher than in the general population. Further studies are needed to clarify the pathophysiology of the less frequent thrombosis in chronic phases. Vigilance must be maintained for this complication [24].

Evidence from randomized clinical trials (RCTs) has confirmed that enoxaparin reduces the risk of DVT from 21.6% to 5.4% in the acute phase of SCI, though some authors have questioned these results and argue that it is more effective in preventing PE compared to no prophylaxis [36, 37]. However, studies comparing low molecular weight heparin (LMWH) with unfractionated heparin (UFH) showed slightly higher thrombotic events with UFH, though without statistical significance, and even higher bleeding events when adjusted UFH was used, also without statistical significance [38]. It is important to note that while LMWH is more expensive than UFH, the incidence of heparin-induced thrombocytopenia is higher with LMWH (2.6% vs. 0.2%) [13].

Anticoagulants are more effective when combined with mechanical therapy, although the evidence supporting this is not strong [39, 40]. The use of an intravenous cava filter for PE prevention is not recommended unless the patient has a contraindication for anticoagulation, as there is no evidence supporting its effectiveness. The optimal time to initiate anticoagulation and intermittent lower limb compression is within the first 72 h, which has been shown to result in lower rates of DVT [17].

Other complications of DVT, besides PE, include post-thrombotic syndrome, ulcerations, trophic skin changes (affecting 20–50% of cases), and, in SCI patients, an increase in spasticity and autonomic dysreflexia [36]. A higher index of suspicion is necessary in these patients, as the lack of symptoms is typical of the disease, and sometimes only complications can be diagnosed.

Summary

The prevention and management of thromboembolic events in SCI require a multi-faceted approach that varies between the acute and chronic phases. In the acute phase, the use of anticoagulation, mechanical therapy, physical therapy, and vena cava filters can significantly reduce the risk of DVT and PE, although these interventions come with potential complications, including bleeding and neurological deficits. The efficacy of enoxaparin in reducing DVT risk has been substantiated by randomized clinical trials, though its superiority in preventing PE compared to no prophylaxis remains debated. The choice between LMWH and UFH involves balancing the slightly higher thrombotic risk of UFH against the increased cost and higher incidence of heparin-induced thrombocytopenia with LMWH.

In the chronic phase, while the risk of thromboembolic events is lower, optimal prevention strategies remain unclear. Physical therapy and electrical stimulation, alongside possible anticoagulation, are recommended, yet further research is needed to better understand the pathophysiology of thrombosis in this phase. Regardless of the phase, vigilance is essential due to the often asymptomatic nature of DVT and the significant complications it can cause, including post-thrombotic syndrome, skin changes, and increased spasticity and autonomic dysreflexia in SCI patients.

The timing of preventive measures is critical, with anticoagulation and intermittent lower limb compression ideally starting within the first 72 h to minimize DVT risk. Although combining anticoagulants with mechanical therapy may enhance efficacy, the evidence remains inconclusive. The use of intravenous cava filters should be reserved for patients with contraindications to anticoagulation, as no solid evidence supports their routine use for PE prevention. Given the complexity and variability of thromboembolic event prevention in SCI, ongoing research and individualized patient care are imperative to optimize outcomes.

15.4 Metabolic Dysfunctions After Spinal Cord Injury

15.4.1 Osseous Metabolism After SCI and Osteoporosis

SCI is a well-known cause of osteoporosis, and patients with SCI have a higher risk of fragility fractures compared to the general population. Estimates suggest that up to 50% of patients may experience a fracture after SCI [41], and these fractures are associated with hospitalization, skin ulcers, amputations, deformities, infections, hypertensive crises, and autonomic dysreflexia [42, 43]. The most common sites of osteoporosis in these patients differ from the typical sites seen in post-menopausal osteoporosis, which usually affect the proximal femur and spine. In SCI patients, osteoporosis predominantly occurs at the distal epiphysis of the femur (DF) and the proximal tibia (PT), making these the most common sites for fractures [44, 45]. The development of osteoporosis in these bones can have devastating consequences, including amputation, infection, pseudoarthrosis, skin scars, and even death.

The main causes of increased osteoporosis risk in SCI patients include mechanical unloading, neurovascular changes, hormonal alterations, poor nutritional status, and hypercortisolism. Hypercortisolism may be secondary to the use of steroids for spinal trauma or due to metabolic changes related to sarcopenia.

Mechanical unloading leads to an imbalance between bone formation by osteoblasts and bone resorption by osteoclasts, resulting in demineralization. According to the mechanostat theory (Wolff's law), a lack of sufficient force applied to bones can lead to bone loss [46]. Bone formation decreases within the first two weeks after injury, and although there may be some improvement after this period, bone resorption continues to increase, leading to a decrease in bone mineral density (BMD) by up to 40% within the first two years [47, 48]. This process is evidenced by hypercalcemia and hypercalciuria, as well as elevated markers of bone resorption during this period.

Compared with other causes of osteoporosis, SCI patients experience a significantly higher rate of bone loss. For instance, post-menopausal patients have a 3–5% annual loss, bedridden patients lose 0.1% per week, and astronauts lose 0.25% per week during space flights. The hypercalcemia present during the first year post-injury inhibits parathyroid hormone activity, leading to decreased levels of 25-hydroxyvitamin D and 1,25-dihydroxyvitamin D, which in turn reduces calcium absorption in the gut and increases renal calcium excretion. Consequently, these patients are at a higher risk of developing urinary tract stones [49]. In the chronic phase, after 1–2 years, calcium levels tend to normalize in both serum and urine.

To understand the mechanisms underlying the mechanostat theory, it's important to grasp the basics of bone metabolism. There are three key types of cells involved in bone health:

1. *Osteoclasts*: These cells are derived from the monocytic lineage and are stimulated by the release of receptor activator of nuclear factor-kappa B ligand (RANKL) from osteocytes under conditions of mechanical unloading, leading to increased bone resorption.
2. *Osteoblasts*: These cells originate from mesenchymal stem cells. Under normal conditions, osteoblasts release osteoprotegerin, an inhibitor of RANKL, which downregulates osteoclast activity and function. Mechanical load stimulates osteoblasts to secrete collagen, osteocalcin, osteonectin, and bone morphogenetic proteins, all of which contribute to the mineralization of the bone matrix.
3. *Osteocytes*: These structural cells play a crucial role in controlling the activity of both osteoblasts and osteoclasts through two main systems. Osteoblastogenesis is regulated by the Wingless (Wnt)/β-catenin signaling pathway, while antagonism is mediated by sclerostin and Dickkopf-1 (Dkk-1). Some studies have found that under mechanical unloading, such as in SCI, RANKL levels are significantly higher [50].

Sclerostin, primarily expressed by osteocytes, plays a crucial role in regulating bone metabolism. Under mechanical unloading, such as in SCI, sclerostin levels increase, leading to the suppression of bone formation by reducing Wnt/β-catenin signaling in osteoblasts. Simultaneously, catabolic activity is promoted by stimulating osteoclast differentiation through the upregulation of RANKL and downregulation of OPG expression in osteocytes [51, 52]. Elevated levels of sclerostin have been observed even five years after SCI and serve as a biomarker for the severity of osteoporosis in these patients [53].

Additionally, several bone resorption biomarkers are significantly elevated in both blood and urine, particularly in the acute and chronic phases of SCI. These include urinary and serum type 1 collagen C-telopeptide (CTx), hydroxyproline, N-telopeptide (NTx), deoxypyridinoline (DPD), and increased calcium concentrations in serum and urine [54–57]. CTx-1 and NTX-1 are specific biomarkers of bone resorption [54, 56] and can be indicative of osteoporosis if chronically elevated. Conversely, markers of bone formation, such as Procollagen 1 intact N-terminal Propeptide (P1NP) and osteocalcin, are typically low in SCI patients [47]. However, the balance between these systems in bone homeostasis remains poorly understood, and further studies are needed to better comprehend the pathophysiology and to establish potential new therapies.

Compromised bone tissue innervation is another contributing factor to osteoporosis, as autonomic nerve fibers and nerve-derived factors such as neuropeptides play a role in modulating and controlling bone metabolism. Although the lack of sympathetic activity, which typically promotes bone formation and suppresses bone resorption, might seem beneficial, the vascular changes caused by vasomotor irregularities are actually linked to bone loss [58–60]. The influence of parasympathetic activity on bone density, however, is not yet well understood [61].

In the acute phase of SCI, hormonal changes include suppressed parathyroid hormone (PTH) levels, resulting from increased bone resorption and the consequent hypercalciuria, as mentioned earlier. This new balance between osteoclasts and osteoblasts also leads to reduced levels of 1,25(OH) vitamin D, driven by bone resorption and PTH suppression [55, 62]. In the chronic phase, the PTH and vitamin D levels tend to normalize [57].

Sarcopenia, caused by muscle inactivity, is further exacerbated by insulin resistance, which is commonly present in chronic SCI and predisposes patients to fat-muscle infiltration [63].

The inhibition of the production and secretion of sex hormones plays a significant role in osteoporosis, as estrogen and androgen both inhibit bone resorption and promote bone formation through various mechanisms [64, 65]. These mechanisms include anti-apoptotic effects, increased cell survival, and a reduction in the inflammatory immune response. Low levels of androgens and estrogens hinder the release of growth factors by osteoblasts and stimulate osteoclastogenesis [64, 65]. In SCI, there is evidence of abnormalities in the hypothalamus-pituitary-gonadal axis [66, 67].

The screening and diagnosis of sublesional osteoporosis (SLOP) are recommended on an annual basis. This includes laboratory evaluations for potentially treatable causes of secondary osteoporosis, bone mineral density testing, and fracture risk assessment using DXA (dual-energy X-ray absorptiometry) or pQCT (peripheral quantitative computed tomography), as recommended by the International Society for Clinical Densitometry. A diagnosis of sublesional osteoporosis (SLOP) is made when the T-score is below −2.5 in men over 50 and postmenopausal women, or if the Z-score is less than −2.0 with three or more risk factors for fractures, or when there is a prior fragility fracture with no identifiable cause of osteoporosis other than SCI [68]. Patients with ASIA A and B classifications typically have more compromised bone density than others [69–71]. Nutritional status, including protein, calcium, and vitamin D intake and serum levels, is a critical parameter for screening osteoporosis and preventing its development. Other systemic diseases such as hyperthyroidism, hypothyroidism, anemia, chronic kidney disease, diabetes, and liver dysfunction are also associated with bone health and should be ruled out.

The treatment of osteoporosis in patients with SCI typically involves vitamin D supplementation when serum levels are below 40 ng/mL. Given that up to 93% of chronic SCI patients have low vitamin D levels, most of these patients require vitamin D therapy [72–76]. Calcium and nutritional supplementation depend on daily intake and serum metabolism. However, they are generally not recommended for SCI patients due to the risk of recurrent urinary tract stones.

Rehabilitation is not contraindicated by any specific bone mineral density (BMD) level, and therapies that allow patients to stand and walk for at least 1 h per day, 5 days per week, have been shown to increase BMD [77]. However, some studies consider this increase insufficient [78–80]. Functional electrical stimulation (FES) and neuromuscular electrical stimulation (NMES) are recommended for 30 min per day or 3–5 h per week with visible muscle contractions. These therapies have been proven to increase BMD and reduce the incidence of fractures, although their effectiveness is only sustained while the therapy is ongoing [81–84].

The most commonly used drugs are alendronate (10 mg/day or 70 mg/week), zoledronic acid (5 mg every 6 months), and denosumab. These are only used when there is osteopenia with a moderate or high risk of fracture or in cases of established osteoporosis. Alendronate is the only drug that has been specifically studied in chronic SCI and has been shown to prevent a decline in trabecular BMD during the first 2 years [85].

Summary

Osteoporosis in SCI

- *Prevalence and Risk*: Osteoporosis is a common complication in SCI patients, leading to a higher risk of fragility fractures. Up to 50% of SCI patients may experience a fracture, with the most common sites being the distal femur and proximal tibia. Fractures can result in severe complications, including hospitalization, skin ulcers, amputations, and increased spasticity.
- *Causes*.

  - *Mechanical unloading*: Lack of mechanical load leads to an imbalance in bone metabolism, favoring bone resorption over formation. This is supported by the mechanostat theory (Wolff's law), which explains how insufficient mechanical force can lead to bone loss.
  - *Hormonal changes*: SCI disrupts the hypothalamus-pituitary-gonadal axis, leading to low levels of sex hormones like estrogen and androgen, which normally inhibit bone resorption and promote bone formation.
  - *Sarcopenia*: Muscle inactivity, compounded by insulin resistance, worsens sarcopenia and leads to fat-muscle infiltration, further compromising bone health.
  - *Nerve function*: Compromised bone tissue innervation, particularly through autonomic nerve fibers, contributes to bone loss. Sclerostin, which inhibits bone formation, is increased in SCI and serves as a biomarker for osteoporosis severity.
- *Screening and Diagnosis.*
  - Annual screening for sublesional osteoporosis (SLOP) is recommended, involving bone mineral density (BMD) testing through DXA or pQCT. A diagnosis of SLOP is made based on specific T-scores or Z-scores, and consideration of fracture risk factors.
- *Treatment.*
  - *Vitamin D supplementation*: Most SCI patients require vitamin D supplementation due to common deficiencies. Calcium supplementation is generally avoided due to the risk of urinary tract stones.
  - *Rehabilitation*: Weight-bearing activities and therapies like functional electrical stimulation (FES) and neuromuscular electrical stimulation (NMES) are recommended to increase BMD, though their benefits are sustained only with ongoing therapy.
  - *Medications*: Alendronate, zoledronic acid, and denosumab are used in cases of osteopenia with a moderate/high fracture risk or established osteoporosis. Alendronate has been shown to prevent trabecular BMD decline in chronic SCI patients.

15.4.2 Glucose, Lipid Metabolism, and Neurogenic Obesity After SCI

Obesity is a significant complication after spinal cord injury (SCI) due to disturbances in glucose and lipid metabolism, which can lead to cardiovascular disease—the leading cause of death in these patients. Paralysis accelerates muscle mass loss and adiposity gain, resulting in peripheral insulin resistance, sarcopenia, and hyperlipidemia. These conditions are well-known contributors to a chronic inflammatory state and atherogenic processes, which are key mediators of metabolic syndrome [19, 64, 65].

Metabolic syndrome is defined as central obesity (waist circumference greater than 94 cm) plus any two of the following criteria: triglycerides (TG) $\geq$150 mg/dl, low high-density lipoprotein (HDL) cholesterol (<40 mg/dl in men and <50 mg/dl in women), elevated blood pressure (systolic >130 mmHg or diastolic >85 mmHg), or fasting plasma glucose >100 mg/dl [86].

In a study by Gater et al. involving 473 veterans from past wars with a mean age of 56 years, 49.6% of the participants were tetraplegic, and 76.7% had a BMI above 22 kg/m^2, the appropriate target in SCI. The study also found that 69.7% had HDL cholesterol levels below 40 mg/dl, 49.8% had fasting glucose levels above 100 mg/dl, 55.1% had hypertension, and nearly 57.5% met the criteria for metabolic syndrome according to the International Diabetes Federation definition [87, 88]. In a typical individual without SCI, a BMI of 25 could correspond to approximately 35% body fat. However, in patients with SCI, a BMI of 27 could correspond to as much as 44% body fat [89].

Many studies involving oral glucose load tests have shown that patients with spinal cord injury (SCI) are often hyperinsulinemic and exhibit insulin resistance. This condition tends to worsen with the duration of the injury, indicating that chronic SCI leads to progressive metabolic alterations directly linked to muscle mass loss and obesity [90, 91]. The incidence of overweight in this population is approximately 50–60%, with 20–30% classified as obese based on body mass index (BMI) criteria. However, BMI underestimates the extent of sarcopenia and adiposity, so the actual prevalence of obesity in this population is likely higher. Additionally, there are elevated levels of low-density lipoprotein (LDL) cholesterol, insulin resistance, and the inflammatory biomarker C-reactive protein (CRP), which is a marker of cardiovascular disease [68, 92–94]. The secretion of pro-inflammatory mediators by adipocytes further increases insulin resistance [95].

Adipose tissue impairs fibrinolysis, which prevents thrombus formation, by secreting thrombin-activatable fibrinolysis inhibitor (TAFI) and plasminogen activator inhibitor-1 (PAI-1), thereby increasing the risk of thromboembolism [96]. Adipocytes are pro-inflammatory, secreting interleukin-6 (IL-6), tumor necrosis factor-alpha (TNF-alpha), and C-reactive protein (CRP). These factors increase nuclear factor kappa B (NF-κB) activity, promote leukocyte adhesion, induce endothelial cell apoptosis, and decrease nitric oxide production, leading to relative vasoconstriction and vascular inflammation [88]. Additionally, the combination of inflammation and obesity contributes to immunosuppression [97].

Adipocytes also contribute to hypertension through the secretion of angiotensin, IL-6, and free fatty acids, which can compress the adrenal glands and promote atherogenesis due to poor arterial compliance. Dyslipidemia is a consequence of increased visceral fat, specifically non-esterified fatty acids (NEFA), which accumulate in the portal circulation, overwhelming the liver and increasing LDL-c and VLDL-c levels while reducing HDL-c levels.

For the reasons previously explained, it is recommended that patients with SCI undergo an oral glucose tolerance test and be referred for endocrinology and nutritional evaluations to calculate the energy balance between expenditure and intake.

Daily energy expenditure is roughly divided into three components: 15–30% from the thermic effect of activity, 7–10% from the thermic effect of meals, and 60–75% from the resting metabolic rate. Resting energy expenditure for a typical person is distributed as follows: 19% for the brain, 29% for the liver, 10% for the heart, 18% for skeletal muscle (with variability in this component), and 10% for the kidneys. A person without disabilities has a total daily energy expenditure (TDEE) of about 2800 kcal/day (including basal metabolism, physical activity, and the thermic effect of food).

Due to the muscle mass loss associated with SCI paralysis, commonly used equations for calculating nitrogen balance may not be entirely appropriate, as resting energy expenditure decreases with nitrogen loss, as noted by Rodrigues et al. [98]. Consequently, a paraplegic patient may have a TDEE of approximately 2240 kcal/day, while a tetraplegic patient may have a TDEE of around 1200 kcal/day.

The prescription of exercise to increase energy expenditure is essential for SCI patients, with goals tailored to their specific limitations. These include considerations for mode, frequency, intensity, duration, and progression, while accounting for potential limitations such as adaptive cardiomyopathy, restrictive or obstructive lung disease, obesity, autonomic dysreflexia, metabolic deficiency, circulatory hypokinesis, osteopenia, peripheral neuropathy, pain, facility access, transportation, temperature, and monitoring expertise.

Exercise is an important part of preventing obesity in SCI patients; however, reducing energy intake is also crucial, as satiety mechanisms are often impaired in individuals with SCI [99].

Summary

1. *Metabolic Changes.*
   - *Glucose metabolism*: Patients with SCI often develop insulin resistance and hyperinsulinemia, which tend to worsen with the duration of the injury. This is largely due to muscle mass loss (sarcopenia) and increased adiposity, leading to a higher prevalence of type 2 diabetes and metabolic syndrome.
   - *Lipid metabolism*: SCI patients frequently experience dyslipidemia, characterized by elevated triglycerides, low HDL cholesterol, and sometimes high LDL cholesterol. This dysregulation contributes to a heightened risk of cardiovascular disease, the leading cause of death in this population.
2. *Neurogenic Obesity.*
   - *Causes*: Neurogenic obesity in SCI is driven by reduced physical activity, changes in body composition (increased fat mass and decreased lean body mass), and disrupted energy balance. Autonomic dysfunction also plays a role in altered energy expenditure and appetite regulation.
   - *Health implications*: Obesity in SCI patients exacerbates metabolic complications such as insulin resistance and dyslipidemia, further increasing the risk of cardiovascular disease. It also contributes to secondary complications like pressure ulcers, sleep apnea, and increased spasticity.
3. *Hormonal and Inflammatory Factors.*
   - *Inflammatory response*: Adipose tissue in SCI patients contributes to chronic inflammation by secreting pro-inflammatory cytokines like IL-6, TNF-alpha, and CRP. These factors promote insulin resistance, vascular inflammation, and atherogenesis, worsening metabolic health.

- *Hormonal changes*: Abnormalities in hormone secretion, such as reduced levels of sex hormones and increased secretion of angiotensin by adipocytes, contribute to hypertension, further complicating the metabolic profile of SCI patients.

4. *Nutritional and Energy Considerations.*
   - *Energy expenditure*: Due to reduced muscle mass, SCI patients have lower resting energy expenditure. For instance, paraplegic patients may have a TDEE of about 2240 kcal/day, and tetraplegic patients about 1200 kcal/day. This necessitates careful nutritional planning to balance energy intake and expenditure.
   - *Exercise and diet*: Regular exercise is essential for increasing energy expenditure and improving metabolic health, but it must be tailored to the patient's physical limitations. Reducing energy intake is also crucial, as satiety mechanisms are often impaired in SCI patients, making weight management more challenging.
5. *Clinical Recommendations.*
   - *Screening and management*: Regular glucose tolerance tests, lipid profiles, and monitoring of inflammatory markers are recommended. Referral to endocrinologists and nutritionists for comprehensive metabolic evaluation and personalized dietary and exercise plans is essential.
   - *Prevention strategies*: Exercise prescription should be designed with specific goals, respecting the patient's limitations and ensuring a balance between energy intake and expenditure to prevent obesity and associated metabolic disorders.

15.4.3 Gonadal Function and Fertility After Spinal Cord Injury

Patients with chronic spinal cord injury (SCI) lasting more than one year frequently exhibit hormonal deficiencies, particularly in testosterone levels among males, compared to healthy controls. Some studies have found a 25% prevalence of low testosterone in men with SCI, compared to just 7% in controls. This deficiency is associated with higher rates of metabolic dysfunction, as low testosterone levels in SCI patients correlate with an increased cardiovascular risk. However, since these findings are based on cross-sectional studies, causality cannot be established [100–107].

Anderson et al. conducted a survey in 2004 to determine the most important functions that quadriplegics and paraplegics wished to regain. For quadriplegics, hand and arm function was the top priority (48.7%), followed by sexual function (13%). Among paraplegics, sexual function was the most important (26.7%), followed by bladder and bowel control (18%) [108].

Genital innervation involves three systems: the somatic nervous system (via the pudendal nerve, S2-S4, which innervates the pelvic floor musculature with afferents from T4-S4), the parasympathetic nervous system (via the pelvic nerve, S2-S5, which mediates reflexogenic arousal), and the sympathetic nervous system (via the hypogastric nerve, T10-L2, which mediates psychogenic arousal). These systems function under the assumption that the central nervous system above these levels remains intact. During the excitement phase, when an erection occurs, the parasympathetic system is primarily active, releasing neurotransmitters such as acetylcholine and vasoactive intestinal peptide. These promote arterial dilation through nitric oxide, leading to penile stiffening in men and vaginal lubrication, as well as increased length, width, and clitoral diameter in women.

Ninety percent of men with SCI cannot father children through sexual intercourse alone. However, women with SCI can conceive and deliver babies similarly to the general population. The primary reason for male infertility is the lack of ejaculation during intercourse and reduced sperm motility post-SCI. Normal ejaculation involves the emission of sperm into the posterior urethra, where it mixes with seminal fluid before being expelled from the penis. This process requires intact reflexes, with the ejaculatory center located at L3-4 (bulbocavernosus spinal nucleus), which regulates parasympathetic, sympathetic, and motor outflow.

Emission is controlled by the sympathetic system between T10 and L2, causing the seminal vesicles and prostate to contract, pushing sperm and seminal fluid into the posterior urethra. Expulsion is mediated by S2–5 radicular nerves, which ensure that the bladder neck closes to prevent retrograde ejaculation, the external urinary sphincter relaxes, and rhythmic contractions expel semen via the parasympathetic pelvic nerve through the pudendal nerve [109].

A psychogenic erection can occur if the central nervous system is intact up to L2, involving the hypogastric nerve (T10-L2), which is sympathetically mediated. In contrast, a reflex erection occurs when the pelvic nerves (S2-S5) are intact and is parasympathetically mediated [110].

Given this understanding of physiology, it can be concluded that patients with SCI may experience various sexual dysfunctions depending on the level of injury. These may include erectile dysfunction, vaginal lubrication issues, retrograde or absent ejaculation, decreased or absent orgasm, reduced libido, male infertility, bladder and bowel incontinence, autonomic dysreflexia, and positioning problems due to contractures and spasticity.

Another common issue in men with SCI is abnormal semen quality and motility. Several factors have been explored as possible causes, including scrotal hyperthermia, urinary tract infections due to frequent bladder management, medications, ejaculation methods, the duration of time since injury, endocrinopathy, semen inflammatory cytokines, and stasis. The conclusion is that bladder management and semen inflammatory cytokines are the primary contributors to compromised semen quality. These cytokines impair sperm motility, though the exact mechanism is unclear and may be linked to obesity, which is common in SCI patients. Additionally, the method of semen collection may also influence its quality [110].

Treatment for these disturbances includes both physical and psychological approaches, involving pharmacological interventions (oral medications, intracavernous injections, transurethral therapies), pumps, implants for erections, in vitro fertilization, and alternative sperm collection methods (masturbation, prostate massage, penile vibrostimulation, electroejaculation, and surgical sperm retrieval) [111]. The use of phosphodiesterase type 5 inhibitors, as described by Wood and Lue in 2000, is common in treating erectile dysfunction in SCI patients [112]. The anterior sacral root stimulator (Finetech-Brindley), combined with posterior root rhizotomy, remains an alternative for treating erectile dysfunction, offering three stimulation patterns: bladder, bowel, and penile erection. However, side effects such as loss of reflexogenic erections, mechanical failure, infection, and autonomic dysreflexia are common [113, 114]. The side effects, indications, and contraindications of these treatments should be carefully studied in the relevant literature before use and prescription.

As mentioned earlier, women with SCI remain fertile, with most regaining menstruation within 3–6 months. Pregnancy should be managed in high-risk centers, as these women have an increased risk of preterm deliveries and lower birth weight infants. The risk of venous thromboembolism (VTE) is higher, along with the potential for undiagnosed autonomic dysreflexia, which can mimic preeclampsia. Labor and delivery are often more challenging, with a cesarean section rate of approximately 50%. Epidural anesthesia is required for SCI patients with injuries above T6, with the epidural catheter remaining in place until uterine contractions resolve and nursing has begun. For women with SCI above T4, nursing can precipitate autonomic dysreflexia, necessitating caution during the process [115].

Summary

1. *Hormonal Deficiency.*
   - *Testosterone Levels in Men*: Men with chronic SCI often exhibit lower testosterone levels compared to healthy controls, with studies indicating a 25% prevalence of low testosterone in SCI patients versus 7% in the general population. This hormonal deficiency is associated with increased metabolic dysfunction and a higher cardiovascular risk, though causality has not been definitively established.
   - *Impact on Women*: While women with SCI can experience disruptions in their menstrual cycle following injury, most regain menstruation within 3–6 months. Estrogen levels may be affected, potentially leading to issues similar to menopause, such as osteoporosis and cardiovascular risk.
2. *Fertility Issues.*
   - *Men.*
     - *Erectile Dysfunction*: A significant number of men with SCI experience erectile dysfunction due to impaired nerve signaling. Treatment options include oral medications, injections, and mechanical devices.
     - *Ejaculation and Sperm Quality*: About 90% of men with SCI are unable to ejaculate naturally during intercourse, leading to fertility challenges. Additionally, sperm quality and motility are often compromised due to factors like scrotal hyperthermia, bladder management, and semen inflammatory cytokines.

  - *Assisted Reproductive Technologies (ART)*: Techniques such as penile vibrostimulation, electroejaculation, and surgical sperm retrieval are used to collect sperm for in vitro fertilization (IVF) or intracytoplasmic sperm injection (ICSI) in cases of male infertility.
- *Women.*
  - *Conception and Pregnancy*: Women with SCI generally retain their fertility and can conceive and deliver babies, although they face higher risks during pregnancy, such as preterm labor, low birth weight, and venous thromboembolism (VTE). Pregnancy should be managed in high-risk centers.
  - *Labor and Delivery*: Labor can be more challenging, with about 50% of deliveries occurring via cesarean section. Epidural anesthesia is often required for women with injuries above T6 to manage pain and prevent autonomic dysreflexia, a serious condition that can occur during labor and nursing.

3. *Management and Treatment*:
   - *Hormone Replacement Therapy (HRT)*: For men with low testosterone, testosterone replacement therapy can help restore hormone levels and improve symptoms. Women may benefit from estrogen replacement therapy if needed.
   - *Psychological Support*: Addressing the emotional and relational impacts of sexual dysfunction and infertility is crucial. Counseling can help SCI patients and their partners navigate these challenges.

15.5 Conclusions

Spinal cord injury (SCI) is a complex condition that disrupts multiple bodily systems, leading to significant hematological and endocrinological complications. The systemic inflammatory response that follows SCI and the autonomic sympathetic nervous system dysfunction plays a central role in the development of infections, impaired healing, and a heightened risk of thromboembolic events, such as deep venous thrombosis (DVT) and pulmonary embolism (PE). In addition, the disruption of the hypothalamic-pituitary-gonadal and thyroid axes contributes to metabolic and hormonal imbalances, exacerbating conditions like obesity, osteoporosis, and muscle loss, while also affecting fertility in men. Hematopoietic dysfunction, a key feature of SCI, underscores the need for vigilant monitoring and intervention, as it significantly increases the risk of blood dyscrasias and infections.

The management of SCI-related complications requires a multidisciplinary approach, with strategies varying between the acute and chronic phases. Preventive measures, including early anticoagulation, physical therapy, and mechanical therapies, are essential to minimize the risk of DVT and PE. However, further research is needed to clarify optimal prevention strategies for chronic phases. Addressing metabolic dysfunctions through nutritional interventions, exercise, and hormonal therapies can mitigate the long-term effects of SCI on bone health and cardiovascular risk. Understanding the complex interplay between the hematological and endocrinological systems in SCI patients is vital for improving their quality of life and preventing secondary complications.

References

1. Carpenter RS, Marbourg JM, Brennan FH, Mifflin KA, Hall JCE, Jiang RR, et al. Spinal cord injury causes chronic bone marrow failure. Nat Commun. 2020;11(1):3702.
2. Huang CT, DeVivo MJ, Stover SL. Anemia in acute phase of spinal cord injury. Arch Phys Med Rehabil. 1990;71(1):3–7.
3. Hirsch GH, Menard MR, Anton HA. Anemia after traumatic spinal cord injury. Arch Phys Med Rehabil. 1991;72(3):195–201.
4. Obayashi K, Ando Y, Terazaki H, Yamashita T, Nakamura M, Suga M, et al. Mechanism of anemia associated with autonomic dysfunction in rats. Auton Neurosci. 2000;82(3):123–9.
5. Fuchs A, Monlish DA, Ghosh S, Chang S-W, Bochicchio GV, Schuettpelz LG, et al. Trauma induces emergency hematopoiesis through IL-1/MyD88-dependent production of G-CSF. J Immunol. 2019;202(10):3020–32.
6. Méndez-Ferrer S, Michurina TV, Ferraro F, Mazloom AR, Macarthur BD, Lira SA, et al. Mesenchymal and haematopoietic stem cells form a unique bone marrow niche. Nature. 2010;466(7308):829–34.
7. Miranda AR, Hassouna HI. Mechanisms of thrombosis in spinal cord injury. Hematol Oncol Clin North Am. 2000;14(2):401–16.
8. Teasell RW, Hsieh JT, Aubut J-AL, Eng JJ, Krassioukov A, Tu L, et al. Venous thromboembolism after spinal cord injury. Arch Phys Med Rehabil. 2009;90(2):232–45.
9. Wei B, Zhou H, Liu G, Zheng Y, Zhang Y, Hao C, et al. Risk factors for venous thromboembolism in patients with spinal cord injury: a systematic review and meta-analysis. J Spinal Cord Med. 2023;46(2):181–93.
10. Sen RK, Kumar A, Tripathy SK, Aggarwal S, Khandelwal N, Manoharan SRR. Risk of postoperative venous thromboembolism in Indian patients sustaining pelvi-acetabular injury. Int Orthop. 2011;35(7):1057–63.
11. Eichinger S, Eischer L, Sinkovec H, Wittgruber G, Traby L, Kammer M, et al. Risk of venous thromboembolism during rehabilitation of patients with spinal cord injury. PLoS One. 2018;13(3):e0193735.
12. Maung AA, Schuster KM, Kaplan LJ, Maerz LL, Davis KA. Risk of venous thromboembolism after spinal cord injury: not all levels are the same. J Trauma. 2011;71(5):1241–5.
13. Cheng JS, Arnold PM, Anderson PA, Fischer D, Dettori JR. Anticoagulation risk in spine surgery. Spine. 2010;35(9 Suppl):S117–24.
14. Szlauer A, Mielimonka A, Głowacki R, Borowczyk K, Stachniuk J, Undas A. Protein N-linked homocysteine is associated with recurrence of venous thromboembolism. Thromb Res. 2015;136(5):911–6.
15. Stein PD, Fowler SE, Goodman LR, Gottschalk A, Hales CA, Hull RD, et al. Multidetector computed tomography for acute pulmonary embolism. N Engl J Med. 2006;354(22):2317–27.
16. Gottschalk A, Juni JE, Sostman HD, Coleman RE, Thrall J, McKusick KA, et al. Ventilation-perfusion scintigraphy in the PIOPED study. Part I. Data collection and tabulation. J Nucl Med. 1993;34(7):1109–18.
17. Aito S, Pieri A, D'Andrea M, Marcelli F, Cominelli E. Primary prevention of deep venous thrombosis and pulmonary embolism in acute spinal cord injured patients. Spinal Cord. 2002;40(6):300–3.
18. DeVivo MJ, Kartus PL, Stover SL, Rutt RD, Fine PR. Cause of death for patients with spinal cord injuries. Arch Intern Med. 1989;149(8):1761–6.

19. Germing A, Schakrouf M, Lindstaedt M, Grewe P, Meindl R, Mügge A. Serial compression B-scan and Doppler sonography for the screening of deep venous thrombosis in patients with spinal cord injuries. J Clin Ultrasound. 2010;38(1):17–20.
20. Boudaoud L, Roussi J, Lortat-Jacob S, Bussel B, Dizien O, Drouet L. Endothelial fibrinolytic reactivity and the risk of deep venous thrombosis after spinal cord injury. Spinal Cord. 1997;35(3):151–7.
21. Frisbie JH, Sasahara AA. Low dose heparin prophylaxis for deep venous thrombosis in acute spinal cord injury patients: a controlled study. Paraplegia. 1981;19(6):343–6.
22. Tribe CR. Causes of death in the early and late stages of paraplegia. Paraplegia. 1963;1:19–47.
23. Wolman L. The disturbance of circulation in traumatic paraplegia in acute and late stages: a pathological study. Paraplegia. 1965;2:213–26.
24. Mackiewicz-Milewska M, Kroszczynski A, Cisowska-Adamiak M, Pyskir J, Rosc D, Hagner W. Hemostatic parameters in patients with spinal cord injury in subacute and chronic phase of the rehabilitation. J Spinal Cord Med. 2021;44(5):782–8.
25. Gando S. Tissue factor in trauma and organ dysfunction. Semin Thromb Hemost. 2006;32(1):48–53.
26. Godat LN, Kobayashi L, Chang DC, Coimbra R. Can we ever stop worrying about venous thromboembolism after trauma? J Trauma Acute Care Surg. 2015;78(3):475–80; discussion 480–1.
27. Mackman N. The role of tissue factor and factor VIIa in hemostasis. Anesth Analg. 2009;108(5):1447–52.
28. Alabed S, de Heredia LL, Naidoo A, Belci M, Hughes RJ, Meagher TM. Incidence of pulmonary embolism after the first 3 months of spinal cord injury. Spinal Cord. 2015;53(11):835–7.
29. Oger E. Incidence of venous thromboembolism: a community-based study in Western France. EPI-GETBP Study Group. Groupe d'Etude de la Thrombose de Bretagne Occidentale. Thromb Haemost. 2000;83(5):657–60.
30. Jones T, Ugalde V, Franks P, Zhou H, White RH. Venous thromboembolism after spinal cord injury: incidence, time course, and associated risk factors in 16,240 adults and children. Arch Phys Med Rehabil. 2005;86(12):2240–7.
31. Furlan JC, Fehlings MG. Role of screening tests for deep venous thrombosis in asymptomatic adults with acute spinal cord injury: an evidence-based analysis. Spine. 2007;32(17):1908–16.
32. Ploumis A, Ponnappan RK, Bessey JT, Patel R, Vaccaro AR. Thromboprophylaxis in spinal trauma surgery: consensus among spine trauma surgeons. Spine J. 2009;9(7):530–6.
33. Lamb GC, Tomski MA, Kaufman J, Maiman DJ. Is chronic spinal cord injury associated with increased risk of venous thromboembolism? J Am Paraplegia Soc. 1993;16(3):153–6.
34. Mackiewicz-Milewska M, Jung S, Kroszczyński AC, Mackiewicz-Nartowicz H, Serafin Z, Cisowska-Adamiak M, et al. Deep venous thrombosis in patients with chronic spinal cord injury. J Spinal Cord Med. 2016;39(4):400–4.
35. Halim TA, Chhabra HS, Arora M, Kumar S. Pharmacological prophylaxis for deep vein thrombosis in acute spinal cord injury: an Indian perspective. Spinal Cord. 2014;52(7):547–50.
36. Green D, Lee MY, Ito VY, Cohn T, Press J, Filbrandt PR, et al. Fixed- vs adjusted-dose heparin in the prophylaxis of thromboembolism in spinal cord injury. JAMA. 1988;260(9):1255–8.
37. Green D, Lee MY, Lim AC, Chmiel JS, Vetter M, Pang T, et al. Prevention of thromboembolism after spinal cord injury using low-molecular-weight heparin. Ann Intern Med. 1990;113(8):571–4.
38. Martel N, Lee J, Wells PS. Risk for heparin-induced thrombocytopenia with unfractionated and low-molecular-weight heparin thromboprophylaxis: a meta-analysis. Blood. 2005;106(8):2710–5.
39. Spinal Cord Injury Thromboprophylaxis Investigators. Prevention of venous thromboembolism in the acute treatment phase after spinal cord injury: a randomized, multicenter trial comparing low-dose heparin plus intermittent pneumatic compression with enoxaparin. J Trauma. 2003;54(6):1116–24; discussion 1125–6.

40. Merli GJ, Herbison GJ, Ditunno JF, Weitz HH, Henzes JH, Park CH, et al. Deep vein thrombosis: prophylaxis in acute spinal cord injured patients. Arch Phys Med Rehabil. 1988;69(9):661–4.
41. Szollar SM, Martin EM, Sartoris DJ, Parthemore JG, Deftos LJ. Bone mineral density and indexes of bone metabolism in spinal cord injury. Am J Phys Med Rehabil. 1998;77(1):28–35.
42. Morse LR, Giangregorio L, Battaglino RA, Holland R, Craven BC, Stolzmann KL, et al. VA-based survey of osteoporosis management in spinal cord injury. PM R. 2009;1(3):240–4.
43. Garland DE, Saucedo T, Reiser TV. The management of tibial fractures in acute spinal cord injury patients. Clin Orthop Relat Res. 1986;213:237–40.
44. Ragnarsson KT, Sell GH. Lower extremity fractures after spinal cord injury: a retrospective study. Arch Phys Med Rehabil. 1981;62(9):418–23.
45. Abderhalden L, Weaver FM, Bethel M, Demirtas H, Burns S, Svircev J, et al. Dual-energy X-ray absorptiometry and fracture prediction in patients with spinal cord injuries and disorders. Osteoporos Int. 2017;28(3):925–34.
46. Frost HM. The mechanostat: a proposed pathogenic mechanism of osteoporoses and the bone mass effects of mechanical and nonmechanical agents. Bone Miner. 1987;2(2):73–85.
47. Uebelhart D, Hartmann D, Vuagnat H, Castanier M, Hachen HJ, Chantraine A. Early modifications of biochemical markers of bone metabolism in spinal cord injury patients. A preliminary study. Scand J Rehabil Med. 1994;26(4):197–202.
48. Dauty M, Perrouin Verbe B, Maugars Y, Dubois C, Mathe JF. Supralesional and sublesional bone mineral density in spinal cord-injured patients. Bone. 2000;27(2):305–9.
49. Stewart AF, Adler M, Byers CM, Segre GV, Broadus AE. Calcium homeostasis in immobilization: an example of resorptive hypercalciuria. N Engl J Med. 1982;306(19):1136–40.
50. Gifre L, Ruiz-Gaspà S, Carrasco JL, Portell E, Vidal J, Muxi A, et al. Effect of recent spinal cord injury on the OPG/RANKL system and its relationship with bone loss and the response to denosumab therapy. Osteoporos Int. 2017;28(9):2707–15.
51. Li X, Ominsky MS, Niu Q-T, Sun N, Daugherty B, D'Agostin D, et al. Targeted deletion of the sclerostin gene in mice results in increased bone formation and bone strength. J Bone Miner Res. 2008;23(6):860–9.
52. Wijenayaka AR, Kogawa M, Lim HP, Bonewald LF, Findlay DM, Atkins GJ. Sclerostin stimulates osteocyte support of osteoclast activity by a RANKL-dependent pathway. PLoS One. 2011;6(10):e25900.
53. Battaglino RA, Lazzari AA, Garshick E, Morse LR. Spinal cord injury-induced osteoporosis: pathogenesis and emerging therapies. Curr Osteoporos Rep. 2012;10(4):278–85.
54. Roberts D, Lee W, Cuneo RC, Wittmann J, Ward G, Flatman R, et al. Longitudinal study of bone turnover after acute spinal cord injury. J Clin Endocrinol Metab. 1998;83(2):415–22.
55. Maïmoun L, Couret I, Mariano-Goulart D, Dupuy AM, Micallef J-P, Peruchon E, et al. Changes in osteoprotegerin/RANKL system, bone mineral density, and bone biochemicals markers in patients with recent spinal cord injury. Calcif Tissue Int. 2005;76(6):404–11.
56. Zehnder Y, Lüthi M, Michel D, Knecht H, Perrelet R, Neto I, et al. Long-term changes in bone metabolism, bone mineral density, quantitative ultrasound parameters, and fracture incidence after spinal cord injury: a cross-sectional observational study in 100 paraplegic men. Osteoporos Int. 2004;15(3):180–9.
57. Vaziri ND, Pandian MR, Segal JL, Winer RL, Eltorai I, Brunnemann S. Vitamin D, parathormone, and calcitonin profiles in persons with long-standing spinal cord injury. Arch Phys Med Rehabil. 1994;75(7):766–9.
58. Dimitri P, Rosen C. The central nervous system and bone metabolism: an evolving story. Calcif Tissue Int. 2017;100(5):476–85.
59. Elefteriou F, Ahn JD, Takeda S, Starbuck M, Yang X, Liu X, et al. Leptin regulation of bone resorption by the sympathetic nervous system and CART. Nature. 2005;434(7032):514–20.
60. Ji-Ye H, Xin-Feng Z, Lei-Sheng J. Autonomic control of bone formation: its clinical relevance. Handb Clin Neurol. 2013;117:161–71.

61. Alexander MS, Biering-Sorensen F, Bodner D, Brackett NL, Cardenas D, Charlifue S, et al. International standards to document remaining autonomic function after spinal cord injury. Spinal Cord. 2009;47(1):36–43.
62. Mechanick JI, Pomerantz F, Flanagan S, Stein A, Gordon WA, Ragnarsson KT. Parathyroid hormone suppression in spinal cord injury patients is associated with the degree of neurologic impairment and not the level of injury. Arch Phys Med Rehabil. 1997;78(7):692–6.
63. Elder CP, Apple DF, Bickel CS, Meyer RA, Dudley GA. Intramuscular fat and glucose tolerance after spinal cord injury–a cross-sectional study. Spinal Cord. 2004;42(12):711–6.
64. Wang YH, Huang TS, Lien IN. Hormone changes in men with spinal cord injuries. Am J Phys Med Rehabil. 1992;71(6):328–32.
65. Tsitouras PD, Zhong YG, Spungen AM, Bauman WA. Serum testosterone and growth hormone/insulin-like growth factor-I in adults with spinal cord injury. Horm Metab Res. 1995;27(6):287–92.
66. Huang TS, Wang YH, Lai JS, Chang CC, Lien IN. The hypothalamus-pituitary-ovary and hypothalamus-pituitary-thyroid axes in spinal cord-injured women. Metabolism. 1996;45(6):718–22.
67. Rahmani A, Shahbandi A, Ghashghaie S, Ghodsi Z, Khazaeipour Z, Abbaszadeh M, et al. Factors affecting sexual health in individuals with spinal cord injury: a systematic scoping review. Chin J Traumatol [Internet]. 2024;28; Available from: https://doi.org/10.1016/j.cjtee.2024.05.002.
68. Morse LR, Biering-Soerensen F, Carbone LD, Cervinka T, Cirnigliaro CM, Johnston TE, et al. Bone mineral density testing in spinal cord injury: 2019 ISCD official position. J Clin Densitom. 2019;22(4):554–66.
69. Gifre L, Vidal J, Carrasco J, Portell E, Puig J, Monegal A, et al. Incidence of skeletal fractures after traumatic spinal cord injury: a 10-year follow-up study. Clin Rehabil. 2014;28(4):361–9.
70. Lala D, Craven BC, Thabane L, Papaioannou A, Adachi JD, Popovic MR, et al. Exploring the determinants of fracture risk among individuals with spinal cord injury. Osteoporos Int. 2014;25(1):177–85.
71. Pelletier CA, Dumont FS, Leblond J, Noreau L, Giangregorio L, Craven BC. Self-report of one-year fracture incidence and osteoporosis prevalence in a community cohort of canadians with spinal cord injury. Top Spinal Cord Inj Rehabil. 2014;20(4):302–9.
72. Farkas GJ, Pitot MA, Berg AS, Gater DR. Nutritional status in chronic spinal cord injury: a systematic review and meta-analysis. Spinal Cord. 2019;57(1):3–17.
73. Javidan AN, Sabour H, Latifi S, Vafa M, Shidfar F, Khazaeipour Z, et al. Calcium and vitamin D plasma concentration and nutritional intake status in patients with chronic spinal cord injury: a referral center report. J Res Med Sci. 2014;19(9):881–4.
74. Koutrakis NE, Goldstein RL, Walia P, Polak MM, Lazzari AA, Tun CG, et al. Vitamin D, diet, and lifestyle in a chronic SCI population. Spinal Cord. 2019;57(2):117–27.
75. Walters JL, Buchholz AC, Martin Ginis KA, SHAPE-SCI Research Group. Evidence of dietary inadequacy in adults with chronic spinal cord injury. Spinal Cord. 2009;47(4):318–22.
76. Flueck JL, Perret C. Vitamin D deficiency in individuals with a spinal cord injury: a literature review. Spinal Cord. 2017;55(5):428–34.
77. Alekna V, Tamulaitiene M, Sinevicius T, Juocevicius A. Effect of weight-bearing activities on bone mineral density in spinal cord injured patients during the period of the first two years. Spinal Cord. 2008;46(11):727–32.
78. Giangregorio LM, Webber CE, Phillips SM, Hicks AL, Craven BC, Bugaresti JM, et al. Can body weight supported treadmill training increase bone mass and reverse muscle atrophy in individuals with chronic incomplete spinal cord injury? Appl Physiol Nutr Metab. 2006;31(3):283–91.
79. Ogilvie C, Bowker P, Rowley DI. The physiological benefits of paraplegic orthotically aided walking. Paraplegia. 1993;31(2):111–5.

80. Thoumie P, Le Claire G, Beillot J, Dassonville J, Chevalier T, Perrouin-Verbe B, et al. Restoration of functional gait in paraplegic patients with the RGO-II hybrid orthosis. A multicenter controlled study. II: physiological evaluation. Paraplegia. 1995;33(11):654–9.
81. Dudley-Javoroski S, Saha PK, Liang G, Li C, Gao Z, Shields RK. High dose compressive loads attenuate bone mineral loss in humans with spinal cord injury. Osteoporos Int. 2012;23(9):2335–46.
82. Frotzler A, Coupaud S, Perret C, Kakebeeke TH, Hunt KJ, Donaldson N d N, et al. High-volume FES-cycling partially reverses bone loss in people with chronic spinal cord injury. Bone. 2008;43(1):169–76.
83. Chen S-C, Lai C-H, Chan WP, Huang M-H, Tsai H-W, Chen J-JJ. Increases in bone mineral density after functional electrical stimulation cycling exercises in spinal cord injured patients. Disabil Rehabil. 2005;27(22):1337–41.
84. Mohr T, Podenphant J, Biering-Sorensen F, Galbo H, Thamsborg G, Kjaer M. Increased bone mineral density after prolonged electrically induced cycle training of paralyzed limbs in spinal cord injured man. Calcif Tissue Int. 1997;61(1):22–5.
85. Zehnder Y, Risi S, Michel D, Knecht H, Perrelet R, Kraenzlin M, et al. Prevention of bone loss in paraplegics over 2 years with alendronate. J Bone Miner Res. 2004;19(7):1067–74.
86. Alberti KGMM, Zimmet P, Shaw J, IDF Epidemiology Task Force Consensus Group. The metabolic syndrome–a new worldwide definition. Lancet. 2005;366(9491):1059–62.
87. Gater DR Jr, Farkas GJ, Berg AS, Castillo C. Prevalence of metabolic syndrome in veterans with spinal cord injury. J Spinal Cord Med. 2019;42(1):86–93.
88. Gater DR Jr, Farkas GJ, Tiozzo E. Pathophysiology of neurogenic obesity after spinal cord injury. Top Spinal Cord Inj Rehabil. 2021;27(1):1–10.
89. Heymsfield SB, Lichtman S, Baumgartner RN, Wang J, Kamen Y, Aliprantis A, et al. Body composition of humans: comparison of two improved four-compartment models that differ in expense, technical complexity, and radiation exposure. Am J Clin Nutr. 1990;52(1):52–8.
90. Bauman WA, Spungen AM. Disorders of carbohydrate and lipid metabolism in veterans with paraplegia or quadriplegia: a model of premature aging. Metabolism. 1994;43(6):749–56.
91. Duckworth WC, Jallepalli P, Solomon SS. Glucose intolerance in spinal cord injury. Arch Phys Med Rehabil. 1983;64(3):107–10.
92. Laughton GE, Buchholz AC, Martin Ginis KA, Goy RE, SHAPE SCI Research Group. Lowering body mass index cutoffs better identifies obese persons with spinal cord injury. Spinal Cord. 2009;47(10):757–62.
93. Gibson AE, Buchholz AC, Martin Ginis KA, SHAPE-SCI Research Group. C-reactive protein in adults with chronic spinal cord injury: increased chronic inflammation in tetraplegia vs paraplegia. Spinal Cord. 2008;46(9):616–21.
94. Liang H, Mojtahedi MC, Chen D, Braunschweig CL. Elevated C-reactive protein associated with decreased high-density lipoprotein cholesterol in men with spinal cord injury. Arch Phys Med Rehabil. 2008;89(1):36–41.
95. Lebovitz HE, Banerji MA. Point: visceral adiposity is causally related to insulin resistance. Diabetes Care. 2005;28(9):2322–5.
96. Aso Y, Wakabayashi S, Yamamoto R, Matsutomo R, Takebayashi K, Inukai T. Metabolic syndrome accompanied by hypercholesterolemia is strongly associated with proinflammatory state and impairment of fibrinolysis in patients with type 2 diabetes: synergistic effects of plasminogen activator inhibitor-1 and thrombin-activatable fibrinolysis inhibitor. Diabetes Care. 2005;28(9):2211–6.
97. Herman P, Stein A, Gibbs K, Korsunsky I, Gregersen P, Bloom O. Persons with chronic spinal cord injury have decreased natural killer cell and increased toll-like receptor/inflammatory gene expression. J Neurotrauma. 2018;35(15):1819–29.
98. Rodriguez DJ, Benzel EC, Clevenger FW. The metabolic response to spinal cord injury. Spinal Cord. 1997;35(9):599–604.

99. Schwartz MW, Woods SC, Porte D Jr, Seeley RJ, Baskin DG. Central nervous system control of food intake. Nature. 2000;404(6778):661–71.
100. Bauman WA, La Fountaine MF, Spungen AM. Age-related prevalence of low testosterone in men with spinal cord injury. J Spinal Cord Med. 2014;37(1):32–9.
101. Sullivan SD, Nash MS, Tefera E, Tinsley E, Blackman MR, Groah S. Prevalence and etiology of hypogonadism in young men with chronic spinal cord injury: a cross-sectional analysis from two university-based rehabilitation centers. PM R. 2017;9(8):751–60.
102. La Fountaine MF, Wecht JM, Cirnigliaro CM, Kirshblum SC, Spungen AM, Bauman WA. Testosterone replacement therapy improves QTaVI in hypogonadal men with spinal cord injury. Neuroendocrinology. 2013;97(4):341–6.
103. Clark MJ, Schopp LH, Mazurek MO, Zaniletti I, Lammy AB, Martin TA, et al. Testosterone levels among men with spinal cord injury: relationship between time since injury and laboratory values. Am J Phys Med Rehabil. 2008;87(9):758–67.
104. Schopp LH, Clark M, Mazurek MO, Hagglund KJ, Acuff ME, Sherman AK, et al. Testosterone levels among men with spinal cord injury admitted to inpatient rehabilitation. Am J Phys Med Rehabil. 2006;85(8):678–84; quiz 685–7.
105. Celik B, Sahin A, Caglar N, Erhan B, Gunduz B, Gultekin O, et al. Sex hormone levels and functional outcomes: a controlled study of patients with spinal cord injury compared with healthy subjects. Am J Phys Med Rehabil. 2007;86(10):784–90.
106. Safarinejad MR. Level of injury and hormone profiles in spinal cord-injured men. Urology. 2001;58(5):671–6.
107. Durga A, Sepahpanah F, Regozzi M, Hastings J, Crane DA. Prevalence of testosterone deficiency after spinal cord injury. PM R. 2011;3(10):929–32.
108. Anderson KD. Targeting recovery: priorities of the spinal cord-injured population. J Neurotrauma. 2004;21(10):1371–83.
109. Ibrahim E, Brackett NL, Lynne CM. Advances in the management of infertility in men with spinal cord injury. Asian J Androl. 2016;18(3):382–90.
110. Ibrahim E, Lynne CM, Brackett NL. Male fertility following spinal cord injury: an update. Andrology. 2016;4(1):13–26.
111. Brackett NL, Ibrahim E, Iremashvili V, Aballa TC, Lynne CM. Treatment for ejaculatory dysfunction in men with spinal cord injury: an 18-year single center experience. J Urol. 2010;183(6):2304–8.
112. Lue TF. Erectile dysfunction. N Engl J Med. 2000;342(24):1802–13.
113. Ehsanian R, Creasey G, Elliott CS, Abu-Eid CA, Ali A, Prutton M, et al. Implantation of sacral nerve stimulator without Rhizotomy for neurogenic bladder in patient with spinal cord injury: 2-dimensional operative video. Oper Neurosurg (Hagerstown). 2020;19(3):E299.
114. Morlière C, Verpillot E, Donon L, Salmi L-R, Joseph P-A, Vignes J-R, et al. A cost-utility analysis of sacral anterior root stimulation (SARS) compared with medical treatment in patients with complete spinal cord injury with a neurogenic bladder. Spine J. 2015;15(12):2472–83.
115. Crane DA, Doody DR, Schiff MA, Mueller BA. Pregnancy outcomes in women with spinal cord injuries: a population-based study. PM R. 2019;11(8):795–806.

16 Gastrointestinal and Genitourinary Dysfunction: Acute and Long-Term Management in Patients with Traumatic Spinal Cord Injury

Gianluca Sampogna, Luigi Rizzato, and Michele Spinelli

16.1 Introduction

Traumatic spinal cord injury (SCI) is a shocking event that may result in a range of physical, psychological, and social changes. Among them, the gastrointestinal (GI) and genitourinary (GU) dysfunctions represent ones of the most impactful modifications, severely altering the quality of life (QoL). These dysfunctions, commonly referred to as neurogenic bowel dysfunction (NBD) and neurogenic lower urinary tract dysfunction (NLUTD), arise due to the disruption of the neural pathways that control bowel and bladder functions. Without proper management, these conditions can lead to serious complications, including ileus, life-threatening urinary tract infections (UTIs), renal failure, and autonomic dysreflexia (AD).

This chapter explores the pathophysiology, acute management strategies, and long-term care for bowel and bladder in patients with traumatic SCI, reporting the issues to consider when dealing with this condition (Table 16.1). We also highlight the latest research and treatment advances, which offer new hope for improving outcomes in this challenging patient population.

G. Sampogna · L. Rizzato · M. Spinelli (✉)
Neuro-Urology Service, Unipolar Spinal Unit, Niguarda Hospital, Milan, Italy
e-mail: michele.spinelli@ospedaleniguarda.it

E. Brogi et al. (eds.), *Traumatic Spinal Cord Injury*, Hot Topics in Acute Care Surgery and Trauma, https://doi.org/10.1007/978-3-031-99890-4_16

Table 16.1 Acute and long-term issues to consider for the bladder and bowel management after spinal cord injury

Bowel	Bladder
Acute management	
Bowel program	Bladder decompression
Parenteral nutrition	Intermittent catheterizations
Prokinetic agents	Bladder outcome
Long-term management	
Bowel program	Bladder emptying techniques
Dietary management	Incontinence products
Pharmacotherapy	Pharmacotherapy
Pelvic floor muscle therapy	Pelvic floor muscle therapy
Transanal irrigation	Botulinum toxin injections
Major surgery	Major surgery
Complications to prevent and diagnose early: Gastrointestinal bleeding, cholelithiasis, small intestinal bacterial overgrowth	Complications to prevent and diagnose early: Urinary tract infections, urolithiasis, vesicoureteral reflux, bladder cancer
Autonomic dysreflexia	
Sexual health and fertility	
Psychological support	
Patient education and empowerment	
Caregiver burden	
Economic sustainability	
Telemedicine and remote monitoring	
Personalized medicine	
Experimental treatments (e.g., neuromodulation, regenerative medicine)	

16.2 Pathophysiology of Gastrointestinal and Genitourinary Dysfunction

16.2.1 Impact of Spinal Cord Injury

The neurogenic control of the GI and GU systems goes beyond the scope of this chapter [1]. The ability to control bladder and bowel emptying is the last function that Homo sapiens learns during development; indeed, children start walking and talking before diaper weaning, so before being able to avoid defecation and micturition at inappropriate times. In this context, the spinal cord plays a critical role in the regulation of GI and GU functions, representing a conduit for neural signals between the brain and the body which are dependent on both the somatic nervous system (SNS) and the autonomic nervous system (ANS) to regulate involuntary functions of the GI and GU systems [2].

16.2.1.1 Gastrointestinal System

The enteric nervous system, sometimes called the "second brain," operates independently of the central nervous system (CNS) but is heavily influenced by the ANS. Sympathetic fibers, originating from the thoracolumbar segments (T5-L2), inhibit GI motility, while parasympathetic fibers from the vagus nerve and sacral spinal segments (S2-S4) promote motility. Disruption of these pathways following SCI results in NBD, characterized by impaired motility, constipation, and fecal incontinence (FI) [3, 4]. Unlike the bladder, the level of the neurological lesion does not determine precisely which sequelae will be produced on bowel function.

16.2.1.2 Genitourinary System

The neurogenic control of the GU system is based on both the SNS and ANS. The physiological bladder cycle encompasses two phases. During the filling phase, bladder distention takes place under low pressures due to the influence of the sympathetic nervous system, via the T10–L2 nerve roots, while the external urinary sphincter remains closed via the pudendal nerves originating from the S2–S4 nerve roots. During the voiding phase, the bladder contracts under the influence of the parasympathetic nervous system, via the S2–S4 nerve roots, and the urinary sphincter relaxes to allow emptying. SCI disrupts these neural pathways, leading to NLUTD, which includes different clinical scenarios: urinary retention (UR), urinary incontinence (UI), detrusor underactivity (DU), detrusor overactivity (DO), detrusor sphincter dyssynergia (DSS), and high post-void residual (PVR) [5, 6]. In particular, the NLUTD-related clinical presentation is predominantly due to the location and the extent of the neurological lesion:

- Suprapontine lesions
  - Examples: Parkinson's disease, Alzheimer's disease, stroke, traumatic brain injury
  - History: predominantly storage symptoms
  - Findings: DO, insignificant PVR
- Spinal lesions between the pons and the sacral cord
  - Examples: SCI, spina bifida
  - History: both storage and voiding symptoms
  - Findings: DO, DSS, usually raised PVR
- Sacral and infrasacral lesions
  - Examples: lumbar degenerative disc disease, iatrogenic pelvic nerve lesions, peripheral neuropathy (e.g., due to diabetes)
  - History: predominantly voiding symptoms
  - Findings: DU, a contractile detrusor, high PVR
- Multiple sclerosis is a disseminated disease, so it can present different and overlapping clinical features based on the extent and localization of demyelination plaques.

16.2.2 Acute Phase

Immediately after SCI, the body often enters a state of *spinal shock*, characterized by the temporary loss of reflex activity below the level of injury. This phase, which can last from days to weeks/months, is associated with several acute GI and GU changes [7, 8].

During the acute phase, patients frequently develop *ileus*, a condition where bowel motility is severely impaired, leading to abdominal distension, pain, and constipation [9]. Additionally, gastroparesis, characterized by delayed gastric emptying, can exacerbate nutritional challenges by causing nausea, vomiting, and a reduced ability to tolerate oral or enteral feeding [10].

UR is a hallmark of the acute phase of SCI, resulting from the disruption of neural pathways that control bladder function [11]. The first description of a patient with SCI is reported in the Edwin Smith papyrus and, among many issues, the patient suffered from overflow incontinence due to bladder overdistension, highlighting visceral alterations as peculiarities of SCI [12]. This can be prevented with the placement of an indwelling catheter, which poses the risk for UTIs [13].

Moreover, bladder distension may trigger AD in people with a neurological level of injury (NLI) above T6; even if it may occur within several weeks since the injury, AD is usually observed in the chronic stage of SCI (i.e., after 1 year since the injury) [14]. AD is a potentially life-threatening condition characterized by the ANS not working properly and is associated with an altered response to stimuli below the NLI. This impairment may manifest as a wide range of symptoms, including headache, tachycardia, tachypnea, hyperthermia, flushing, nasal congestion, piloerection, sweating, pallor, chills, convulsions, severe hypertension, retinal detachments, myocardial ischemia, arrhythmias, pulmonary oedema, and hemorrhagic stroke. Systolic blood pressure over a baseline of at least 20 mmHg is the cardinal finding of AD. Besides bladder distension, other triggers for AD are represented by bowel distension, pain, acute abdominal pathology, UTIs, skeletal fractures, pressure ulcers, tight clothing or footwear, ingrown toenail, urolithiasis, hemorrhoids, sexual activity, and uterine contractions.

16.3 Acute Management Strategies

16.3.1 Gastrointestinal Management

Effective management of GI dysfunction during the acute phase of SCI is crucial to prevent complications and support the patient's recovery.

Early initiation of a *bowel care regimen* is essential to prevent complications like fecal impaction. This typically involves the use of stool softeners, laxatives, and enemas to encourage bowel movements [15, 16]. High-fiber diets and adequate fluid intake are recommended as soon as they can be safely implemented, although care must be taken to avoid exacerbating symptoms of ileus or gastroparesis. The aim is to guarantee 3–4 evacuations per week.

In cases where severe ileus or gastroparesis limits the ability to provide adequate nutrition enterally, *parenteral nutrition* may be necessary to maintain nutritional status and prevent further complications [17]. However, this approach carries risks, including infections associated with central lines, which must be carefully managed.

The *prokinetic agents*, such as metoclopramide, may help to stimulate GI motility and reduce the duration of ileus or gastroparesis: they can improve the patient's tolerance to oral or enteral feeding and promote earlier nutritional support [18].

16.3.2 Genitourinary Management

The primary objective in managing GU dysfunction during the acute phase is to prevent UR and its associated complications, like UTIs and renal failure.

Immediate *bladder decompression*, typically with the placement of an indwelling bladder catheter, is critical in preventing bladder distension [19]. Regular monitoring of urine output and bladder volumes is essential to ensure that bladder emptying is adequate and to prevent complications like bladder overdistension.

As spinal shock resolves, transitioning to *intermittent catheterization* (IC) can help reduce the risk of UTIs and maintain bladder function [20, 21]. The IC, which involves scheduled bladder emptying at regular intervals, is generally preferred over continuous catheterization with indwelling catheters due to the lower risk of UTIs and bladder defunctionalization. The number of voids per day should be 4–6, avoiding a bladder filling >500 ml each time.

Bladder overdistension may trigger AD, so vigilant monitoring for its signs is mandatory: in this case, early intervention is essential through bladder decompression and the use of antihypertensive agents if necessary [22].

16.4 Long-Term Management of Gastrointestinal Dysfunction

16.4.1 Chronic Neurogenic Bowel Dysfunction

NBD is a chronic condition in patients with SCI, characterized by constipation, FI, or both, that requires a long-term management to establish a consistent bowel routine by adopting the following solutions:

- *Bowel Program*: A structured bowel program, tailored to the individual needs of the patient, is essential. This typically includes dietary modifications, regular bowel movements, and the use of pharmacologic agents. Manual techniques, like digital rectal stimulation, may also be necessary, even if not encouraged [23]. The Monitoring Efficacy of NBD Treatment On Response (MENTOR) tool can be used to monitor the NBD treatment and change it according to the patient's status [24].
- *Diet*: A diet high in fiber, combined with adequate hydration and regular physical activity, can enhance bowel motility and reduce the risk of constipation [25]. However, dietary recommendations must be individualized based on the patient's overall health status and any other comorbidities.

- *Pharmacotherapy*: Chronic NBD often requires the use of medications like the following ones [26–29]:
  - *Bulk-Forming Laxatives*: They increase the bulk of the stool and promote peristalsis. Examples: psyllium, methylcellulose, and polycarbophil.
  - *Osmotic Laxatives*: They draw water into the bowel, soften the stool, and ease its transit. Examples: polyethylene glycol (PEG), lactulose, and magnesium citrate.
  - *Stimulant Laxatives*: They stimulate the intestinal wall to increase muscle contractions, accelerating the stool transit. Examples: bisacodyl, senna, and cascara.
  - *Stool Softeners*: They reduce the surface tension of stool, allowing water and fats to penetrate, finally softening the stool. Example: docusate sodium.
  - *Lubricant Laxatives*: They coat the stool and the bowel with a waterproof film, making stool easier to pass. Example: mineral oil.
  - *Others*: Peripherally acting mu-opioid receptor antagonists (PAMORAs) or prokinetic agents may be considered in patients not responding to previous therapies [30, 31].
  - ***Standard Approach:*** Dietary fibers with bulking properties (e.g., psyllium) and osmotically active substances (e.g., PEG) should be used regularly to modulate stool and support bowel function, while stimulant laxatives (e.g., bisacodyl) should only be used for short periods in case of worsened constipation. If the patient takes PEG in the afternoon, we encourage evacuation in the next morning, with the use of glycerin suppositories and/or microenemas to start and/or to complete evacuation, limiting digitation to reduce the risk of lacerations/traumas.
- *Pelvic Floor Muscle Therapy*: Pelvic floor muscle therapy (PFMT) helps improve anorectal control, reduce FI, and enhance bowel evacuation. The exercises target the muscles involved in sphincter control, increasing their strength and endurance. Regular PFMT with the use of biofeedback proved to improve the symptoms of FI and constipation in individuals with SCI [32].
- *Transanal Irrigation*: Transanal irrigation (TAI) is a highly effective method for managing NBD in people with SCI [33]. TAI involves the introduction of water into the rectum through a catheter to stimulate bowel movements, facilitating the evacuation of stool from the last colon tract at a predictable time [34]. This technique can significantly improve bowel evacuation, reduce the frequency of FI episodes, moderate the risk for bowel-related AD, and enhance the overall QoL [35]. Several types of TAI systems are available, ranging from simple enema kits to more sophisticated devices that allow for controlled water flow and pressure. The system choice depends on the patient's NLI, manual dexterity, and individual preferences. Some systems are designed for self-administration, while others may require assistance from a caregiver. However, TAI may be associated with severe complications, including abdominal discomfort, rectal irritation, and, in rare cases, bowel perforation. Therefore, preventive coloscopy, proper training in the use of TAI systems, and regular follow-up with a healthcare provider are essential to ensure safe and effective use.

- *Surgical Interventions*: In cases of severe and refractory NBD, surgical options such as a colostomy or Malone antegrade continence enema (MACE) may be necessary [36]. The MACE requires an appendicostomy, i.e., a surgically created channel between the abdomen and the colon through the appendix use. In case of an unavailable appendix for previous appendicectomy or inadequate morphology, an ileum tract may be used as in the Monti-Mitrofranoff procedure. This allows an increased bowel emptying with an enema at the beginning of the colon instead of at the end through the rectum. These procedures can provide significant relief and improve the QoL for patients who have not responded to conservative treatments [37]. The decision to pursue surgical intervention should be based on a thorough discussion of the risks and benefits [38].

16.4.2 Gastrointestinal Complications

NBD May Be Associated with Several Long-Term Complications

- *Gastrointestinal Bleeding*: GI bleeding is a serious complication in SCI patients, particularly those who are taking NSAIDs or have other risk factors (e.g., peptic ulcer disease). We advocate regular monitoring for signs of bleeding through occult blood in stool and endoscopic evaluation [39].
- *Cholelithiasis*: The risk of gallstone formation is elevated in patients with SCI due to altered bile composition and reduced physical activity. Preventive measures, like maintaining a healthy weight and avoiding rapid weight loss, can help reduce this risk. Surgical intervention, typically cholecystectomy, may be required for symptomatic gallstones, even if some authors advocate this procedure prophylactically in people with SCI [40].
- *Small Intestinal Bacterial Overgrowth (SIBO)*: SIBO can occur due to impaired motility and altered gut flora in patients with SCI. This condition is often characterized by symptoms such as bloating, diarrhea, and malabsorption. Treatment typically involves the use of antibiotics to reduce bacterial overgrowth, along with dietary modifications and the use of probiotics to restore gut balance [41].

16.5 Long-Term Management of Genitourinary Dysfunction

16.5.1 Neurogenic Lower Urinary Tract Dysfunction

NLUTD presents ongoing challenges for patients with SCI, necessitating a comprehensive approach to long-term management through different strategies:

- *Bladder Emptying Techniques*: Various methods are available for long-term management of NLUTD, including IC, indwelling catheters, and suprapubic catheters [42]. The choice of technique should be based on the patient's NLI, hand function, and personal preferences. The IC is preferred due to its lower risk of UTI, besides preserving bladder integrity and function.

- *Pharmacotherapy*: Medications play a key role in managing NLUTD. Anticholinergics (e.g., oxybutynin, tolterodine) and beta-3-agonists are commonly used to reduce DO and increase storage capacity. Other drugs, such as alpha-blockers, may be used to facilitate bladder emptying and reduce symptoms related to chronic UR [43, 44].
- *Pelvic Floor Muscle Therapy*: PFMT may help in managing stress UI and OAB [45]. Studies demonstrated that PFMT could improve bladder control and reduce the frequency of UI episodes [46]. It involves exercises that focus on the contraction and relaxation of the pelvic floor muscles, which can be guided by a healthcare provider or through telerehabilitation platforms.
- *Botulinum Toxin Injections*: For patients with refractory DO, intradetrusor injections of botulinum toxin under direct endoscopic vision can provide significant relief by reducing involuntary detrusor contractions and increasing bladder capacity [47]. This procedure may be performed on an outpatient basis and needs to be repeated periodically, as the effects usually last 9–10 months. In case of DSD, botulinum toxin may be injected into the external urinary sphincter, inducing patients to empty their bladder by reflex voiding usually into a urinary condom.
- *Surgical Interventions*: In some cases, surgical options such as bladder augmentation, urinary diversion, or sphincterotomy may be necessary to improve bladder management and prevent upper urinary tract deterioration. These procedures are generally reserved for patients who have not responded to more conservative treatments [48, 49].

16.5.2 Complications

Patients with chronic SCI are at increased risk for various GU complications, necessitating ongoing monitoring and management:

- *Urinary Tract Infections*: UTIs are a frequent and serious complication in patients with NLUTD. Long-term management strategies focus on prevention, early detection, and appropriate treatment. Preventive strategies include maintaining a regular bladder emptying schedule, ensuring adequate hydration, keeping a bowel routine, and using ICs with a proper technique and device. Prophylactic antibiotics may be considered in patients with recurrent UTIs, although their use must be weighed against the risk of developing antibiotic resistance [50]. A meta-analysis by Lenger et al. (2020) reported that D-mannose was protective for recurrent UTIs in adult women, possibly with similar effectiveness as antibiotics [51]. Patients and caregivers should be educated on recognizing the early signs of UTIs, such as cloudy urine, foul odor, or increased spasticity [52]. Prompt treatment with appropriate antibiotics is mandatory to prevent complications such as pyelonephritis or urosepsis [53].

- *Urolithiasis*: Patients with SCI are at increased risk of developing bladder, ureteral, or renal stones due to urinary stasis and recurrent UTIs. Regular imaging studies, such as ultrasound or CT scans, may be required for early detection. Surgical intervention may be necessary for the removal of symptomatic stones; in these cases, patient-specific challenges (e.g., the risk for AD in case of high-level SCI) should be considered during pre-operative planning [54].
- *Vescicoureteral Reflux*: Vesicoureteral reflux (VUR) occurs in more than 20% of patients with NLUTD [8]. This condition is more common when the lesion is suprasacral. High detrusor pressure and reflux are responsible for renal damage that may lead to renal failure. Besides treating the VUR itself (e.g., with endoscopic or open techniques), the treatment for reflux also requires the normalization of the detrusor pressure in case of associated DO [55].
- *Bladder Cancer*: The risk of bladder cancer is higher in SCI patients compared to the general population, with squamous cell cancer occurring more commonly than in able-bodied people [56]. The risk factors are UTIs, bladder stones, and indwelling catheters. Unfortunately, the diagnosis is usually made in the more advanced stages, also because macrohematuria episodes are underestimated and thought to be due to inappropriate IC maneuvers.

16.6 Sexual and Reproductive Health

16.6.1 Introduction

Besides GI and GU functions, SCI can severely disrupt the neural pathways that coordinate the organs and structures involved in sexual health and fertility, due to the loss of sensory and motor control, as well as ANS dysfunction. Sexual health is often overlooked in SCI, although it is considered one of the most important areas affecting the QoL of this population [57]. Sexuality in people with SCI may be affected by the new body image, sensory-motor changes, culture, emotions, pain, spasticity, drugs (e.g., baclofen, antidepressants), AD, FI, and UR. The degree of sexual dysfunction largely depends on the NLI and its completeness [58].

Addressing sexual health early, even in the acute phase, is important for setting realistic expectations and initiating early interventions. Patients should be informed about the potential changes in sexual function and the available medical or mechanical aids that can help manage these changes [59]. The psychological impact of these changes can be profound, affecting self-esteem, relationships, and overall QoL. A multidisciplinary approach is essential and may include pharmacological treatments, mechanical aids, counseling, psychotherapy, and, when necessary, assisted reproductive technology (ART).

16.6.2 Sexual Dysfunction

Sexual functions are often compromised in SCI people [60]. They may report alterations in the sensitivity of external genitalia, so healthcare professionals should inform about stimulation of other erogenous zones (e.g., nipples, neck, ear lobes). After SCI, orgasm is compromised in about 50% cases. While women may face challenges with lubrication, men may experience erectile dysfunction (ED) and/or ejaculation disorders. Indeed, antegrade ejaculation is preserved in 15% men, with the other ones experiencing anejaculation or retrograde ejaculation.

Treatment options for sexual dysfunction vary according to the patient's individual needs and preferences. For men, ED may be treated with oral phosphodiesterase inhibitors (e.g., sildenafil, tadalafil), intracavernosal injections, vacuum erection devices, or penile prosthesis implant. Women may benefit from vaginal lubricants, vibratory stimulation, clitoral suction devices, and counseling on alternative sexual practices. Counseling is mandatory and should assess specific topics: besides the ones previously described, indications about sex positions that can be easily adopted with a reduced motor effort, drugs that limit sexual life (e.g., baclofen, antidepressants), the risk for AD during sex, and the importance of looking for initial skin ulcers after sex.

16.6.3 Fertility

SCI can impact fertility, particularly in men, so counseling and reproductive health care should be offered to patients who wish to conceive [61].

Ejaculatory reflex may be induced by penile vibratory stimulation or electroejaculation. If these methods fail, the patient can be referred to the surgical retrieval of spermatozoa through different techniques.

In case of women, menstruations disappear after SCI for a variable time, from 2 weeks to 6 months; later, they resume, and women may be impregnated. Pregnancy in women with SCI is considered high risk because it may exacerbate many of their existing problems, including AD, spasticity, skin ulcers, UTIs, and respiratory infections [62]. Childbirth may be challenging due to many issues (e.g., difficulty with recognizing impending labor, reduced abdominal contractions), so a cesarean section may be safely performed in these cases.

16.7 Psychological and Social Considerations

16.7.1 Impact on Quality of Life

The QoL of people with SCI may be more impacted by the GI and GU dysfunctions than others [57]. Indeed, issues like FI and UI, the need for IC, and chronic constipation can lead to significant physical discomfort, embarrassment, and social isolation [58, 63].

People with SCI requires psychological support and counseling from the very beginning of their rehabilitation to learn how to cope with the challenges of living with these chronic conditions. Overall well-being will benefit from addressing patient-specific concerns such as body image, self-esteem, and anxiety related to bowel and bladder management [64]. Education of patients and caregivers is essential to promote independence while fostering a valid management of GI and GU dysfunctions, which is associated with a valid QoL; similarly, the empowerment of patients to take an active role in their care may improve adherence to treatment regimens and enhance QoL [65, 66].

16.7.2 Socio-economic Impact

The long-term management of NBD and NLUTD may be associated with a significant social and economic impact [67].

A significant burden on caregiver may be provoked by the bowel care through TAI, the bladder management with regular ICs, the prevention of complications, and their management, like UTIs and pressure sores. Therefore, providing support and resources for caregivers is mandatory to prevent burnout and ensure that patients receive adequate care [68, 69].

The cost of long-term management can be substantial to furnish the required medications, supplies, and surgical procedures [70]. In countries without a universally public healthcare system, access to the necessary care may be a significant challenge for people with SCI, with the risk of exposing them to life-threatening complications [46]. Therefore, we advocate improved access to care and support services for people with SCI.

16.8 Advances in NBD and NLUTD Management

16.8.1 Ongoing Research

Ongoing research holds promise for improving outcomes and reducing the burden of NBD and NLUTD in people with SCI. Among many areas of research, the authors selected three innovations that showed high potential.

- *Neurostimulation*: By restoring neural control and improving functions of pelvic organs, sacral neuromodulation (i.e., the stimulation of spinal nerves at the S3 foramen) and epidural spinal cord stimulation may represent potential treatments for NBD and NLUTD, particularly in patients with refractory symptoms not responding to conventional treatments [71–73].
- *Regenerative Medicine*: Stem cell therapy and tissue engineering represent probably the largest hope for people with SCI, as they could potentially offer long-term solutions to NBD and NLUTD by regenerating damaged neural tissue or creating new pathways for neural control [74–76]. Therefore, they have

been investigated over the last decades with high expectations, even if we are still far from a safe application to restore GI and GU functions on a large scale so far.

- *Pharmacologic Innovations*: Current drugs for NBD and NLUTD may be associated with significant side effects besides representing a valid solution only for a part of patients with SCI. Therefore, new drugs targeting specific pathways involved in GI and GU dysfunctions are being investigated to offer directed treatment options with fewer side effects. An example of this approach is represented by the use of agents modulating neurotransmitter activity (e.g., selective serotonin reuptake inhibitors), which proved to enhance GI and GU functions [77, 78].

16.8.2 Personalized Medicine

The patient-specific genetic and physiological profile may lead to a significant improvement in the management of GI and GU dysfunctions in SCI patients [79]. Future research may focus on identifying biomarkers that predict response to specific treatments to reduce the incidence of adverse effects and offer a more individualized and effective care [80, 81].

16.8.3 Telemedicine

Telemedicine is defined as the long-distance distribution of health-related services via information and communication technology. Considering the shortage of healthcare professionals who are experts in the peculiarities of people with SCI, the use of telemedicine could revolutionize the long-term management of GI and GU dysfunctions in this population, as it may ease regular follow-up, detect complications at early stages, and advocate a timely intervention, particularly for patients in remote or underserved areas [19, 82]. Moreover, telemedicine proved to be a system to enhance patient education and advocate prevention, as it provides access to healthcare providers regularly and promotes a proactive management [46, 83].

16.9 Conclusion

Traumatic SCI may be commonly associated with GI and GU dysfunctions, whose effective management requires a comprehensive understanding of the underlying pathophysiology and a multidisciplinary approach that addresses both the acute and long-term needs of the patient. Healthcare professionals can significantly improve the QoL of patients with SCI by implementing evidence-based strategies for the management of NBD and NLUTD. In the next years, we will face a significant outcome improvement thanks to ongoing research and technological advancement. In the meantime, we should remain committed to providing compassionate and patient-centered care that addresses the unique challenges faced by individuals living with SCI.

References

1. Rodriguez G, Cameron AP, Bush-Arnold M. Neurogenic bowel dysfunction. In: Liao L, Madersbacher H, editors. Handbook of Neurourology. Singapore: Springer; 2022. https://doi.org/10.1007/978-981-16-7939-1_55-1.
2. Kirshblum SC, Burns SP, Biering-Sorensen F, Donovan W, Graves DE, Jha A, Johansen M, Jones L, Krassioukov A, Mulcahey MJ, Schmidt-Read M, Waring W. International standards for neurological classification of spinal cord injury (revised 2011). J Spinal Cord Med. 2011;34(6):535–46. https://doi.org/10.1179/204577211X13207446293695.
3. American Gastroenterological Association, Bharucha AE, Dorn SD, Lembo A, Pressman A. American Gastroenterological Association medical position statement on constipation. Gastroenterology. 2013;144(1):211–7. https://doi.org/10.1053/j.gastro.2012.10.029.
4. Di Nardo G, Blandizzi C, Volta U, Colucci R, Stanghellini V, Barbara G, Del Tacca M, Tonini M, Corinaldesi R, De Giorgio R. Review article: molecular, pathological and therapeutic features of human enteric neuropathies. Aliment Pharmacol Ther. 2008;28(1):25–42. https://doi.org/10.1111/j.1365-2036.2008.03707.x.
5. Groen J, Pannek J, Castro Diaz D, Del Popolo G, Gross T, Hamid R, Karsenty G, Kessler TM, Schneider M, 't Hoen L, Blok B. Summary of European Association of Urology (EAU) guidelines on neuro-urology. Eur Urol. 2016;69(2):324–33. https://doi.org/10.1016/j.eururo.2015.07.071.
6. Panicker JN, Fowler CJ, Kessler TM. Lower urinary tract dysfunction in the neurological patient: clinical assessment and management. Lancet Neurol. 2015;14(7):720–32. https://doi.org/10.1016/S1474-4422(15)00070-8.
7. Rodriguez GM, Gater DR. Neurogenic bowel and management after spinal cord injury: a narrative review. J Pers Med. 2022;12(7):1141. https://doi.org/10.3390/jpm12071141.
8. Taweel WA, Seyam R. Neurogenic bladder in spinal cord injury patients. Res Rep Urol. 2015;7:85–99. https://doi.org/10.2147/RRU.S29644.
9. Christensen P, Kvitzau B, Krogh K, Buntzen S, Laurberg S. Neurogenic colorectal dysfunction – use of new antegrade and retrograde colonic wash-out methods. Spinal Cord. 2000;38(4):255–61. https://doi.org/10.1038/sj.sc.3100991.
10. Holmes GM, Blanke EN. Gastrointestinal dysfunction after spinal cord injury. Exp Neurol. 2019;320:113009. https://doi.org/10.1016/j.expneurol.2019.113009.
11. Wyndaele JJ. The management of neurogenic lower urinary tract dysfunction after spinal cord injury. Nat Rev Urol. 2016;13(12):705–14. https://doi.org/10.1038/nrurol.2016.206.
12. van Middendorp JJ, Sanchez GM, Burridge AL. The Edwin Smith papyrus: a clinical reappraisal of the oldest known document on spinal injuries. Eur Spine J. 2010;19(11):1815–23. https://doi.org/10.1007/s00586-010-1523-6.
13. Lightner DJ, Gomelsky A, Souter L, Vasavada SP. Diagnosis and treatment of overactive bladder (non-neurogenic) in adults: AUA/SUFU Guideline Amendment 2019. J Urol. 2019;202(3):558–63. https://doi.org/10.1097/JU.0000000000000309.
14. Eldahan KC, Rabchevsky AG. Autonomic dysreflexia after spinal cord injury: systemic pathophysiology and methods of management. Auton Neurosci. 2018;209:59–70. https://doi.org/10.1016/j.autneu.2017.05.002.
15. Benevento BT, Sipski ML. Neurogenic bladder, neurogenic bowel, and sexual dysfunction in people with spinal cord injury. Phys Ther. 2002;82(6):601–12.

16. Kurze I, Geng V, Böthig R. Guideline for the management of neurogenic bowel dysfunction in spinal cord injury/disease. Spinal Cord. 2022;60(5):435–43. https://doi.org/10.1038/s41393-022-00786-x.
17. Farkas GJ, Sneij A, Gater DR Jr. Dietetics after spinal cord injury: current evidence and future perspectives. Top Spinal Cord Inj Rehabil. 2021;27(1):100–8. https://doi.org/10.46292/sci20-00031.
18. Johns JS, Krogh K, Ethans K, Chi J, Querée M, Eng JJ, Spinal Cord Injury Research Evidence Team. Pharmacological management of neurogenic bowel dysfunction after spinal cord injury and multiple sclerosis: a systematic review and clinical implications. J Clin Med. 2021;10(4):882. https://doi.org/10.3390/jcm10040882.
19. Rapidi CA, Kontaxakis A, Del Popolo G, et al. Telerehabilitation in neurogenic bladder and bowel dysfunction. In: Alexander M, editor. Telerehabilitation: principles and practice. Elsevier; 2022. p. 225–49, ISBN 9780323824866.
20. Sampogna G, Barbosa F, Brambillasca PM, Montanari E, Rampoldi A, Spinelli M. Prostatic artery embolization in people with spinal cord injury: a safe and effective technique to ease intermittent catheterization in case of concomitant benign prostatic hyperplasia. Spinal Cord Ser Cases. 2022;8(1):34. https://doi.org/10.1038/s41394-022-00499-6.
21. Stoffel JT, Van der Aa F, Wittmann D, Yande S, Elliott S. Neurogenic bowel management for the adult spinal cord injury patient. World J Urol. 2018;36(10):1587–92. https://doi.org/10.1007/s00345-018-2388-2.
22. Karlsson AK. Autonomic dysreflexia. Spinal Cord. 1999;37(6):383–91. https://doi.org/10.1038/sj.sc.3100867.
23. Magnuson FS, Christensen P, Krassioukov A, Rodriguez G, Emmanuel A, Kirshblum S, Krogh K. Neurogenic bowel dysfunction in patients with spinal cord injury and multiple sclerosis-an updated and simplified treatment algorithm. J Clin Med. 2023;12(22):6971. https://doi.org/10.3390/jcm12226971.
24. Emmanuel A, Krogh K, Kirshblum S, Christensen P, Spinelli M, van Kuppevelt D, Abel R, Leder D, Santacruz BG, Bain K, Passananti V. Creation and validation of a new tool for the monitoring efficacy of neurogenic bowel dysfunction treatment on response: the MENTOR tool. Spinal Cord. 2020;58(7):795–802. https://doi.org/10.1038/s41393-020-0424-8.
25. Johns J, Krogh K, Rodriguez GM, Eng J, Haller E, Heinen M, Laredo R, Longo W, Montero-Colon W, Wilson C, Korsten M. Management of neurogenic bowel dysfunction in adults after spinal cord injury: clinical practice guideline for health care providers. Top Spinal Cord Inj Rehabil. 2021;27(2):75–151. https://doi.org/10.46292/sci2702-75.
26. Ford AC, Suares NC. Effect of laxatives and pharmacological therapies in chronic idiopathic constipation: systematic review and meta-analysis. Gut. 2011;60(2):209–18. https://doi.org/10.1136/gut.2010.227132.
27. McRorie JW, Chey WD. Fermented fiber supplements are no better than placebo for a laxative effect. Dig Dis Sci. 2016;61:3140–6. https://doi.org/10.1007/s10620-016-4304-1.
28. Müller-Lissner SA, Kamm MA, Scarpignato C, Wald A. Myths and misconceptions about chronic constipation. Am J Gastroenterol. 2005;100(1):232–42. https://doi.org/10.1111/j.1572-0241.2005.40885.x.
29. Sayuk GS, Yu QT, Shy C. Management of Constipation in hospitalized patients. J Clin Med. 2023;12(19):6148. https://doi.org/10.3390/jcm12196148.
30. Camilleri M, Bharucha AE, di Lorenzo C, Hasler WL, Prather CM, Rao SS, Wald A. American Neurogastroenterology and Motility Society consensus statement on intraluminal measurement of gastrointestinal and colonic motility in clinical practice. Neurogastroenterol Motil. 2008;20(12):1269–82. https://doi.org/10.1111/j.1365-2982.2008.01230.x.
31. Holzer P. New approaches to the treatment of opioid-induced constipation. Eur Rev Med Pharmacol Sci. 2008;12(Suppl 1):119–27.
32. Mazor Y, Jones M, Andrews A, Kellow JE, Malcolm A. Anorectal biofeedback for neurogenic bowel dysfunction in incomplete spinal cord injury. Spinal Cord. 2016;54(12):1132–8. https://doi.org/10.1038/sc.2016.67.

33. Hultling C. Neurogenic bowel management using Transanal irrigation by persons with spinal cord injury. Phys Med Rehabil Clin N Am. 2020;31(3):305–18. https://doi.org/10.1016/j.pmr.2020.04.003.
34. Emmanuel A, Krogh K, Bazzocchi G, et al. Consensus review of best practice of transanal irrigation in adults. Spinal Cord. 2013;51:732–8. https://doi.org/10.1038/sc.2013.86.
35. Mekhael M, Kristensen HØ, Larsen HM, Juul T, Emmanuel A, Krogh K, Christensen P. Transanal irrigation for neurogenic bowel disease, low anterior resection syndrome, Faecal incontinence and chronic constipation: a systematic review. J Clin Med. 2021;10(4):753. https://doi.org/10.3390/jcm10040753.
36. Spinelli M, Sampogna G, Rizzato L, Spinelli A, Sammartano F, Cimbanassi S, Montanari E, Chiara O. The Malone antegrade continence enema adapting a transanal irrigation system in patients with neurogenic bowel dysfunction. Spinal Cord Ser Cases. 2021;7(1):34. https://doi.org/10.1038/s41394-021-00397-3.
37. Knowles CH, De Giorgio R, Kapur RP, Bruder E, Farrugia G, Geboes K, Lindberg G, Martin JE, Meier-Ruge WA, Milla PJ, Smith VV, Vandervinden JM, Veress B, Wedel T. The London classification of gastrointestinal neuromuscular pathology: report on behalf of the Gastro 2009 International Working Group. Gut. 2010;59(7):882–7. https://doi.org/10.1136/gut.2009.200444.
38. Alenezi A, McGrath I, Kimpton A, Livesay K. Quality of life among ostomy patients: a narrative literature review. J Clin Nurs. 2021;30(21–22):3111–23. https://doi.org/10.1111/jocn.15840.
39. Siau K, Chapman W, Sharma N, Tripathi D, Iqbal T, Bhala N. Management of acute upper gastrointestinal bleeding: an update for the general physician. J R Coll Physicians Edinb. 2017;47(3):218–30. https://doi.org/10.4997/JRCPE.2017.303.
40. Viana FB, Viana JB, Seabra Beraldo PS. Prophylactic cholecystectomy in individuals with spinal cord injury: a systematic review. J Spinal Cord Med. 2023;46(4):649–57. https://doi.org/10.1080/10790268.2022.2144026.
41. Pimentel M, Saad RJ, Long MD, Rao SSC. ACG clinical guideline: small intestinal bacterial overgrowth. Am J Gastroenterol. 2020;115(2):165–78. https://doi.org/10.14309/ajg.0000000000000501.
42. Sampogna G, Forgione A, Chevallard G, Spinelli M. Perioperative management and surgical challenges in patients with spinal cord dysfunction. In: Aseni P, Grande AM, Leppäniemi A, Chiara O, editors. The high-risk surgical patient. Cham: Springer; 2023. https://doi.org/10.1007/978-3-031-17273-1_29.
43. Cameron AP. Pharmacologic therapy for the neurogenic bladder. Urol Clin North Am. 2010;37(4):495–506. https://doi.org/10.1016/j.ucl.2010.06.004.
44. Elkhashab MM, Alqahtani AM, Kim MH, Kim J, Kim JH, Jung JH. Safety and efficacy of beta-3 adrenergic agonists in treating neurogenic lower urinary tract dysfunction: a systematic review and meta-analysis. Investig Clin Urol. 2024;65(3):217–29. https://doi.org/10.4111/icu.20230271.
45. Manaila AI, Roman NA, Baseanu ICC, Minzatanu D, Tuchel VI, Basalic EB, Miclaus RS. The efficiency of rehabilitation therapy in patients diagnosed with neurogenic bladder: a systematic review. Medicina (Kaunas). 2024;60(7):1152. https://doi.org/10.3390/medicina60071152.
46. Sampogna G, Pelizzari L, Lombardo R, De Nunzio C, Li Marzi V. Young research Group of the Italian Society of Urodynamics. Pelvic floor muscle training: novel versus traditional remote rehabilitation methods-A systematic review and meta-analysis on their effectiveness for women with urinary incontinence. Neurourol Urodyn. 2023;42(8):1863–4. https://doi.org/10.1002/nau.25265.
47. Herschorn S, Gajewski J, Ethans K, Corcos J, Carlson K, Bailly G, Bard R, Valiquette L, Baverstock R, Carr L, Radomski S. Efficacy of botulinum toxin A injection for neurogenic detrusor overactivity and urinary incontinence: a randomized, double-blind trial. J Urol. 2011;185(6):2229–35. https://doi.org/10.1016/j.juro.2011.02.004.
48. Cameron AP, Rodriguez GM, Schomer KG. Systematic review of urological followup after spinal cord injury. J Urol. 2012;187(2):391–7. https://doi.org/10.1016/j.juro.2011.10.020.

49. Çetinel B, Kocjancic E, Demirdağ Ç. Augmentation cystoplasty in neurogenic bladder. Investig Clin Urol. 2016;57(5):316–23. https://doi.org/10.4111/icu.2016.57.5.316.
50. Vigil HR, Hickling DR. Urinary tract infection in the neurogenic bladder. Transl Androl Urol. 2016;5(1):72–87. https://doi.org/10.3978/j.issn.2223-4683.2016.01.06.
51. Lenger SM, Bradley MS, Thomas DA, Bertolet MH, Lowder JL, Sutcliffe S. D-mannose vs other agents for recurrent urinary tract infection prevention in adult women: a systematic review and meta-analysis. Am J Obstet Gynecol. 2020;223(2):265.e1–265.e13. https://doi.org/10.1016/j.ajog.2020.05.048.
52. Pannek J, Wöllner J. Management of urinary tract infections in patients with neurogenic bladder: challenges and solutions. Res Rep Urol. 2017;9:121–7. https://doi.org/10.2147/RRU.S113610.
53. Dinh A, Hallouin-Bernard MC, Davido B, Lemaignen A, Bouchand F, Duran C, Even A, Denys P, Perrouin-Verbe B, Sotto A, Lavigne JP, Bruyère F, Grall N, Tavernier E, Bernard L. Weekly sequential Antibioprophylaxis for recurrent urinary tract infections among patients with neurogenic bladder: a randomized controlled trial. Clin Infect Dis. 2020;71(12):3128–35. https://doi.org/10.1093/cid/ciz1207.
54. Sampogna G, Maltagliati M, Rocco B, Micali S, Montanari E, Spinelli M. Shock wave lithotripsy for a renal stone in a tetraplegic patient as a trigger for life-threatening posterior reversible encephalopathy syndrome. Urol Case Rep. 2020;31:101204. https://doi.org/10.1016/j.eucr.2020.101204.
55. Blais AS, Bolduc S, Moore K. Vesicoureteral reflux: from prophylaxis to surgery. Can Urol Assoc J. 2017;11(1-2 Suppl 1):S13–8. https://doi.org/10.5489/cuaj.4342.
56. Sampogna G, Maltagliati M, Galfano A, Bocciardi A, Rocco B, Micali S, Montanari E, Spinelli M. Experience of a tertiary referral center in managing bladder cancer in conjunction with neurogenic bladder. Spinal Cord Ser Cases. 2020;6(1):61. https://doi.org/10.1038/s41394-020-0302-9.
57. Simpson LA, Eng JJ, Hsieh JT, Wolfe DL, Spinal Cord Injury Rehabilitation Evidence Scire Research Team. The health and life priorities of individuals with spinal cord injury: a systematic review. J Neurotrauma. 2012;29(8):1548–55. https://doi.org/10.1089/neu.2011.2226.
58. Alexander MS, Sampogna G. Telerehabilitation for treatment of sexual concerns. In: Alexander M, editor. Telerehabilitation: principles and practice. Elsevier; 2022. p. 251–61. ISBN 9780323824866.
59. Anderson KD, Borisoff JF, Johnson RD, Stiens SA, Elliott SL. The impact of spinal cord injury on sexual function: concerns of the general population. Spinal Cord. 2007;45(5):328–37. https://doi.org/10.1038/sj.sc.3101977.
60. Longoni M, Degano M, Sampogna G. An integrated vision of sexuality after spinal cord injury. Phys Med Rehabil Clin. 2024;36 https://doi.org/10.1016/j.pmr.2024.07.008.
61. Ibrahim E, Lynne CM, Brackett NL. Male fertility following spinal cord injury: an update. Andrology. 2016;4(1):13–26. https://doi.org/10.1111/andr.12119.
62. Robertson K, Ashworth F. Spinal cord injury and pregnancy. Obstet Med. 2022;15(2):99–103. https://doi.org/10.1177/1753495X211011918.
63. Kennedy P, Rogers BA. Anxiety and depression after spinal cord injury: a longitudinal analysis. Arch Phys Med Rehabil. 2000;81(7):932–7. https://doi.org/10.1053/apmr.2000.5580.
64. Pollard C, Kennedy P. A longitudinal analysis of emotional impact, coping strategies and post-traumatic psychological growth following spinal cord injury: a 10-year review. Br J Health Psychol. 2007;12(Pt 3):347–62. https://doi.org/10.1348/135910707X197046.
65. Zhao C, Liang S, Wang X, Gao L, Lai Y, Huang Y, Li J, Chen L, Cai W. User experience of a self-management WeChat applet for patients with neurogenic bladder: a qualitative approach. Int J Nurs Sci. 2022;10(1):89–96. https://doi.org/10.1016/j.ijnss.2022.12.009.
66. Kuipers P, Kendall MB, Amsters D, Pershouse K, Schuurs S. Descriptions of community by people with spinal cord injuries: concepts to inform community integration and community rehabilitation. Int J Rehabil Res. 2011;34(2):167–74. https://doi.org/10.1097/MRR.0b013e3283460e39.

67. Diop M, Epstein D. A systematic review of the impact of spinal cord injury on costs and health-related quality of life. Pharmacoecon Open. 2024;8 https://doi.org/10.1007/s41669-024-00517-3.
68. Blanes L, Carmagnani MI, Ferreira LM. Health-related quality of life of primary caregivers of persons with paraplegia. Spinal Cord. 2007;45(6):399–403. https://doi.org/10.1038/sj.sc.3102038.
69. Bökel A, Dierks ML, Gutenbrunner C, Weidner N, Geng V, Kalke YB, Liebscher T, Abel FR, Sturm C. Perceived environmental barriers for people with spinal cord injury in Germany and their influence on quality of life. J Rehabil Med. 2020;52(8):jrm00090. https://doi.org/10.2340/16501977-2717.
70. Merritt CH, Taylor MA, Yelton CJ, Ray SK. Economic impact of traumatic spinal cord injuries in the United States. Neuroimmunol Neuroinflamm. 2019;6:9. https://doi.org/10.20517/2347-8659.2019.15.
71. Hassouna M, Elmayergi N, Abdelhady M. Update on sacral neuromodulation: indications and outcomes. Curr Urol Rep. 2003;4(5):391–8. https://doi.org/10.1007/s11934-003-0014-2.
72. Samejima S, Shackleton C, McCracken L, Malik RN, Miller T, Kavanagh A, Ghuman A, Elliott S, Walter M, Nightingale TE, Berger MJ, Lam T, Sachdeva R, Krassioukov AV. Effects of non-invasive spinal cord stimulation on lower urinary tract, bowel, and sexual functions in individuals with chronic motor-complete spinal cord injury: protocol for a pilot clinical trial. PLoS One. 2022;17(12):e0278425. https://doi.org/10.1371/journal.pone.0278425.
73. Liechti MD, van der Lely S, Knüpfer SC, Abt D, Kiss B, Leitner L, Mordasini L, Tornic J, Wöllner J, Mehnert U, Bachmann LM, Burkhard FC, Engeler DS, Pannek J, Kessler TM. Sacral neuromodulation for neurogenic lower urinary tract dysfunction. NEJM Evid. 2022;1(11):EVIDoa2200071. https://doi.org/10.1056/EVIDoa2200071.
74. Sampogna G, Guraya SY, Forgione A. Regenerative medicine: historical roots and potential strategies in modern medicine. J Microsc Ultrastruct. 2015;3(3):101–7. https://doi.org/10.1016/j.jmau.2015.05.002.
75. Assinck P, Duncan GJ, Hilton BJ, Plemel JR, Tetzlaff W. Cell transplantation therapy for spinal cord injury. Nat Neurosci. 2017;20(5):637–47. https://doi.org/10.1038/nn.4541.
76. Kawai M, Nagoshi N, Okano H, Nakamura M. A review of regenerative therapy for spinal cord injury using human iPS cells. N Am Spine Soc J. 2022;13:100184. https://doi.org/10.1016/j.xnsj.2022.100184.
77. Sikander A, Rana SV, Prasad KK. Role of serotonin in gastrointestinal motility and irritable bowel syndrome. Clin Chim Acta. 2009;403(1–2):47–55. https://doi.org/10.1016/j.cca.2009.01.028.
78. Valiyeva S, Tiso D, Cerri P, Pisciaroli A, Pietroletti R. Results of medical treatment with psyllium, lactobacillus, and tryptophan (Plurilac® Trio) in obstructive defecation syndrome. Front Surg. 2024;11:1361049. https://doi.org/10.3389/fsurg.2024.1361049.
79. Garrino L, Curto N, Decorte R, Felisi N, Matta E, Gregorino S, Actis MV, Marchisio C, Carone R. Towards personalized care for persons with spinal cord injury: a study on patients' perceptions. J Spinal Cord Med. 2011;34(1):67–75. https://doi.org/10.1179/107902610x12883422813741.
80. Jameson JL, Longo DL. Precision medicine–personalized, problematic, and promising. N Engl J Med. 2015;372(23):2229–34. https://doi.org/10.1056/NEJMsb1503104.
81. Karabacak M, Margetis K. Precision medicine for traumatic cervical spinal cord injuries: accessible and interpretable machine learning models to predict individualized in-hospital outcomes. Spine J. 2023;23(12):1750–63. https://doi.org/10.1016/j.spinee.2023.08.009.
82. Duplaga M. Digital divide among people with disabilities: analysis of data from a nationwide study for determinants of Internet use and activities performed online. PLoS One. 2017;12(6):e0179825. https://doi.org/10.1371/journal.pone.0179825.
83. Cason J. Telehealth: a rapidly developing service delivery model for occupational therapy. Int J Telerehabil. 2014;6(1):29–35. https://doi.org/10.5195/ijt.2014.6148.

Infectious Complications

17

Rodrigo Kuromoto and Wellingson Silva Paiva

17.1 Introduction

Besides the devastating consequences of losing motor, sensory, and autonomic function, Spinal Cord Injury (SCI) is often followed by other multiple systemic complications. These complications justify the fact that survival rates in subjects with spinal cord injury (SCI) are significantly lower compared to the healthy population [1, 2], with infectious complications as the primary cause of death [3–5]. Infections also lengthen hospital stays, elevate costs, induce antibiotic resistance, worsen rehabilitation, and may also induce further non-infectious morbidities. In this chapter, we will discuss the different infectious complications, their management, and strategies for prevention.

17.2 Physiopathology of Infections in Spinal Cord Injury

Patients with SCI are at risk for infections due to multiple factors. Major trauma causes a pro-inflammatory response, and an accompanying anti-inflammatory response leads to a state of immunosuppression [6]. SCI is accompanied by a neurological injury that further aggravates the immunosuppression due to the occurrence of a phenomenon called "SCI-induced immune deficiency syndrome" (SCI-IDS) [7–12]. Emerging data suggest that SCI affects autonomic and neuroendocrine control over lymphoid tissues, adrenal glands, and bone marrow, causing cellular immunodeficiency. SCI-IDS also diminishes humoral immunity via

R. Kuromoto
Division of Neurosurgery, Hospital das Clinicas – University of Sao Paulo Medical School, São Paulo, SP, Brazil

W. S. Paiva (✉)
Division of Neurosurgery, Hospital das Clinicas – University of Sao Paulo Medical School, São Paulo, SP, Brazil

E. Brogi et al. (eds.), *Traumatic Spinal Cord Injury*, Hot Topics in Acute Care Surgery and Trauma, https://doi.org/10.1007/978-3-031-99890-4_17

immunoglobulins. The level of injury and severity of neurological impairment are the main factors related to the grade of immunosuppression [7, 10]. The neurological injury seems to alter not only susceptibility to infections but also the way the body responds to them. Patients with tetraplegia may not be able to mount a fever and tachycardia to the same degree as patients with paraplegia and may also be more prone to develop altered mental status during sepsis [13, 14].

In addition to immunosuppression, other factors place SCI patients at risk for infectious complications [15–21]. Limitations in clearing the airway may lead to pneumonia. Frequent insertion of urologic, vascular, orthopedic, respiratory, gastrointestinal, and neurosurgical devices predisposes to various prosthesis-related infections. Motor and sensory impairments lead to immobility and predispose to pressure injuries, skin and soft tissue infection, and osteomyelitis. Prolonged or repetitive hospitalizations make them vulnerable to multidrug-resistant organisms. Typical physical and psychosocial elements such as nutrition difficulties, depression, and lack of social support are other fragilities found in this population.

17.3 Thermo(dys)regulation and SCI

Diagnosis of infection in patients with SCI can often be challenging. One of the main reasons is the thermoregulation impairment that affects this population in both acute and chronic phases. In the acute phase (< 3 months postinjury) of SCI, the mean incidence of fever ranges from 47% to 85% and is most common in neurological lesions above T6 level and complete injuries [22–26] However, approximately 4–5% of fevers in this period are defined as "neurogenic" fever or fever of unknown origin in a person with SCI [27]. The pathophysiology of "neurogenic fever" is not fully understood, but some authors believe it to be caused partially by autonomic dysfunction, loss of afferent thermal sensing, and loss of central hypothalamic control over peripheral functions such as vasoconstriction, vasodilatation, and sweating [23, 27, 28]. There is also a condition described in 1982 by Sugarman et al. and called "quadriplegic fever", which is an idiopathic extreme elevation of core temperature in patients with SCI that can be prolonged for weeks and carries a poor prognosis [22, 27, 29, 30]. Rarely, fever can occur in the context of autonomic dysreflexia, another condition associated with SCI.

On the other hand, patients with SCI may also present with hypothermia, and the primary explanation for it is the loss of afferent thermal sensing and vasomotor reaction [31]. It is also described that patients with chronic SCI cannot mount a febrile response to infection and inflammation to the same degree as the able-bodied population [13, 14]. Song et al. found that patients with tetraplegia may not be able to mount a fever and tachycardia to the same degree as patients with paraplegia and may be more prone to developing altered mental status during sepsis [14]. Anas et al. analyzed septic SCI patients and found that procalcitonin (PCT) values were elevated in all patients, C-reactive protein (CRP) was raised in 80%, white blood cells (WBC) were elevated in 30% of the population, and only 80% of the population had a raised body temperature [32].

17.4 Infectious Complications Following SCI

17.4.1 Urinary Tract Infection (UTI)

Bladder function differs according to the anatomic level of the SCI, but the correlation between the level of neurological injury and bladder dysfunction type is not always exactly as theoretically expected. During spinal shock, patients present with detrusor and sphincter areflexia, requiring catheterization. After recovery from spinal shock, a complete urodynamic study should be undertaken to determine the type of bladder and sphincter dysfunction [33].

SCI patients have multiple risk factors for UTI as reduced sensation of UTI symptoms, incomplete bladder emptying, frequent catheterizations, or chronic urinary tract catheters [34]. The listed risk factors justify UTI as the most common infection in patients with SCI and a common cause of hospitalization, with an estimated incidence of 0.68 episodes per 100 patients daily. In other words, the overall rate of urinary infection in SCI patients is about 2.5 episodes per patient per year [35, 36]. Despite improved methods of treatment, UTI still ranks as a significant cause of death in SCI patients [4, 37].

UTI is defined as the presence of signs and/or symptoms of UTI with laboratory findings (bacteriuria, leukocyturia, and positive urine culture). However, there is no clear consensus regarding the diagnosis of UTI in persons with SCI [38]. Clinically, the diagnosis of ITU can be difficult, and professionals should always raise suspicion. Loss of sensation masks dysuria, and the abnormal voiding interferes with polyuria evaluation. Abnormal-smelling urine, worsening of muscular spasticity, and/or aggravation of autonomic dysreflexia are often the only clinical clues to the presence of UTI [20]. A study found that patient self-diagnosis was only 48% sensitive and 71% specific for UTI, and those specific individual symptoms, such as cloudy urine or foul smell, showed poor sensitivity and specificity. The most sensitive objective sign of UTI was pyuria at 83%, whereas fever was 99% specific in this cohort [39]. The most common identifiable cause of fever is urinary tract infection in the SCI population. Another confounder in the evaluation of ITU is the high prevalence of asymptomatic bacteriuria (ASB), which is almost universal in patients with chronic catheterization, and ASB should not be treated [20, 38, 40–42]. Leucocytes in the urine (pyuria) is a nonspecific finding also observed in uninfected individuals whose urinary tract is inflamed by catheter manipulations, renal calculi, and interstitial nephritis [20].

Most cases are caused by bacteria derived from the patient's bowel and perineum flora, particularly gram-negative bacilli and enterococci. If the patient carries a catheter for more than 30 days, the risk of infection with multiple organisms will increase. SCI patients are at risk for resistant organisms because of recurrent and/or prolonged hospitalizations and frequent use of antibiotics [20, 21]. UTI and bacteriuria are strongly related to vesical catheterization. Historically, Intermittent catheterization was preferred over indwelling catheterization since it is supposed to cause fewer UTIs. Recent publications that do not support its superiority have questioned the recommendation favoring intermittent catheterization based on UTI risk

[43, 44]. Studies have found lower rates of infection and urethral trauma using hydrophilic-coated catheters for intermittent catheterization [45–48]. There is no strong evidence for antibiotic-impregnated catheters. Antibiotic prophylaxis is generally discouraged to avoid antibiotic resistance [18, 38, 49–52]. There isn't strong evidence to support the use of cranberry products either [21, 38, 48].

Patients with neurogenic bladder after SCI have an elevated risk for urinary tract stone formation for multiple reasons [53, 54]. The lack of sensation can make obstructed renal stones with associated infection challenging to diagnose and sepsis treatment to be delayed [55, 56]. Recurrent infections are also associated with bladder cancer, and frequent urinary infections or purulent urethral discharge may also be a presentation of bladder cancer [57, 58].

17.4.2 Pneumonia

Although the incidence of pneumonia varies significantly between studies, there is a consensus among them that respiratory complications and pneumonia are the leading causes of morbidity and mortality following SCI. It is estimated that approximately one-third of the mortality after SCI is attributable to respiratory complications, with two-thirds of them due to pneumonia [4, 5, 59–66]. Most cases of pneumonia occur in the acute setting, with a median of 6 days post-injury [61].

Besides the immunosuppression caused by SCI, it causes multiple dysfunctions in the respiratory system that facilitate infections, not only elevating its incidence but also the chances of mortality. First and obvious is the weakness of the respiratory muscles. Lesions above C5 can compromise the diaphragm, the main muscle responsible for the predicted vital capacity. Lesions from C5 to thoracic levels can compromise the inspiratory accessory muscles. Respiratory muscle weakness requires mechanical ventilation, making them susceptible to ventilator-associated pneumonia (VAP). Reduced inspiratory muscle strength also predisposes to atelectasis. One study showed that for every 10 cmH2O increase in inspiratory muscle strength, pneumonia risk was reduced by 13% [61]. Expiratory muscle weakness results in low voluntary cough peak expiratory flow, which means ineffective clearance of bronchial secretions. Another point is the unopposed vagal parasympathetic input in patients with tetraplegia, leading to bronchoconstriction and increased bronchial mucus secretion [67, 68]. Besides the level of injury, grade of neurological injury, and the need for mechanical ventilation, dysphagia is another relevant risk factor for pneumonia, and a study by Shem et al. reported that 75% of SCI patients with dysphagia developed pneumonia compared to 29% without dysphagia [69]. Poor nutritional status is another condition these patients face, and there is a statistical relationship between nutritional status and pneumonia [60].

As with other infections, pneumonia may also be a challenging diagnosis. Respiratory muscle fatigue and chest pain perception may be altered in this population. Other conditions can also mimic pneumonia. Atelectasis can cause mild fever and leukocytosis. Pulmonary embolism, which is facilitated by mobility restriction, can also cause respiratory impairments and mild fever. In the acute setting, a fracture of a long bone can lead to fat embolism, and pulmonary contusions can also make pneumonia a differential diagnosis. Aspiration of gastric contents in the presence of paralytic ileus and an ineffective cough reflex can lead to chemical pneumonitis that mimics bacterial pneumonia [20].

Pneumonia and postoperative wound infections are significantly associated with lower gains in motor scores [66], and efforts to prevent these infections must be a priority in the SCI population by treating the risk factors. Although there is no strong evidence for the use of S. pneumoniae and influenza viruses vaccination in the SCI scenario, it is discussed by a few articles [70–72], and a good percentage of the patients are eligible for it by other indications. Secretion management and timing for intubation are essential aspects of prevention.

The causative pathogens differ in acute and chronic settings. Antibiotics are chosen according to endotracheal secretion cultures, which are usually not positive and require empirical treatment. In the acute setting, nosocomial pneumonia and VAP present with the most common organisms as *Pseudomonas aeruginosa*, *Klebsiella pneumoniae*, *Acinetobacter baumannii*, *Serratia marcescens,* and methicillin-resistant *Staphylococcus aureus* [21]. In the outpatient population, pneumococcus, as in the general population, is the leading cause of pneumonia. Pseudomonas, an uncommon pathogen in the general population, is a commonly identified pathogen due to the colonization of the perineum, lower urinary tract, and urine collection system, which is common in persons with SCI [67].

17.4.3 Infection of Pressure Injuries

Pressure injuries are one of the most severe chronic complications of spinal cord injury, being estimated to happen in one in three patients with SCI [73]. SCI breaks the physiological response to changing the position by lacking sensation and mobility. The soft tissues are compressed between bony prominences and external surfaces, which causes hypoxia, ischemia, and subsequent necrosis. Besides compression, shearing forces may also play an important role in these injuries. For example, when lying at an angle, the downward force of gravity is countered by friction, which prevents the person from sliding down the bed. Though the skin may not move down the bed, internal structures like muscle and bone, not in contact with an external surface, are displaced downward because of gravity. These shearing forces can disrupt blood flow as vessels caught between the skin and bone are distorted or compressed [74–76]. Risk factors for pressure lesions include impaired mobility and sensation, sedation, immobilization, poor nutrition, and natural skin aging. Since 1996, SCI Pressure Ulcer Scale (SCIPUS) has considered 15 risk factors for risk assessment: level of activity, mobility, presence of complete SCI, urine incontinence or moisture, autonomic dysreflexia/severe spasticity, age, tobacco use, pulmonary disease, cardiac disease/abnormal ECG, diabetes or glucose $\geq$110 mg/dL, renal disease, impaired cognitive function, living in a nursing home or hospital, albumin <3.4 or total protein <6.4, and hematocrit <36.0% or hemoglobin

<12.0 g/dL [77]. The National Pressure Ulcer Advisory Panel (NPUAP) has provided a widely accepted staging system for pressure injuries [76].

Pressure injuries are at risk of infections since they break the integrity of the skin barrier, worsen skin perfusion, and are frequently contiguous to dirty areas. The sacrum, ischial tuberosity, trochanteric area, and malleolus are common sites for developing ulcers. In paralyzed individuals who cannot directly visualize the injuries and have a severe loss of sensation, infection is usually advanced by the time they seek medical care. Staphylococcus aureus, Proteus mirabilis, Pseudomonas aeruginosa, and Enterococcus faecalis are the most frequent infection-associated pathogens [78]. Some authors advocate that for advanced-stage pressure injuries, the cultures of a superficial ulcer swab are not helpful in either the diagnosis of infection or the prediction of the role of involved micro-organisms, requiring deep tissue biopsy [20, 79]. Clinical signs can be remembered by the acronyms NERDS (non-healing wound, exudative wound, red and bleeding wound, debris in the wound, and smell from the wound) or STONES (size is bigger, temperature is increased, osteomyelitis, new areas of breakdown, exudate, erythema, or edema, and smell) [80]. Deeper infections can result in Fournier's gangrene, which is the most severe form of necrotizing fasciitis that affects the perineal and genital regions.

Prevention of pressure injury formation is the first step for pressure injury infection prevention. Since it happens, pressure or shear avoidance and soft tissue offloading are cornerstones of treatment. A combined treatment with surgical debridement and antibiotic therapy is usually needed for deeper lesions. Multiple strategies to enhance skin cicatrization have also been proposed. Skin closure may be challenging when primary closure is not achievable, requiring complex fasciocutaneous, cutaneous, or musculocutaneous flaps. Infected ulcers' lack of response to treatment may result from inadequate antibiotic therapy targeted at the wrong organisms, an undrained abscess, communication of the ulcer with an infected bone or joint, or a fistula communicating with the gastrointestinal or urinary tract [20].

17.4.4 Osteomyelitis

Extension of infection from pressure injury is the leading cause of osteomyelitis. Other presentations are post-operative infections and after hematogenous spread. The definitive diagnosis of osteomyelitis requires a histopathologic examination of bone tissue. There is a lot of debate on investigating osteomyelitis caused by pressure injuries. Magnetic resonance imaging (MRI) for diagnosis of pelvic pressure ulcer osteomyelitis has very low specificity but very high sensitivity, also showing information as the extension of infection, abscesses, fluid collections, and sinus tracts [81–84]. Nuclear scintiscans are usually not used in pressure injury-associated osteomyelitis due to the low specificity attributed to the capacity of the injected technetium to concentrate in areas of bone that have pressure-induced changes or heterotopic ossification as confounder [85], being helpful only in case of a negative result that excludes the diagnosis.

The most common isolated organisms are *Staphylococcus aureus*, *Peptostreptococcus*, and *Bacteroides*. Coagulase-negative staphylococci, group B *Streptococcus*, *Proteus*, and group milleri *Streptococcus* may also be isolated as less common agents [81]. Treatment of osteomyelitis is based on prolonged antibiotic therapy; when indicated, a surgical approach may be needed. The most relevant action is the prevention of pressure injuries.

17.4.5 Bloodstream Infection

Bloodstream infections (BSI) are an important cause of infection in the SCI population. Evans et al. found about 7 episodes of BSI per 100 admissions in SCI patients, with less than 10% of the cases being community-acquired infections [86].

Most cases of BSI are secondary to another site of infection. Urinary tract infection and pressure injuries are the main sources of secondary BSI. Primary BSIs are most catheter-related bloodstream infections. The most frequent pathogens are Enterobacteriaceae, Staphylococcus aureus, Pseudomonas aeruginosa, Streptococcus spp., and Enterococcus spp., with elevated rates of Multidrug-resistant organisms. The prognosis is worse when BSI is secondary to respiratory tract infections, Pseudomonas aeruginosa infections, or when related to immunosuppressive therapy, or initial severity signs [87]. Although often with a severe presentation, mortality associated with BSI is relatively low [87–90].

17.4.6 Clostridium Difficile

Clostridium difficile infection (CDI) is the most common cause of healthcare-associated diarrhea in developed countries [91]. Prolonged hospitalization and frequent use of antibiotics are reasons why CDI is a genuine concern in the SCI population. The use of antibiotics for urinary tract infections has been associated with elevated risk for CDI or recurrence of CDI [92, 93]. Clostridium difficile is also frequently found in asymptomatic SCI patients [94]. Neurogenic bowel and lack of sensation may mask the diagnosis, and CDI may be clinically undetected until severe complications occur.

17.5 Conclusion

Infectious complications are significant causes of morbidity and mortality among the SCI population. Immunosuppression, hospitalizations, medical device insertion, and other infection risk factors are often inevitable consequences of SCI. There is no doubt that efforts should be made not only to improve infection prevention and treatment but also to prevent SCI occurrence and improve neurological outcomes after it, which is strongly related to the rates of complications. Particular attention should be given to the unique characteristics of SCI patients when an infection is suspected. The occurrence of infections also affects neurological outcomes, making them even more critical in the care of SCI patients.

References

1. Hagen EM, Lie SA, Rekand T, Gilhus NE, Gronning M. Mortality after traumatic spinal cord injury: 50 years of follow-up. J Neurol Neurosurg Psychiatry. 2010;81(4):368–73. https://doi.org/10.1136/jnnp.2009.178798.
2. Di Marco AF, Dawson NV. Risk factors for mortality in spinal cord injury. J Spinal Cord Med. 2014;37(6):670–1. https://doi.org/10.1179/2045772314Y.0000000208.
3. van den Berg MEL, Castellote JM, de Pedro-Cuesta J, Mahillo-Fernandez I. Survival after spinal cord injury: A systematic review. J Neurotrauma. 2010;27(8):1517–28. https://doi.org/10.1089/neu.2009.1138.
4. Savic G, De Vivo MJ, Frankel HL, Jamous MA, Soni BM, Charlifue S. Causes of death after traumatic spinal cord injury—a 70-year British study. Spinal Cord. 2017;55(10):891–7. https://doi.org/10.1038/sc.2017.64.
5. De Vivo MJ, Chen Y, Wen H. Cause of death trends among persons with spinal cord injury in the United States: 1960–2017. Arch Phys Med Rehabil. 2022;103(4):634–41. https://doi.org/10.1016/j.apmr.2021.09.019.
6. Cheron A, Floccard B, Allaouchiche B, et al. Lack of recovery in monocyte human leukocyte antigen-DR expression is independently associated with the development of sepsis after major trauma. Crit Care. 2010;14(6):R208. https://doi.org/10.1186/cc9331.
7. Kopp MA, Meisel C, Liebscher T, et al. The spinal cord injury-induced immune deficiency syndrome: results of the SCIentinel study. Brain. 2023;146(8):3500–12. https://doi.org/10.1093/brain/awad092.
8. Brommer B, Engel O, Kopp MA, et al. Spinal cord injury-induced immune deficiency syndrome enhances infection susceptibility dependent on lesion level. Brain. 2016;139(Pt 3):692–707. https://doi.org/10.1093/brain/awv375.
9. Prüss H, Tedeschi A, Thiriot A, et al. Spinal cord injury-induced immunodeficiency is mediated by a sympathetic-neuroendocrine adrenal reflex. Nat Neurosci. 2017;20(11):1549–59. https://doi.org/10.1038/nn.4643.
10. Rodgers KA, Kigerl KA, Schwab JM, Popovich PG. Immune dysfunction after spinal cord injury – a review of autonomic and neuroendocrine mechanisms. Curr Opin Pharmacol. 2022;64:102230. https://doi.org/10.1016/j.coph.2022.102230.
11. Riegger T, Conrad S, Liu K, Schluesener HJ, Adibzahdeh M, Schwab JM. Spinal cord injury-induced immune depression syndrome (SCI-IDS). Eur J Neurosci. 2007;25(6):1743–7. https://doi.org/10.1111/j.1460-9568.2007.05447.x.
12. Lucin K, Sanders V, Jones T, Malarkey W, Popovich P. Impaired antibody synthesis after spinal cord injury is level dependent and is due to sympathetic nervous system dysregulation. Exp Neurol. 2007;207(1):75–84. https://doi.org/10.1016/j.expneurol.2007.05.019.
13. Trbovich M, Li C, Lee S. Does the CDC definition of fever accurately predict inflammation and infection in persons with SCI? Top Spinal Cord Inj Rehabil. 2016;22(4):260–8. https://doi.org/10.1310/sci2016-00049.
14. Song SH, Sankary KM, Burns SP. Vital sign differences between septic patients with tetraplegia and paraplegia. Spinal Cord Ser Cases 2022;8(1):87. https://doi.org/10.1038/s41394-022-00553-3.

15. Cardenas DD, Hoffman JM, Kirshblum S, McKinley W. Etiology and incidence of rehospitalization after traumatic spinal cord injury: a multicenter analysis11No commercial party having a direct financial interest in the results of the research supporting this article has or will confer a benefit upon the author(s) or upon any organization with which the author(s) is/are associated. Arch Phys Med Rehabil. 2004;85(11):1757–63. https://doi.org/10.1016/j.apmr.2004.03.016.
16. Haisma J, van der Woude L, Stam H, et al. Complications following spinal cord injury: occurrence and risk factors in a longitudinal study during and after inpatient rehabilitation. J Rehabil Med 2007;39(5):393–398. https://doi.org/10.2340/16501977-0067.
17. Evans CT, LaVela SL, Weaver FM, et al. Epidemiology of hospital-acquired infections in veterans with spinal cord injury and disorder. Infect Control Hosp Epidemiol. 2008;29(3):234–42. https://doi.org/10.1086/527509.
18. Garcia-Arguello LY, O'Horo JC, Farrell A, et al. Infections in the spinal cord-injured population: a systematic review. Spinal Cord. 2017;55(6):526–34. https://doi.org/10.1038/sc.2016.173.
19. Dinh A, Saliba M, Saadeh D, et al. Blood stream infections due to multidrug-resistant organisms among spinal cord-injured patients, epidemiology over 16 years and associated risks: a comparative study. Spinal Cord. 2016;54(9):720–5. https://doi.org/10.1038/sc.2015.234.
20. Darouiche RO. Infections in persons with spinal cord injury. In: Spinal cord medicine. Springer Publishing Company; 2018. https://doi.org/10.1891/9780826137753.0019.
21. Abbasi F, Korooni S. Infectious complications after spinal cord injury. In: Essentials of spinal cord injury medicine. InTech; 2018. https://doi.org/10.5772/intechopen.72783.
22. Sugarman B, Brown D, Musher D. Fever and infection in spinal cord injury patients. JAMA. 1982;248(1):66–70.
23. Colachis SC, Otis SM. Occurrence of fever associated with thermoregulatory dysfunction after acute traumatic spinal cord injury. Am J Phys Med Rehabil. 1995;74(2):114–9.
24. McKinley W, McNamee S, Meade M, Kandra K, Abdul N. Incidence, etiology, and risk factors for fever following acute spinal cord injury. J Spinal Cord Med. 2006;29(5):501–6. https://doi.org/10.1080/10790268.2006.11753899.
25. Unsal-Delialioglu S, Kaya K, Sahin-Onat S, Kulakli F, Culha C, Ozel S. Fever during rehabilitation in patients with traumatic spinal cord injury: analysis of 392 cases from a National Rehabilitation Hospital in Turkey. J Spinal Cord Med. 2010;33(3):243–8. https://doi.org/10.1080/10790268.2010.11689701.
26. PSS B, Neves EDC, Alves CMF, Khan P, Cirilo ACM, Alencar MRB. Pyrexia in hospitalised spinal cord injury patients. Spinal Cord. 1993;31(3):186–91. https://doi.org/10.1038/sc.1993.35.
27. Savage KE, Oleson CV, Schroeder GD, Sidhu GS, Vaccaro AR. Neurogenic fever after acute traumatic spinal cord injury: a qualitative systematic review. Glob Spine J. 2016;6(6):607–14. https://doi.org/10.1055/s-0035-1570751.
28. Attia M, Engel P. Thermoregulatory set point in patients with spinal cord injuries (spinal man). Spinal Cord. 1983;21(4):233–48. https://doi.org/10.1038/sc.1983.37.
29. Goyal J, Jha R, Bhatia P, Mani RK. QUAD fever: beware of non-infectious fever in high spinal cord injuries. BMJ Case Rep. 2017; https://doi.org/10.1136/bcr-2017-219937. Published online June 18, 2017:bcr-2017-219937
30. Watson CCL, Shaikh D, JC DG, et al. Unraveling quad fever: severe hyperthermia after traumatic cervical spinal cord injury. Chin J Traumatol. 2023;26(1):27–32. https://doi.org/10.1016/j.cjtee.2022.01.006.
31. Khan S, Plummer M, Martinez-Arizala A, Banovac K. Hypothermia in patients with chronic spinal cord injury. J Spinal Cord Med. 2007;30(1):27–30. https://doi.org/10.1080/10790268.2007.11753910.

32. Anas M, Hasan T, Raja U, Raza WA. Is procalcitonin a reliable indicator of sepsis in spinal cord injury patients: an observational cohort study. Eur Spine J. 2023;32(5):1591–7. https://doi.org/10.1007/s00586-023-07609-4.
33. Agrawal M, Joshi M. Urodynamic patterns after traumatic spinal cord injury. J Spinal Cord Med. 2015;38(2):128–33. https://doi.org/10.1179/2045772313Y.0000000136.
34. Tofte N, Nielsen ACY, Trøstrup H, et al. Chronic urinary tract infections in patients with spinal cord lesions—biofilm infection with need for long-term antibiotic treatment. APMIS. 2017;125(4):385–91. https://doi.org/10.1111/apm.12685.
35. Esclarín De Ruz A, García Leoni E, Herruzo Cabrera R. Epidemiology and risk factors for urinary tract infection in patients with spinal cord injury. J Urol. 2000;164(4):1285–9.
36. Adriaansen J, Post M, Groot S, et al. Secondary health conditions in persons with spinal cord injury: a longitudinal study from one to five years post-discharge. J Rehabil Med. 2013;45(10):1016–22. https://doi.org/10.2340/16501977-1207.
37. Siroky MB. Pathogenesis of bacteriuria and infection in the spinal cord injured patient. Am J Med 2002;113(1):67–79. https://doi.org/10.1016/S0002-9343(02)01061-6.
38. Milligan J, Goetz LL, Kennelly MJ. A primary care provider's guide to management of neurogenic lower urinary tract dysfunction and urinary tract infection after spinal cord injury. Top Spinal Cord Inj Rehabil. 2020;26(2):108–15. https://doi.org/10.46292/sci2602-108.
39. Massa LM, Hoffman JM, Cardenas DD. Validity, accuracy, and predictive value of urinary tract infection signs and symptoms in individuals with spinal cord injury on intermittent catheterization. J Spinal Cord Med. 2009;32(5):568–73. https://doi.org/10.1080/10790268.2009.11754562.
40. Nicolle L. The paradigm shift to non-treatment of asymptomatic bacteriuria. Pathogens 2016;5(2):38. https://doi.org/10.3390/pathogens5020038.
41. Nicolle LE, Gupta K, Bradley SF, et al. Clinical practice guideline for the Management of Asymptomatic Bacteriuria: 2019 update by the infectious diseases Society of Americaa. Clin Infect Dis. 2019; https://doi.org/10.1093/cid/ciy1121. Published online March 21, 2019
42. Darouiche RO, Green BG, Donovan WH, et al. Multicenter randomized controlled trial of bacterial interference for prevention of urinary tract infection in patients with neurogenic bladder. Urology. 2011;78(2):341–6. https://doi.org/10.1016/j.urology.2011.03.062.
43. Davis M, Jethani L, Robbins E, Kaner M. Is it really the Foley? A systematic review of bladder management and infection risk. Top Spinal Cord Inj Rehabil. 2023;29(1):94–107. https://doi.org/10.46292/sci22-00009.
44. Neumeier V, Stangl FP, Borer J, et al. Indwelling catheter vs intermittent catheterization: is there a difference in UTI susceptibility? BMC Infect Dis. 2023;23(1):507. https://doi.org/10.1186/s12879-023-08475-7.
45. Cardenas DD, Moore KN, Dannels-McClure A, et al. Intermittent catheterization with a hydrophilic-coated catheter delays urinary tract infections in acute spinal cord injury: a prospective, randomized, multicenter trial. PM&R. 2011;3(5):408–17. https://doi.org/10.1016/j.pmrj.2011.01.001.
46. Spinu A, Onose G, Daia C, et al. Intermittent catheterization in the management of post spinal cord injury (SCI) neurogenic bladder using new hydrophilic, with lubrication in close circuit devices--our own preliminary results. J Med Life. 2012;5(1):21–8.
47. De Ridder DJMK, Everaert K, Fernández LG, et al. Intermittent catheterisation with hydrophilic-coated catheters (SpeediCath) reduces the risk of clinical urinary tract infection in spinal cord injured patients: a prospective randomised parallel comparative trial. Eur Urol. 2005;48(6):991–5. https://doi.org/10.1016/j.eururo.2005.07.018.
48. Salameh A, AI Mohajer M, Daroucihe RO. Prevention of urinary tract infections in patients with spinal cord injury. Can Med Assoc J 2015;187(11):807–811. https://doi.org/10.1503/cmaj.141044.

49. Kennelly M, Thiruchelvam N, Averbeck MA, et al. Adult neurogenic lower urinary tract dysfunction and intermittent catheterisation in a community setting: risk factors model for urinary tract infections. Adv Urol. 2019;2019(2019):1–13. https://doi.org/10.1155/2019/2757862.
50. Goetz LL, Klausner AP. Strategies for prevention of urinary tract infections in neurogenic bladder dysfunction. Phys Med Rehabil Clin N Am. 2014;25(3):605–18. https://doi.org/10.1016/j.pmr.2014.04.002.
51. Kranz J, Bartoletti R, Bruyère F, et al. European Association of Urology guidelines on urological infections: summary of the 2024 guidelines. Eur Urol. 2024;86(1):27–41. https://doi.org/10.1016/j.eururo.2024.03.035.
52. LE N. Urinary tract infections in patients with spinal injuries. Curr Infect Dis Rep. 2014;16(1):390. https://doi.org/10.1007/s11908-013-0390-9.
53. Chen Y, DeVivo MJ, Stover SL, Lloyd LK. Recurrent kidney stone: a 25-year follow-up study in persons with spinal cord injury. Urology. 2002;60(2):228–32. https://doi.org/10.1016/S0090-4295(02)01734-X.
54. Ramsey S, C MI. Evidence-based management of upper tract urolithiasis in the spinal cord-injured patient. Spinal Cord. 2011;49(9):948–54. https://doi.org/10.1038/sc.2011.50.
55. Todd J, Murden M, Brooks E. A report of two cases of sepsis in patients with spinal cord injuries. J R Coll Physicians Edinb. 2023;53(1):40–3. https://doi.org/10.1177/14782715221148055.
56. Yang JH, Shin JY, Roh SG, Chang SC, Lee NH. Delayed diagnosis of xanthogranulomatous pyelonephritis in a quadriplegic patient with uncontrolled cutaneous fistula. Medicine 2018;97(2):e9659. https://doi.org/10.1097/MD.0000000000009659.
57. Kalisvaart JF, Katsumi HK, Ronningen LD, Hovey RM. Bladder cancer in spinal cord injury patients. Spinal Cord. 2010;48(3):257–61. https://doi.org/10.1038/sc.2009.118.
58. Welk B, McIntyre A, Teasell R, Potter P, Loh E. Bladder cancer in individuals with spinal cord injuries. Spinal Cord. 2013;51(7):516–21. https://doi.org/10.1038/sc.2013.33.
59. Burns SP, Weaver FM, Parada JP, et al. Management of community-acquired pneumonia in persons with spinal cord injury. Spinal Cord. 2004;42(8):450–8. https://doi.org/10.1038/sj.sc.3101600.
60. Hayashi T, Fujiwara Y, Irie M, et al. Effect of nutritional status on occurrence of pneumonia after traumatic cervical spinal cord injury. Sci Rep. 2024;14(1):13286. https://doi.org/10.1038/s41598-024-64121-5.
61. Mueller G, Berlowitz DJ, Raab AM, et al. Incidence and risk factors of pneumonia in individuals with acute spinal cord injury: a multi-national, multi-center, prospective cohort study. Arch Phys Med Rehabil. 2024;105(5):884–91. https://doi.org/10.1016/j.apmr.2023.11.002.
62. Agostinello J, Battistuzzo CR, Batchelor PE. Early clinical predictors of pneumonia in critically ill spinal cord injured individuals: a retrospective cohort study. Spinal Cord. 2019;57(1):41–8. https://doi.org/10.1038/s41393-018-0196-6.
63. Hayashi T, Fujiwara Y, Kawano O, et al. Incidence and risk factors of pneumonia following acute traumatic cervical spinal cord injury. J Spinal Cord Med. 2023;46(5):725–31. https://doi.org/10.1080/10790268.2022.2027323.
64. Ushiku C, Suda K, Michikawa T, et al. Incidence and risk factors for pneumonia in the chronic phase of cervical spinal cord injury with complete motor paralysis. Spine Surg Relat Res. 2023;7(4):2022–0254. https://doi.org/10.22603/ssrr.2022-0254.
65. DeVivo MJ. Epidemiology of traumatic spinal cord injury: trends and future implications. Spinal Cord. 2012;50(5):365–72. https://doi.org/10.1038/sc.2011.178.
66. Kopp MA, Watzlawick R, Martus P, et al. Long-term functional outcome in patients with acquired infections after acute spinal cord injury. Neurology. 2017;88(9):892–900. https://doi.org/10.1212/WNL.0000000000003652.
67. Burns SP. Acute respiratory infections in persons with spinal cord injury. Phys Med Rehabil Clin N Am. 2007;18(2):203–16. https://doi.org/10.1016/j.pmr.2007.02.001.

68. Schilero GJ, Grimm DR, Bauman WA, Lenner R, Lesser M. Assessment of airway caliber and bronchodilator responsiveness in subjects with spinal cord injury. Chest. 2005;127(1):149–55. https://doi.org/10.1378/chest.127.1.149.
69. Shem K, Castillo K, Wong S, Chang J. Dysphagia in individuals with tetraplegia: incidence and risk factors. J Spinal Cord Med. 2011;34(1):85–92. https://doi.org/10.1179/107902610X12911165974981.
70. Waites KB, Canupp KC, Chen Y Ying, DeVivo MJ, Nahm MH. Revaccination of adults with spinal cord injury using the 23-Valent pneumococcal polysaccharide vaccine. J Spinal Cord Med 2008;31(1):53–59. https://doi.org/10.1080/10790268.2008.11753981.
71. Waites KB, Canupp KC, Edwards K, Palmer P, Gray BM, De Vivo MJ. Immunogenicity of pneumococcal vaccine in persons with spinal cord injury. Arch Phys Med Rehabil 1998;79(12):1504–1509. https://doi.org/10.1016/S0003-9993(98)90410-5.
72. Darouiche RO, Groover J, Rowland J, Musher DM. Pneumococcal vaccination for patients with spinal cord injury. Arch Phys Med Rehabil 1993;74(12):1354–1357. https://doi.org/10.1016/0003-9993(93)90092-O.
73. Shiferaw WS, Akalu TY, Mulugeta H, Aynalem YA. The global burden of pressure ulcers among patients with spinal cord injury: a systematic review and meta-analysis. BMC Musculoskelet Disord. 2020;21(1):334. https://doi.org/10.1186/s12891-020-03369-0.
74. Mervis JS, Phillips TJ. Pressure ulcers: pathophysiology, epidemiology, risk factors, and presentation. J Am Acad Dermatol. 2019;81(4):881–90. https://doi.org/10.1016/j.jaad.2018.12.069.
75. Vecin NM, Gater DR. Pressure injuries and management after spinal cord injury. J Pers Med. 2022;12(7):1130. https://doi.org/10.3390/jpm12071130.
76. Edsberg LE, Black JM, Goldberg M, McNichol L, Moore L, Sieggreen M. Revised national pressure ulcer advisory panel pressure injury staging system. J Wound Ostomy Continence Nurs. 2016;43(6):585–97. https://doi.org/10.1097/WON.0000000000000281.
77. Salzberg CA, Byrne DW, Cayten CG, van Niewerburgh P, Murphy JG, Viehbeck M. A new pressure ulcer risk assessment SCALE for individuals with spinal cord INJURY1. Am J Phys Med Rehabil. 1996;75(2):96–104. https://doi.org/10.1097/00002060-199603000-00004.
78. Dana AN, Bauman WA. Bacteriology of pressure ulcers in individuals with spinal cord injury: what we know and what we should know. J Spinal Cord Med. 2015;38(2):147–60. https://doi.org/10.1179/2045772314Y.0000000234.
79. Tedeschi S, Negosanti L, Sgarzani R, et al. Superficial swab versus deep-tissue biopsy for the microbiological diagnosis of local infection in advanced-stage pressure ulcers of spinal-cord-injured patients: a prospective study. Clin Microbiol Infect. 2017;23(12):943–7. https://doi.org/10.1016/j.cmi.2017.04.015.
80. Sibbald RG, Woo K, Ayello EA. Increased bacterial burden and infection. Adv Skin Wound Care. 2006;19(8):447–61. https://doi.org/10.1097/00129334-200610000-00012.
81. Brunel AS, Lamy B, Cyteval C, et al. Diagnosing pelvic osteomyelitis beneath pressure ulcers in spinal cord injured patients: a prospective study. Clin Microbiol Infect. 2016;22(3):267.e1–8. https://doi.org/10.1016/j.cmi.2015.11.005.
82. Huang AB, Schweitzer ME, Hume E, Batte WG. Osteomyelitis of the pelvis/hips in paralyzed patients: accuracy and clinical utility of MRI. J Comput Assist Tomogr. 1998;22(3):437–43. https://doi.org/10.1097/00004728-199805000-00017.
83. Hauptfleisch J, Meagher TM, Hughes RJ, Singh JP, Graham A, López de Heredia L. Interobserver agreement of magnetic resonance imaging signs of osteomyelitis in pelvic pressure ulcers in patients with spinal cord injury. Arch Phys Med Rehabil 2013;94(6):1107–1111. https://doi.org/10.1016/j.apmr.2012.11.012.
84. Ruan CM, Escobedo E, Harrison S, Goldstein B. Magnetic resonance imaging of nonhealing pressure ulcers and myocutaneous flaps. Arch Phys Med Rehabil 1998;79(9):1080–1088. https://doi.org/10.1016/S0003-9993(98)90175-7.
85. Lewis VL, Bailey MH, Pulawski G, Kind G, Bashioum RW, Hendrix RW. The diagnosis of osteomyelitis in patients with pressure sores. Plast Reconstr Surg. 1988;81(2):229–32. https://doi.org/10.1097/00006534-198802000-00016.

86. Evans CT, Hershow RC, Chin A, Foulis PR, Burns SP, Weaver FM. Bloodstream infections and setting of onset in persons with spinal cord injury and disorder. Spinal Cord. 2009;47(8):610–5. https://doi.org/10.1038/sc.2009.2.
87. Saliba M, Saadeh D, Bouchand F, et al. Outcome of bloodstream infections among spinal cord injury patients and impact of multidrug-resistant organisms. Spinal Cord. 2017;55(2):148–54. https://doi.org/10.1038/sc.2016.176.
88. Waites KB, Canupp KC, Chen Y, DeVivo MJ, Moser SA. Bacteremia after spinal cord injury in initial versus subsequent hospitalizations. J Spinal Cord Med 2001;24(2):96–100. https://doi.org/10.1080/10790268.2001.11753562.
89. Bhatt K, Cid E, Maiman D. Bacteremia in the spinal cord injury population. J Am Paraplegia Soc 1987;10(1):11–14. https://doi.org/10.1080/01952307.1987.11719628.
90. Montgomerie JZ, Chan E, Gilmore DS, Canawati HN, Sapico FL. Low mortality among patients with spinal cord injury and bacteremia. Clin Infect Dis 1991;13(5):867–871. https://doi.org/10.1093/clinids/13.5.867.
91. Poutanen SM. Clostridium difficile-associated diarrhea in adults. Can Med Assoc J 2004;171(1):51–58. https://doi.org/10.1503/cmaj.1031189.
92. Liu B, Reid J, Silverman M, Welk B. High risk of Clostridium difficile infection among spinal cord injured patients after the use of antibiotics commonly used to treat urinary tract infections. Neurourol Urodyn. 2020;39(8):2401–8. https://doi.org/10.1002/nau.24502.
93. Ramanathan S, Johnson S, Burns SP, et al. Recurrence of Clostridium difficile infection among veterans with spinal cord injury and disorder. Am J Infect Control. 2014;42(2):168–73. https://doi.org/10.1016/j.ajic.2013.08.009.
94. Dumford DM III, Nerandzic M, Chang S, Richmond MA, Donskey C. Epidemiology of Clostridium difficile and vancomycin-resistant enterococcus colonization in patients on a spinal cord injury unit. J Spinal Cord Med. 2011;34(1):22–7. https://doi.org/10.1179/107902610x12883422813822.

Metabolism, Nutrition, and Muscle Wasting in Critically Ill Spinal Cord Injury Patients

18

Paolo Formenti, Elda Sterchele, Alessandro Menozzi, and Michele Umbrello

18.1 Introduction

Spinal cord injury (SCI) refers to damage inflicted upon the spinal cord, leading to alterations, which may be temporary or permanent, in its typical motor, sensory, or autonomic functions [3]. This injury can be classified into two main categories: tetraplegia, affecting the upper limbs and trunk, and paraplegia, affecting the lower limbs [26]. The prevalence of SCI varies globally, affecting approximately 11.5–57.8 individuals per million people worldwide [32]. Damage at the cervical level (CSCI) constitutes a significant portion, accounting for approximately 41.6–76.0% of all SCI cases [4]. Critically ill patients with SCI encounter a variety of challenges related to metabolism, nutrition, and muscle wasting [63]. These alterations have insightful implications for energy expenditure, nutrient requirements, and muscle metabolism, necessitating a comprehensive understanding to provide tailored nutritional support and prevent complications in this vulnerable population. Patients may experience hypermetabolism, characterized by increased resting energy expenditure (REE) and higher energy requirements, particularly during the acute phase of injury. This increased metabolic demand is driven by factors such as inflammation, tissue repair, and the energy cost of maintaining physiological functions in the face of injury-induced stress. As a result, patients require higher caloric intake to meet their metabolic needs and support the healing process. The trauma itself triggers a cascade of events, including inflammation, oxidative stress, and hormonal imbalances,

P. Formenti (✉)
SC Anestesia, Rianimazione e Terapia Intensiva, ASST Nord Milano, Ospedale Bassini, Cinisello Balsamo, Italy

E. Sterchele · M. Umbrello
Department of Intensive Care, ASST Ovest Milanese, New Hospital of Legnano, Milan, Italy
e-mail: michele.umbrello@asst-ovestmi.it

A. Menozzi
School of Medicine and Surgery, University of Milano-Bicocca, Milan, Italy

E. Brogi et al. (eds.), *Traumatic Spinal Cord Injury*, Hot Topics in Acute Care Surgery and Trauma, https://doi.org/10.1007/978-3-031-99890-4_18

all of which contribute to alterations in metabolic homeostasis [31]. The sympathetic nervous system, responsible for regulating many metabolic functions, becomes dysregulated following SCI, further exacerbating metabolic disturbances [69]. Moreover, muscle metabolism is profoundly affected by SCI, leading to muscle wasting and loss of lean body mass [70]. This is the result of a combination of events, which, however, find a connection at the cellular level and particularly mitochondrial. Few studies have evaluated in vivo mitochondrial function in paralyzed skeletal muscle, showing how oxidative metabolism was reduced in paralyzed muscle [41]. Furthermore, disuse atrophy, a common consequence of immobility following injury, accelerates muscle breakdown and impairs muscle protein synthesis [25]. Additionally, alterations in hormonal signaling, such as increased levels of cortisol and pro-inflammatory cytokines, further contribute to muscle catabolism [45]. As a result, patients with SCI are at heightened risk of developing sarcopenia and functional impairment, which can significantly impact their overall prognosis and quality of life. In this chapter, we will address these complexities, providing clinical suggestions to deliver tailored nutritional support and improve outcomes in critically ill patients with SCI.

18.2 Metabolic Changes in Critically Ill SCI Patients

Clinical observations showed that 44.3% of patients with cervical spinal cord injury were either at risk for malnutrition or were already malnourished at the time of admission. The risk was higher in cases of acute high cervical SCI compared to those with lower SCI (60.7% versus 34.5%), and it was more common in patients with additional complications such as ventilator support (56.3% with tracheotomy versus 38.7%) [67]. Critically ill SCI patients experience metabolic alterations that significantly impact their overall health and recovery. These changes encompass shifts in energy expenditure, substrate utilization, and hormonal regulation [26]. Like all type of trauma, the initial changes in metabolism start with elevated circulating levels of glucagon, cortisol, catecholamine, and cytokines [58], but in the acute phase post-injury, patients with SCI undergo metabolic changes, including reduced basal energy expenditure due to paralysis, coupled with increased nitrogen excretion. This increased state of stress leads to amplified catabolism, accelerated breakdown of muscle tissue and other metabolic substrates, contributing to muscle wasting and loss of lean body mass. In addition to alterations in energy metabolism, SCI also affects substrate utilization. The increased catabolic state induced by SCI leads to accelerated breakdown of metabolic substrates, including carbohydrates, fats, and proteins [6]. This results in a shift towards gluconeogenesis and lipolysis, as the body mobilizes energy from alternative sources to meet increased metabolic demands.

In trauma patients, it is estimated that the REE is approximately 140% of the predicted normal basal energy expenditure. However, in SCI patients, this response appears to be blunted, with reductions in REE ranging from 20% to 30% [42]. Basal metabolic rate, typically assessed via indirect calorimetry after an overnight fast and prolonged bed rest, constitutes approximately 65% of total daily energy expenditure, significantly impacting energy balance [10, 55]. Studies have primarily focused on REE measurement due to its feasibility without extensive bed rest, highlighting its susceptibility to muscle loss and potential disruption of energy balance. Individuals with complete SCI often exhibit BMR ranging from 900 to 1500 kcal/day, with variations likely attributed to the extent of injury, whether tetraplegia or paraplegia [22, 40]. The influence of regional body composition changes on basal metabolic rate or REE in SCI individuals remains unclear. A reduced REE (14–27% lower than able-bodied controls) and physical activity energy expenditure (PAEE, up to 14% lower than able-bodied controls) determine a reduction in total energy expenditure in SCI patients [11]. This reduction in REE is partially attributed to decreased fat-free mass (FFM) and attenuated autonomic responses post-SCI. Discrepancies in total energy expenditure estimation between studies may stem from variations in methodology and individual characteristics, potentially exceeding the typical 2200 kcal/day observed in able-bodied controls [6]. Kearns et al. found that in a study involving 10 patients, the mean REE after acute injury was only 67% of the basal energy expenditure predicted by the Harris-Benedict formula [30]. Interestingly, REE increased by 5% with the return of muscle tone. During the acute stage, there's often a negative nitrogen balance, measured by urinary nitrogen, which can increase up to 27% (0.18 to 0.23 g/kg/day). These nitrogen losses persist for at least 7 weeks following the injury. Despite the provision of sufficient quantities of calories and protein during acute injury, a negative nitrogen balance typically occurs, peaking during the third week after injury. In a study involving twelve patients with acute SCI, none of the SCI patients achieved a positive nitrogen balance during the 7 week period following injury, despite receiving an average delivery of 2.4 g of protein/kg IBW and 120% of the predicted energy expenditure [50]. As a consequence, in the initial 4 weeks following SCI, patients commonly experience weight loss, estimated at 10–20% of their body weight with approximately 85% of this weight loss consists of lean mass [21].

Elevated levels of stress hormones, such as cortisol and catecholamines, contribute to insulin resistance and impaired glucose metabolism. This phenomenon is exacerbated by factors such as inflammation, oxidative stress, and hormonal imbalances, all of which are prevalent in critically ill SCI patients [14]. Disruptions in sympathetic nervous system activity following SCI contribute to metabolic disturbances observed in critically ill patients [53]. Dysregulation of sympathetic activity can lead to insulin resistance, impaired glucose uptake, and alterations in lipid metabolism, further complicating the metabolic profile of SCI patients.

In summary, critically ill spinal cord injury patients undergo significant metabolic changes characterized by increased catabolism, muscle wasting, and dysregulation of metabolic pathways. These alterations are driven by the stress response to injury, immobilization, and disruptions in sympathetic nervous system activity. Understanding these metabolic complexities is essential for providing optimal care and nutritional support to SCI patients, to mitigate muscle loss, promoting healing, and improving overall outcomes.

18.3 Nutritional Considerations in Critically Ill SCI Patients

Nutritional support is crucial in the management of critically ill SCI patients, requiring attention to address their distinctive metabolic and physiological needs mentioned above. Wong et al. [68] showed how the median length of stay was significantly longer in patients with cervical spinal injury compared to those without (129 days vs. 85 days), with a greater 12-month mortality rate observed in the CSIC group (9.2% deceased vs. 1.4%). Furthermore, declining dynamic nutritional status, as indicated by low serum protein levels in the 2 weeks following initial treatment for CSIC, was associated with early mortality in CSIC patients. This finding underscores the importance of nutritional support in improving outcomes for this patient population. In a study by Jiang Shao et al. [57], nearly 80% of patients in the early mortality group were found to be malnourished compared to only 27% of patients who survived beyond 30 days. Rowan et al. [52] suggest that a hypermetabolic reaction could be prevalent yet diverse among individuals in this group. In their retrospective study, caloric intake swiftly increased to a stable level of 2300–2400 kcal per day within the initial 4 days. Initially, the median measured total energy expenditure via indirect calorimetry was notably high, starting at 3472 kcal/day and gradually decreasing to 2784 kcal/day by the third week. However, there was considerable diversity in energy expenditure among patients. Consequently, there's a risk of both under- and overfeeding if nutrition goals aren't informed by indirect calorimetry.

Adequate protein intake is of greatest importance in critically ill SCI patients to preserve muscle mass and promote wound healing. Despite aggressive nutritional support, patients number of patients experience an obligatory negative nitrogen balance which persists for up to 2 months post-injury [29, 36, 49]. While some patients exhibit a positive nitrogen balance in the first week post-injury, this is believed to be a delay in protein losses rather than genuine incorporation of protein into body stores [50]. Thus, individualized assessments are necessary to determine optimal protein requirements, considering factors such as injury severity, metabolic rate, and clinical status.

The proportion of carbohydrates and fats in the diet should be carefully balanced to prevent complications such as hyperglycemia or excessive weight gain. For these two macronutrients, there is no specific evidence providing indications regarding types and quantities. Therefore, we would prefer to refer to the ESPEN guidelines [59]. However, it should be borne in mind that the prevalence of neurogenic obesity in adults with SCI varies widely, ranging from 22% to 97%, compared to 42% in the non-disabled population [18]. Neurogenic obesity stems from factors such as disrupted energy metabolism, physical deconditioning, a sedentary lifestyle, reduced fitness, dysfunction of the sympathetic nervous system, hormonal imbalances, alterations in satiety, and loss of lean body mass following SCI. All these considerations are summarized in Fig. 18.1.

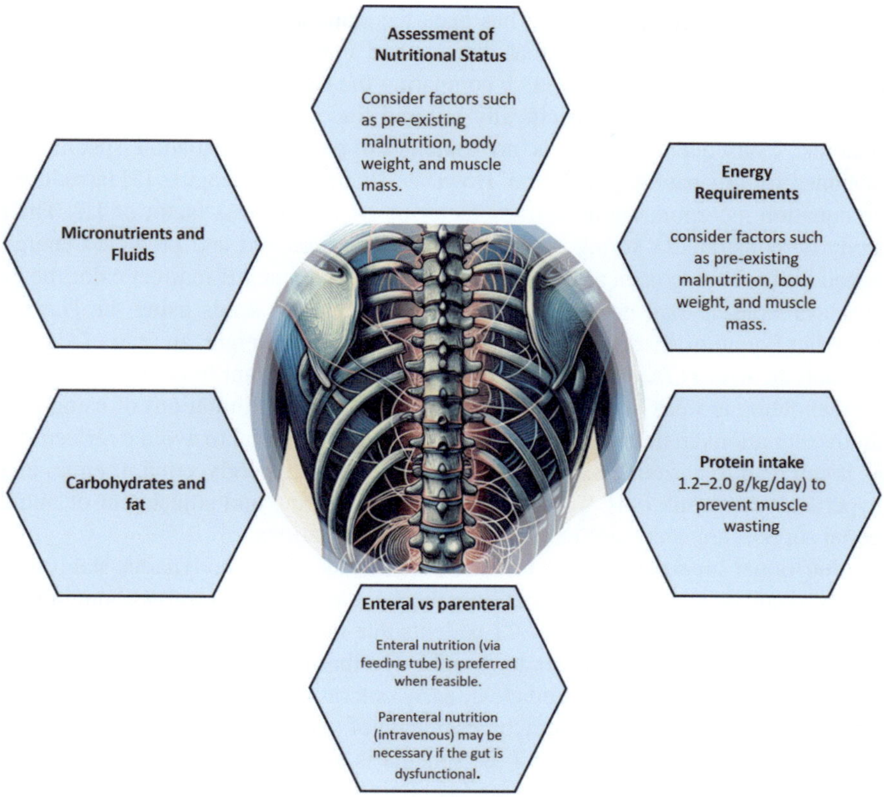

Fig. 18.1 Nutritional management for critically ill patients with spinal cord injuries

18.4 Determining Energy Requirements

In the acute care setting, nutrition assessment should be conducted within the first 48 h post-injury to promptly identify and address any nutritional needs. Assessing metabolic needs through biochemical and anthropometric tests can provide valuable insights [15, 29, 36]. In SCI patients with quadriplegia, a reduction of 10–15% below their ideal body weight is recommended, while in those with paraplegia, a reduction of 5–10% below their ideal body weight is advised. These recommendations emphasize the importance of maintaining appropriate body weight to support overall health and function in individuals with quadriplegia or paraplegia. Indirect calorimetry is more accurate than estimating energy needs in critically ill patients. This recommendation is based on strong evidence with conditional support. Additionally, the traditional method of estimating energy needs using resting energy expenditure calculated by multiplying the Harris–Benedict Equation by an activity factor and an injury factor of 1.6 has been the standard criterion for many years. However, studies have shown that this method may overestimate energy needs. Currently, there is a lack of research comparing the Harris–Benedict Equation with other predictive equations specifically tailored for critically ill spinal cord injury patients. Consequently, there is no established predictive equation specifically designed for this patient population. However, Barco and colleagues [5] introduced an equation incorporating an activity factor of 1.1 and a stress factor of 1.2. Their study demonstrated a strong correlation between measured and predicted energy expenditures among critically ill spinal cord injury patients. If indirect calorimetry is unavailable, it may be considered to estimate energy needs using the Harris–Benedict Equation, incorporating the patient's admission weight, an injury factor of 1.2, and an activity factor of 1.1 [46]. However, it's important to note that this recommendation is weak and conditional due to the potential limitations of using predictive equations in this population. Furthermore, it is crucial to avoid overfeeding, as it can lead to various risks, including hypercapnia, hyperglycemia, uremia, and hypertriglyceridemia [44]. Therefore, careful monitoring and adjustment of nutritional support are necessary to prevent these complications.

Nutritional support should be initiated early, as soon as hemodynamic stability is achieved and deemed feasible. Traditionally, there have been concerns about initiating enteral feeding promptly in SCI patients due to worries about ileus and other complications. However, studies have indicated that feeding these patients within the first 72 h is safe [63]. Nonetheless, early enteral feeding has not been demonstrated to impact neurological outcomes, length of stay, or the incidence of complications in patients with acute SCI. Dysphagia is a common issue following SCI, particularly with higher-level injuries [1]. Thus, enteral feeding is considered the preferred route for administering nutritional requirements following SCI. Similarly to the general critical care population, among the enteral feeding options, nasogastric feeding is commonly initiated, followed by nasojejunal feeding if gastric intolerance occurs, and percutaneous endoscopic gastrostomy if longer-term feeding is required. The advantages of enteral nutrition over parenteral nutrition include the maintenance of gut integrity and function, a lower risk of infection, and avoidance of complications associated with intravenous catheterization. If enteral feeds are unable to meet the metabolic demands due to conditions such as bowel injury, mechanical bowel obstruction, or prolonged ileus within 5 days of injury, total parenteral nutrition should be initiated.

18.5 Peculiar Clinical Scenarios Associated with Spinal Cord Injury

18.5.1 Pressure Ulcers

Due to immobility, individuals with spinal cord injury are at an elevated risk of developing pressure ulcers (Table 18.1). The Spinal Cord Injury Pressure Ulcer Scale (SCIPUS) is a valuable tool for assessing pressure ulcer risk and identifying

Table 18.1 Management of pressure ulcers in critically ill patients with spinal cord injuries

Pressure ulcers		
Energy	30–40 kcal/kg per day	
Protein	Stage II ulcers	1.2–1.5 g/kg per day
	Stage III-IV ulcers	1.5–2.0 g/kg per day
UCR	Below 20:1 mg/dl	
Vitamin C	Stage I–II ulcers	100–200 mg per day
	Stage III–IV ulcers	1000–2000 mg per day
Zinc	50 mg twice per day (until 2–3 weeks)	
Vitamin A	10,000–50,000 IU per day (until 10 days)	
Vitamin E	800 IU per day	

potential nutritional issues [24]. Potential nutritional risk factors associated with spinal cord injury include patients with albumin levels below 3.5 g/dl, who were nearly five times as likely to develop a pressure ulcer [34]. Other risk factors include hematocrit levels below 36% and hemoglobin levels below 12 g/dl, negative nitrogen balance, low body mass index/thinness, inadequate fluid intake/dehydration, poor nutritional intake, obesity, inadequate serum ascorbic acid, inadequate serum zinc, triceps skinfold thickness below normal, inadequate protein intake, and general vitamin deficiencies. Assessment for individuals with spinal cord injury and pressure ulcers includes determining their energy needs using indirect calorimetry. If it is not available, an estimate of 30–40 kcal per kg of body weight per day can be used, adjusted according to the Harris-Benedict equation and specific stress factor (such as 1.2 for stage II ulcers, 1.5 for stage III and IV ulcers) [35]. Protein needs for individuals with pressure ulcers are recommended at 1.2–1.5 g of protein per kg of body weight per day for Stage II ulcers, and 1.5–2.0 g of protein per kg of body weight per day for Stage III and IV ulcers [54]. It is important to calculate these requirements using actual body weight and closely monitor patients for signs and symptoms of overfeeding or underfeeding. Fluid needs should be assessed by evaluating hydration status through various indicators such as input and output measurements, urine color, skin integrity, blood urea nitrogen, and serum sodium levels. A urea nitrogen/creatinine ratio greater than 20:1 mg/dl may indicate dehydration, although this measure can be inaccurate in individuals with renal impairment. Micronutrient supplementation should be re-evaluated by the dietitian every seven to 10 days to ensure adequacy. For Vitamin C supplementation, a dosage of 100–200 mg per day for Stage I and II pressure ulcers, and 1000–2000 mg per day for Stage III and IV ulcers [43]. However, caution should be exercised in individuals with renal failure due to the potential risk of renal oxalate stone formation. For Zinc supplementation, a recommended dosage is 50 mg elemental Zinc twice per day. However, it is important to note that high-dose supplementation can have adverse effects on copper status, immune response, and lipid profiles. Some authors have suggested limiting high-dose supplementation to 2–3 weeks to mitigate these risks. As for Vitamin A supplementation, documented recommendations for promoting enhanced wound healing in injured patients range from 10,000 IU to 50,000 IU per day [71]. However, caution should be exercised due to the potential for toxicity. It is advisable to implement Vitamin A supplementation cautiously, with a limit of

10 days. Acute spinal cord compression injury in cats swiftly depletes endogenous tissue vitamin E levels, plummeting by 80% compared to non-injured spinal tissue within 4 h post-injury [63, 64]. This rapid decline is attributed to the intensive consumption of vitamin E during the vigorous post-SCI lipid peroxidation reactions [2]. Vitamin E deficiency has been demonstrated to exacerbate post-SCI lipid peroxidation and impede motor functional recovery [61]. However, the immediate utility of vitamin E as an acute treatment for SCI is hindered by the time it takes weeks to achieve a significant increase in parenchymal central nervous system tissue levels [39]. For potential application in human use of vitamin E supplementation to mitigate post-SCI neurological impairment, research indicates that a dosage of 800 I.U./day is necessary to reduce baseline lipid peroxidation product levels in human plasma after 20 weeks of daily supplementation [47].

18.5.2 Neurogenic Bowel

Neurogenic bowel dysfunction presents a significant problem for those living with SCI, profoundly affecting both their well-being and health outcomes. This condition manifests through a range of lower gastrointestinal symptoms, including loss of voluntary bowel control, diminished awareness of stool passage, and challenges with stool evacuation [48]. Additionally, individuals may contend with upper intestinal symptoms like abdominal discomfort, bloating, epigastric burning, and premature feelings of fullness. Over time, these intestinal issues tend to exacerbate, contributing to a decline in overall health and necessitating more frequent hospitalization. The sympathetic nervous system provides innervation to the upper gastrointestinal (GI) tract, descending colon, and rectal vault, with increased activation during crises, reducing GI function to prioritize skeletal muscle activity [7]. Parasympathetic nervous system innervation extends from the upper GI tract to the mid-transverse colon via the vagus nerve, and to the remainder of the large bowel, including the internal anal sphincter, via pelvic nerves. Gut reflexes, including the gastrocolic, colocolonic, rectocolic, and anorectal reflexes, assist in defecation and can be suppressed voluntarily. Injury to the terminal portion of the spinal cord (conus medullaris) may affect both upper and lower motor neurons [38]. Oral medications like bowel stimulants and osmotic agents are commonly used to facilitate stool movement. Dietary choices, including high-fiber foods and adequate fluid intake, play a significant role in maintaining stool consistency and transit times (Fig. 18.2). However, caution is needed with fiber intake to avoid exacerbating constipation [27]. Regarding fiber intake, it's recommended to start with an initial intake of 15 g per day, gradually increasing to 30 g per day as tolerated [28]. In terms of fluid intake, it's crucial to ensure adequate hydration for bowel movement. The recommendation is to consume one milliliter of fluid per kilocalorie of estimated energy intake, with a minimum of 1.5 liters per day [8]. Relative newer medications, such as lubiprostone, linaclotide, plecanatide, prucalopride, methylnaltrexone, and alvimopan, offer additional options for improving neurogenic bowel care when standard medications are ineffective [17, 62]. Lubiprostone enhances

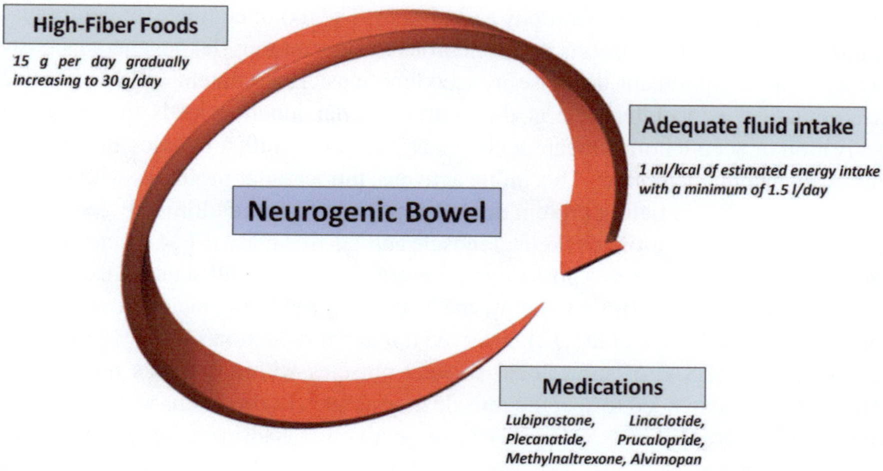

Fig. 18.2 Schematic representation of neurogenic bowel management in critically ill spinal cord injury patients

intestinal fluid secretion, aiding stool passage, while linaclotide and plecanatide promote intestinal transit by activating guanylate cyclase-C receptors. Prucalopride stimulates colonic transit and segmental contractions, improving constipation. Methylnaltrexone and alvimopan act as peripherally acting μ-opioid receptor antagonists, alleviating constipation caused by high-dose opioids without affecting central nervous system function.

18.6 Muscle Wasting and Functional Implications

Muscle wasting is a common complication in critically ill SCI patients, driven by a combination of factors including disuse atrophy, inflammation, and protein breakdown. ICU-acquired weakness (ICUAW) encompasses a range of neuromuscular disorders stemming from ICU admission and severe illness [19]. While its exact pathophysiology remains unclear, it seems to be induced by critical illness itself rather than the underlying condition. Characterized by inflammatory responses, bioenergetic dysfunction, altered protein balance, neuronal degeneration, changes in muscle histology, and muscle wasting, ICUAW is exacerbated by factors like immobilization and disrupted neuroendocrine responses during critical illness [33]. Muscle wasting is driven by negative protein balance, while muscle dysfunction arises from microcirculatory disturbances, mitochondrial impairment, and disruptions in ion channels. These factors, combined with immobilization and malnutrition, contribute to muscle wasting as the predominant feature of acquired muscle weakness in critically ill patients.

After spinal cord injury, motor neurons undergo apoptosis, leading to changes in morphology and function [70]. Synapses shorten, and skeletal muscles innervated by these neurons experience atrophy and fibrosis. The motor endplate, or neuromuscular junction, which connects motor neurons to skeletal muscle, degenerates post-injury, with a significant decrease in acetylcholinesterase content [37]. Excessive accumulation of acetylcholine at the neuromuscular junction leads to prolonged activation of acetylcholine receptor channels, causing an influx of calcium ions into the postsynaptic membrane. This influx activates intracellular proteases within skeletal muscle cells, initiating protein degradation pathways and ultimately leading to apoptosis [64]. Alterations in skeletal muscle and fat-free mass (FFM) occur following SCI. In the initial stages post-injury, there is a rapid and substantial decrease in skeletal muscle mass, primarily below the level of injury. Using magnetic resonance imaging (MRI), Castro et al. [12] observed a notable reduction (18–46%) in cross-sectional area (CSA) of sublesional skeletal muscles within 6 weeks post-injury. This reduction extended to specific muscle groups such as the soleus and gastrocnemius, with decreases of 12% and 24%, respectively. Quadriceps, hamstrings, and hip adductor muscles also experienced a decline (14–16%) within the initial 24 weeks post-SCI, with CSA reaching 45–80% smaller compared to able-bodied controls at 24 weeks [56]. Incomplete SCI individuals exhibit a 30% reduction in CSA of knee extensors 6 weeks post-injury compared to controls. Muscle atrophy persists, with a 43% decrease in original muscle size noted 4.5 months post-SCI, accompanied by an increase in intramuscular fat levels [20], which can contribute to glucose intolerance [16]. Moreover, SCI alters the balance between fast and slow-twitch muscle fibers, primarily due to paralysis below the injury level. Over time, muscle fibers transition predominantly to fast-twitch fibers, rendering the muscles more fatigable and prone to damage [23]. This decline in muscle mass is paralleled by changes in FFM, as noted by studies comparing SCI individuals with their able-bodied counterparts. Spungen et al. [60] reported a significant decline in FFM over time in SCI individuals, particularly in areas below the level of injury. Moreover, individuals with SCI exhibit higher fat mass (FM) percentages and lower FFM percentages compared to able-bodied twins [66]. The decline in FFM is associated with the level and completeness of injury, with tetraplegia resulting in greater FFM loss compared to paraplegia. Decreases in muscle mass, particularly in the upper extremities, may contribute to impaired upper limb function post-SCI. Few studies have employed methods such as whole-body potassium counts and predictive equations to estimate FFM in SCI individuals. Reduced muscle mass and resting energy expenditure are consistently observed in SCI individuals compared to able-bodied controls. Predictive equations developed by Gorgey et al. [22] offer a practical approach for estimating FFM in SCI populations, aiding in monitoring longitudinal adaptations post-injury. Then, systemic muscle loss can exacerbate when the adrenal glands lose central nervous system regulation, leading to a hormonal imbalance [9]. In such cases, hypercortisolism, marked by excessive cortisol release, may occur following spinal cord injury. This hypercortisolism affects muscle tissue throughout the body via specific receptors, resulting in muscle loss [13]. Interventions targeting this pathway could potentially preserve muscle tissue and enhance the response to rehabilitation efforts. SCI triggers a secondary injury cascade, affecting hormones like testosterone and glucocorticoids [65]. Testosterone treatment can prevent oxidative neural stress damage and skeletal muscle atrophy post-SCI, while estradiol improves motor function and has anti-inflammatory effects. Hormone therapy shows promise in reducing muscle atrophy by increasing myogenic fibronectin DNA transcription and activating muscle satellite cells. Synthetic steroid hormones, including testosterone and insulin-like growth factor, combat muscle atrophy by promoting muscle cell proliferation and differentiation. Current strategies for preventing and treating skeletal muscle atrophy after SCI primarily focus on exercise and hormone therapy. Both approaches have demonstrated positive therapeutic effects through diverse molecular mechanisms. Clinical interventions for managing skeletal muscle atrophy following SCI often involve exercise training as a cornerstone of treatment. Table 18.2 describes in detail the characteristics of the main studies published on the current topic.

Table 18.2 Key clinical studies on nutritional support in critically ill patients with spinal cord injuries

Study	Patients	Design	Main findings
[67]	150 patients	Cross-sectional multicenter study	Upon admission, 44.3% of patients were either malnourished or at risk of undernutrition. Nutritional risk was more prevalent among patients with acute high cervical SCI compared to those with lower SCI. Additionally, 45% of patients were at risk of overnutrition. The prevalence of malnutrition in SCI patients admitted to SCIC is higher than the national average for general hospitalized patients, indicating a particular vulnerability to malnutrition in this group
[42]	69 patients	Case-control study	Patients with spinal cord injury exhibited a significantly reduced 24-h energy expenditure compared to control subjects. This variance may be attributed to decreased levels of physical activity, as well as lower resting metabolic rate and reduced thermic effect of food values observed in individuals with SCI
[51]	30 patients	Case-control study	Paralysis resulting from spinal cord injury (SCI) leads to obligatory nitrogen losses, preventing the attainment of positive nitrogen balance (NB) regardless of calorie and protein intake levels. Achieving positive NB in these patients necessitates an average protein delivery of 2.3 grams per kilogram of ideal body weight (IBW) and an intake equivalent to 110% of predicted energy expenditure (PEE)
[57]	Medical records for 1163	Retrospective observational study	Among 1163 patients, early mortality was observed in 109 cases. Several factors influenced this rate, including the level and severity of spinal cord injury, the performance of surgical intervention, the duration between SCI occurrence and surgery, malnutrition status, and the presence of tracheotomy

(continued)

Table 18.2 (continued)

Study	Patients	Design	Main findings
[52]	16 patients	Retrospective observational study	This study indicates the likelihood of a widespread yet varied hypermetabolic response within this cohort. Caloric intake rapidly escalated to a consistent range of 2300–2400 kcal per day within the initial 4 days. Initially, the median total energy expenditure, as measured through indirect calorimetry, was notably elevated, starting at 3472 kcal/day and gradually declining to 2784 kcal/day by the third week
[5]	11 patients	Case series	The authors developed an equation that includes an activity factor of 1.1 and a stress factor of 1.2. They discovered a correlation between the measured and predicted energy expenditures in critically ill spinal cord injured patients
[46]	20 patients	Retrospective review	The Weir formula had the strongest correlation to measured energy expenditure followed by Penn State. Correlations were similar among Harris-Benedict formula Mifflin St. Jeor, and Ireton Jones, and weakest with 24 kcal/kg. In this study, the Weir formula emerged as the most accurate predictive energy equation
[34]	34 patients	Retrospective observational study	Potential nutritional risk factors for spinal cord injury include albumin levels below 3.5 g/dl, a critical parameter in the Spinal Cord Injury Pressure Ulcer Scale (SCIPUS). The SCIPUS can predict the occurrence of pressure ulcers within 2–3 days after assessment during acute care, but it is not effective for long-term predictions
[35]	Data from 13,254 patients	Retrospective multicenter	The overall prevalence of pressure ulcers in ICU patients was 26.6%. Identified risk factors included older age, male sex, being underweight, admission for emergency surgery, lower Braden scores, prolonged ICU stay, chronic obstructive pulmonary disease, immunodeficiency, renal replacement therapy, mechanical ventilation upon ICU admission, higher SAPS II scores, and residing in low or lower-middle-income economies
[47]	35 patients	Double blind randomized placebo-controlled study	For potential application in human use of vitamin E supplementation to mitigate post-SCI neurological impairment, research indicates that a dosage of 800 I.U./day is necessary to reduce baseline lipid peroxidation product levels in human plasma after 20 weeks of daily supplementation

18.7 Conclusion

Metabolism, nutrition, and muscle wasting are intricately linked in critically ill spinal cord injury patients. Understanding the underlying metabolic changes and nutritional requirements is essential for providing effective care and optimizing patient outcomes. A multidisciplinary approach that integrates nutrition therapy, rehabilitation, and pharmacological interventions is necessary to address the complex needs of this population and minimize the impact of muscle wasting on functional recovery and long-term prognosis.

References

1. Abel R, Ruf S, Spahn B. Cervical spinal cord injury and deglutition disorders. Dysphagia. 2004;19(2):87–94. https://doi.org/10.1007/s00455-003-0511-y.
2. Anderson DK, Saunders RD, Demediuk P, Dugan LL, Braughler JM, Hall ED, Means ED, Horrocks LA. Lipid hydrolysis and peroxidation in injured spinal cord: partial protection with methylprednisolone or vitamin E and selenium. Cent Nerv Syst Trauma. 1985;2(4):257–67. https://doi.org/10.1089/cns.1985.2.257.
3. Anjum A, Yazid MD, Fauzi Daud M, Idris J, Ng AMH, Selvi Naicker A, Ismail OHR, Athi Kumar RK, Lokanathan Y. Spinal cord injury: pathophysiology, multimolecular interactions, and underlying recovery mechanisms. Int J Mol Sci. 2020;21(20):7533. https://doi.org/10.3390/ijms21207533.
4. Barbiellini Amidei C, Salmaso L, Bellio S, Saia M. Epidemiology of traumatic spinal cord injury: a large population-based study. Spinal Cord. 2022;60(9):812–9. https://doi.org/10.1038/s41393-022-00795-w.
5. Barco KT, Smith RA, Peerless JR, Plaisier BR, Chima CS. Energy expenditure assessment and validation after acute spinal cord injury. Nut in Clin Pract. 2002;17(5):309–13. https://doi.org/10.1177/0115426502017005309.
6. Bauman WA, Spungen AM. Metabolic changes in persons after spinal cord injury. Phys Med Rehabil Clin N Am. 2000;11(1):109–40.
7. Benarroch EE. Physiology and pathophysiology of the autonomic nervous system. Continuum (Minneap Minn). 2020;26(1):12–24. https://doi.org/10.1212/CON.0000000000000817.
8. Bernardi M, Fedullo AL, Bernardi E, Munzi D, Peluso I, Myers J, Lista FR, Sciarra T. Diet in neurogenic bowel management: a viewpoint on spinal cord injury. World J Gastroenterol. 2020;26(20):2479–97. https://doi.org/10.3748/wjg.v26.i20.2479.
9. Braun TP, Zhu X, Szumowski M, Scott GD, Grossberg AJ, Levasseur PR, Graham K, Khan S, Damaraju S, Colmers WF, Baracos VE, Marks DL. Central nervous system inflammation induces muscle atrophy via activation of the hypothalamic–pituitary–adrenal axis. J Exp Med. 2011;208(12):2449–63. https://doi.org/10.1084/jem.20111020.
10. Buchholz AC, Pencharz PB. Energy expenditure in chronic spinal cord injury. Curr Opin Clin Nutr Metab Care. 2004;7(6):635–9. https://doi.org/10.1097/00075197-200411000-00008.
11. Buchholz AC, McGillivray CF, Pencharz PB. Physical activity levels are low in free-living adults with chronic paraplegia. Obes Res. 2003;11(4):563–70. https://doi.org/10.1038/oby.2003.79.
12. Castro MJ, Apple DF, Hillegass EA, Dudley GA. Influence of complete spinal cord injury on skeletal muscle cross-sectional area within the first 6 months of injury. Eur J Appl Physiol Occup Physiol. 1999;80(4):373–8. https://doi.org/10.1007/s004210050606.
13. Delivanis DA, Iñiguez-Ariza NM, Zeb MH, Moynagh MR, Takahashi N, McKenzie TJ, Thomas MA, Gogos C, Young WF, Bancos I, Kyriazopoulou V. Impact of hypercortisolism on skeletal muscle mass and adipose tissue mass in patients with adrenal adenomas. Clin Endocrinol. 2018;88(2):209–16. https://doi.org/10.1111/cen.13512.
14. Duckworth WC, Solomon SS, Jallepalli P, Heckemeyer C, Finnern J, Powers A. Glucose intolerance due to insulin resistance in patients with spinal cord injuries. Diabetes. 1980;29(11):906–10. https://doi.org/10.2337/diab.29.11.906.
15. Dvorak MF, Noonan VK, Bélanger L, Bruun B, Wing PC, Boyd MC, Fisher C. Early versus late enteral feeding in patients with acute cervical spinal cord injury: a pilot study. Spine (Phila Pa 1976). 2004;29(9):E175–80. https://doi.org/10.1097/00007632-200405010-00020.

16. Elder CP, Apple DF, Bickel CS, Meyer RA, Dudley GA. Intramuscular fat and glucose tolerance after spinal cord injury–a cross-sectional study. Spinal Cord. 2004;42(12):711–6. https://doi.org/10.1038/sj.sc.3101652.
17. Eswaran S, Guentner A, Chey WD. Emerging pharmacologic therapies for constipation-predominant irritable bowel syndrome and chronic constipation. J Neurogastroenterol Motil. 2014;20(2):141–51. https://doi.org/10.5056/jnm.2014.20.2.141.
18. Farkas GJ, Sneij A, Gater DR. Dietetics after spinal cord injury: current evidence and future perspectives. Top Spinal Cord Inj Rehabil. 2021;27(1):100–8. https://doi.org/10.46292/sci20-00031.
19. Formenti P, Umbrello M, Coppola S, Froio S, Chiumello D. Clinical review: peripheral muscular ultrasound in the ICU. Ann Intensive Care. 2019;9(1):57. https://doi.org/10.1186/s13613-019-0531-x.
20. Gorgey AS, Dudley GA. Skeletal muscle atrophy and increased intramuscular fat after incomplete spinal cord injury. Spinal Cord. 2007;45(4):304–9. https://doi.org/10.1038/sj.sc.3101968.
21. Gorgey AS, Chiodo AE, Zemper ED, Hornyak JE, Rodriguez GM, Gater DR. Relationship of spasticity to soft tissue body composition and the metabolic profile in persons with chronic motor complete spinal cord injury. J Spinal Cord Med. 2010;33(1):6–15. https://doi.org/10.1080/10790268.2010.11689669.
22. Gorgey AS, Dolbow DR, Dolbow JD, Khalil RK, Castillo C, Gater DR. Effects of spinal cord injury on body composition and metabolic profile – Part I. J Spinal Cord Med. 2014;37(6):693–702. https://doi.org/10.1179/2045772314Y.0000000245.
23. Grimby G, Broberg C, Krotkiewska I, Krotkiewski M. Muscle fiber composition in patients with traumatic cord lesion. Scand J Rehabil Med. 1976;8(1):37–42.
24. Higgins J, Laramée M-T, Harrison KR, Delparte JJ, Scovil CY, Flett HM, Burns AS. The spinal cord injury pressure ulcer scale (SCIPUS): an assessment of validity using Rasch analysis. Spinal Cord. 2019;57(10):874–80. https://doi.org/10.1038/s41393-019-0287-z.
25. Howard EE, Pasiakos SM, Fussell MA, Rodriguez NR. Skeletal muscle disuse atrophy and the rehabilitative role of protein in recovery from musculoskeletal injury. Adv Nutr. 2020;11(4):989–1001. https://doi.org/10.1093/advances/nmaa015.
26. Hunt A, McQuillan KA. Acute management of cervical spinal cord injuries. Crit Care Nurs Clin North Am. 2023;35(2):119–28. https://doi.org/10.1016/j.cnc.2023.02.004.
27. Johns J, Krogh K, Rodriguez GM, Eng J, Haller E, Heinen M, Laredo R, Longo W, Montero-Colon W, Wilson C, Korsten M. Management of neurogenic bowel dysfunction in adults after spinal cord injury. Top Spinal Cord Inj Rehabil. 2021;27(2):75–151. https://doi.org/10.46292/sci2702-75.
28. Jones JM. Dietary fiber future directions: integrating new definitions and findings to inform nutrition research and communication. Adv Nutr. 2013;4(1):8–15. https://doi.org/10.3945/an.112.002907.
29. Kaufman HH, Rowlands BJ, Stein DK, Kopaniky DR, Gildenberg PL. General metabolism in patients with acute paraplegia and quadriplegia. Neurosurgery. 1985;16(3):309–13. https://doi.org/10.1227/00006123-198503000-00005.
30. Kearns PJ, Thompson JD, Werner PC, Pipp TL, Wilmot CB. Nutritional and metabolic response to acute spinal-cord injury. JPEN J Parenter Enteral Nutr. 1992;16(1):11–5. https://doi.org/10.1177/014860719201600111.
31. Khatri N, Sumadhura B, Kumar S, Kaundal RK, Sharma S, Datusalia AK. The complexity of secondary Cascade consequent to traumatic brain injury: pathobiology and potential treatments. Curr Neuropharmacol. 2021;19(11):1984–2011. https://doi.org/10.2174/1570159X19666210215123914.
32. Kim HS, Lim K-B, Kim J, Kang J, Lee H, Lee SW, Yoo J. Epidemiology of spinal cord injury: changes to its cause amid aging population, a single center study. Ann Rehabil Med. 2021;45(1):7–15. https://doi.org/10.5535/arm.20148.
33. Kress JP, Hall JB. ICU-acquired weakness and recovery from critical illness. N Engl J Med. 2014;370(17):1626–35. https://doi.org/10.1056/NEJMra1209390.

34. Krishnan S, Brick RS, Karg PE, Tzen Y-T, Garber SL, Sowa GA, Brienza DM. Predictive validity of the Spinal Cord Injury Pressure Ulcer Scale (SCIPUS) in acute care and inpatient rehabilitation in individuals with traumatic spinal cord injury. NeuroRehabilitation. 2016;38(4):401–9. https://doi.org/10.3233/NRE-161331.
35. Labeau SO, Afonso E, Benbenishty J, Blackwood B, Boulanger C, Brett SJ, Calvino-Gunther S, Chaboyer W, Coyer F, Deschepper M, François G, Honore PM, Jankovic R, Khanna AK, Llaurado-Serra M, Lin F, Rose L, Rubulotta F, Saager L, Williams G, Blot SI. Prevalence, associated factors and outcomes of pressure injuries in adult intensive care unit patients: the DecubICUs study. Intensive Care Med. 2021;47(2):160–9. https://doi.org/10.1007/s00134-020-06234-9.
36. Laven GT, Huang CT, DeVivo MJ, Stover SL, Kuhlemeier KV, Fine PR. Nutritional status during the acute stage of spinal cord injury. Arch Phys Med Rehabil. 1989;70(4):277–82.
37. Lin CS-Y, Macefield VG, Elam M, Wallin BG, Engel S, Kiernan MC. Axonal changes in spinal cord injured patients distal to the site of injury. Brain. 2007;130(Pt 4):985–94. https://doi.org/10.1093/brain/awl339.
38. Lynch AC, Frizelle FA. Colorectal motility and defecation after spinal cord injury in humans. Prog Brain Res. 2006;152:335–43. https://doi.org/10.1016/S0079-6123(05)52022-3.
39. Machlin LJ, Gabriel E. Kinetics of tissue alpha-tocopherol uptake and depletion following administration of high levels of vitamin E. Ann N Y Acad Sci. 1982;393:48–60. https://doi.org/10.1111/j.1749-6632.1982.tb31231.x.
40. Maggioni M, Bertoli S, Margonato V, Merati G, Veicsteinas A, Testolin G. Body composition assessment in spinal cord injury subjects. Acta Diabetol. 2003;40(Suppl 1):S183–6. https://doi.org/10.1007/s00592-003-0061-7.
41. McCully KK, Mulcahy TK, Ryan TE, Zhao Q. Skeletal muscle metabolism in individuals with spinal cord injury. J Appl Physiol (1985). 2011;111(1):143–8. https://doi.org/10.1152/japplphysiol.00094.2011.
42. Monroe MB, Tataranni PA, Pratley R, Manore MM, Skinner JS, Ravussin E. Lower daily energy expenditure as measured by a respiratory chamber in subjects with spinal cord injury compared with control subjects. Am J Clin Nutr. 1998;68(6):1223–7. https://doi.org/10.1093/ajcn/68.6.1223.
43. Moores J. Vitamin C: a wound healing perspective. Br J Community Nurs Suppl. 2013:S6, S8-11. https://doi.org/10.12968/bjcn.2013.18.sup12.s6.
44. Patkova A, Joskova V, Havel E, Kovarik M, Kucharova M, Zadak Z, Hronek M. Energy, protein, carbohydrate, and lipid intakes and their effects on morbidity and mortality in critically ill adult patients: a systematic review. Adv Nutr. 2017;8(4):624–34. https://doi.org/10.3945/an.117.015172.
45. Priego T, Martín AI, González-Hedström D, Granado M, López-Calderón A. Role of hormones in sarcopenia. Vitam Horm. 2021;115:535–70. https://doi.org/10.1016/bs.vh.2020.12.021.
46. Ramirez CL, Pelekhaty S, Massetti JM, Galvagno S, Harmon L, Botwinick I, Scalea TM, Stein DM. Validation of predictive equations to assess energy expenditure in acute spinal cord injury. J Trauma Acute Care Surg. 2018;85(5):984–91. https://doi.org/10.1097/TA.0000000000001959.
47. Roberts LJ, Oates JA, Linton MF, Fazio S, Meador BP, Gross MD, Shyr Y, Morrow JD. The relationship between dose of vitamin E and suppression of oxidative stress in humans. Free Radic Biol Med. 2007;43(10):1388–93. https://doi.org/10.1016/j.freeradbiomed.2007.06.019.
48. Rodriguez GM, Gater DR. Neurogenic bowel and management after spinal cord injury: a narrative review. J Pers Med. 2022;12(7):1141. https://doi.org/10.3390/jpm12071141.
49. Rodriguez DJ, Clevenger FW, Osler TM, Demarest GB, Fry DE. Obligatory negative nitrogen balance following spinal cord injury. JPEN J Parenter Enteral Nutr. 1991;15(3):319–22. https://doi.org/10.1177/0148607191015003319.
50. Rodriguez DJ, Benzel EC, Clevenger FW. The metabolic response to spinal cord injury. Spinal Cord. 1997;35(9):599–604. https://doi.org/10.1038/sj.sc.3100439.

51. Rodriguez NR, Vislocky LM, Gaine PC. Dietary protein, endurance exercise, and human skeletal-muscle protein turnover. Curr Opin Clin Nutr Metab Care. 2007;10(1):40–5. https://doi.org/10.1097/MCO.0b013e328011 5e3b.
52. Rowan C, Kazemi A. An observational study of feeding practice in ventilated patients with spinal cord injury. Clin Nutr ESPEN. 2020;37:107–13. https://doi.org/10.1016/j.clnesp.2020.03.010.
53. Sacino A, Rosenblatt K. Critical care management of acute spinal cord injury—part II: intensive care to rehabilitation. J Neuroanaesth Crit Care. 2019;6(3):222–35. https://doi.org/10.1055/s-0039-1694686.
54. Saghaleini SH, Dehghan K, Shadvar K, Sanaie S, Mahmoodpoor A, Ostadi Z. Pressure ulcer and nutrition. Indian J Crit Care Med. 2018;22(4):283–9. https://doi.org/10.4103/ijccm.IJCCM_277_17.
55. Sedlock DA, Laventure SJ. Body composition and resting energy expenditure in long term spinal cord injury. Paraplegia. 1990;28(7):448–54. https://doi.org/10.1038/sc.1990.60.
56. Shah PK, Stevens JE, Gregory CM, Pathare NC, Jayaraman A, Bickel SC, Bowden M, Behrman AL, Walter GA, Dudley GA, Vandenborne K. Lower-extremity muscle cross-sectional area after incomplete spinal cord injury. Arch Phys Med Rehabil. 2006;87(6):772–8. https://doi.org/10.1016/j.apmr.2006.02.028.
57. Shao J, Zhu W, Chen X, Jia L, Song D, Zhou X, Yan W, Zhang Y. Factors associated with early mortality after cervical spinal cord injury. J Spinal Cord Med. 2011;34(6):555–62. https://doi.org/10.1179/2045772311Y.0000000024.
58. Şimşek T, Şimşek HU, Cantürk NZ. Response to trauma and metabolic changes: post-traumatic metabolism. Ulus Cerrahi Derg. 2014;30(3):153–9. https://doi.org/10.5152/UCD.2014.2653.
59. Singer P, Blaser AR, Berger MM, Alhazzani W, Calder PC, Casaer MP, Hiesmayr M, Mayer K, Montejo JC, Pichard C, Preiser J-C, van Zanten ARH, Oczkowski S, Szczeklik W, Bischoff SC. ESPEN guideline on clinical nutrition in the intensive care unit. Clin Nutr. 2019;38(1):48–79. https://doi.org/10.1016/j.clnu.2018.08.037.
60. Spungen AM, Wang J, Pierson RN, Bauman WA. Soft tissue body composition differences in monozygotic twins discordant for spinal cord injury. J Appl Physiol (1985). 2000;88(4):1310–5. https://doi.org/10.1152/jappl.2000.88.4.1310.
61. Taoka Y, Ikata T, Fukuzawa K. Influence of dietary vitamin E deficiency on compression injury of rat spinal cord. J Nutr Sci Vitaminol (Tokyo). 1990;36(3):217–26. https://doi.org/10.3177/jnsv.36.217.
62. Thayalasekeran S, Ali H, Tsai H-H. Novel therapies for constipation. World J Gastroenterol. 2013;19(45):8247–51. https://doi.org/10.3748/wjg.v19.i45.8247.
63. Thibault-Halman G, Casha S, Singer S, Christie S. Acute management of nutritional demands after spinal cord injury. J Neurotrauma. 2011;28(8):1497–507. https://doi.org/10.1089/neu.2009.1155.
64. Tintignac LA, Brenner H-R, Rüegg MA. Mechanisms regulating neuromuscular junction development and function and causes of muscle wasting. Physiol Rev. 2015;95(3):809–52. https://doi.org/10.1152/physrev.00033.2014.
65. Wang H, Zhou W, Huang J, Zheng X, Tian H, Wang B, Fu W, Wu A. Endocrine therapy for the functional recovery of spinal cord injury. Front Neurosci. 2020;14:590570. https://doi.org/10.3389/fnins.2020.590570.
66. Wilmet E, Ismail AA, Heilporn A, Welraeds D, Bergmann P. Longitudinal study of the bone mineral content and of soft tissue composition after spinal cord section. Paraplegia. 1995;33(11):674–7. https://doi.org/10.1038/sc.1995.141.

67. Wong S, Derry F, Jamous A, Hirani SP, Grimble G, Forbes A. The prevalence of malnutrition in spinal cord injuries patients: a UK multicentre study. Br J Nutr. 2012;108(5):918–23. https://doi.org/10.1017/S0007114511006234.
68. Wong JJ, Côté P, Quesnele JJ, Stern PJ, Mior SA. The course and prognostic factors of symptomatic cervical disc herniation with radiculopathy: a systematic review of the literature. Spine J. 2014;14(8):1781–9. https://doi.org/10.1016/j.spinee.2014.02.032.
69. Wulf MJ, Tom VJ. Consequences of spinal cord injury on the sympathetic nervous system. Front Cell Neurosci. 2023;17:999253. https://doi.org/10.3389/fncel.2023.999253.
70. Xu X, Talifu Z, Zhang C-J, Gao F, Ke H, Pan Y-Z, Gong H, Du H-Y, Yu Y, Jing Y-L, Du L-J, Li J-J, Yang D-G. Mechanism of skeletal muscle atrophy after spinal cord injury: a narrative review. Front Nutr. 2023;10:1099143. https://doi.org/10.3389/fnut.2023.1099143.
71. Zinder R, Cooley R, Vlad LG, Molnar JA. Vitamin a and wound healing. Nutr Clin Pract. 2019;34(6):839–49. https://doi.org/10.1002/ncp.10420.

Clinical Consequences of Disrupted Feedback Control and Abnormal Circuit Reorganization After Spinal Cord Injury

19

James Guest, Pedro P. Saraiva, J. Ceisler, and N. Datta

19.1 Introduction

SCI can result in multiple physiologic abnormalities, generally in proportion to its severity. It is not just a condition of loss but also gain of aberrant responses within the neural circuits of the spinal cord, brain, brainstem, cerebellum, and peripherally innervated organs. These neuroplastic responses dysregulate spinal cord circuits that are normally feedback-modulated within the neural axis. SCI-related disordering of feedback control affects BP, muscle tone, and spasticity and causes disordered pain and sensory signaling as well as impaired thermoregulation. The circuit "rewiring" undermines the normally well regulated processes.

Chapter Organization

I. Feedback and setpoint control in physiological systems
II. Sensory, motor, autonomic, and inhibitory circuits of the spinal cord
III. Phases of spinal cord injury and impact of neuroplasticity
IV. Disordered cardiovascular function and blood pressure regulation
V. Autonomic dysreflexia
VI. Spasticity
VII. Neuropathic pain

J. Guest (✉)
The Miami Project to Cure Paralysis at the Lynn Center for Rehabilitation, The Miller School of Medicine, Miami, FL, USA

Neurological Surgery, The Miller School of Medicine, Miami, FL, USA
e-mail: jguest@med.miami.edu

P. P. Saraiva · J. Ceisler · N. Datta
The Miami Project to Cure Paralysis at the Lynn Center for Rehabilitation, The Miller School of Medicine, Miami, FL, USA
e-mail: pmpsaraiva@med.miami.edu; jac89459@miami.edu; nxd693@med.miami.edu

E. Brogi et al. (eds.), *Traumatic Spinal Cord Injury*, Hot Topics in Acute Care Surgery and Trauma, https://doi.org/10.1007/978-3-031-99890-4_19

VIII. Thermoregulation
IX. Treatment targets and therapy for disrupted feedback regulation

19.2 Feedback and Setpoint Control in Physiological Systems

Feedback regulation is essential in biological systems such as the endocrine and nervous systems to maintain stability and return to setpoints following perturbations (Fig. 19.1). Within the nervous system, feedback mechanisms involve filtering sensory input, segmental and hierarchical processing, and regulated output through balanced excitation and inhibition of synaptic activities [35, 111]. This feedback system enables homeostasis across immediate and extended timeframes and functions largely without conscious input, encapsulated in Langley's term "autonomic nervous system" [105].

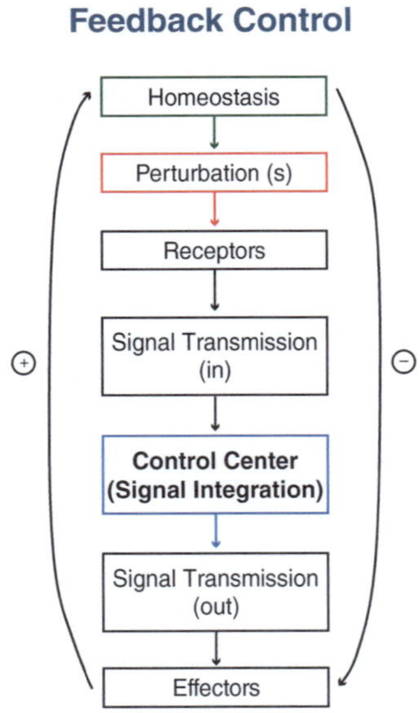

Fig. 19.1 A schematic representation of a biological feedback control system highlights the key components and their interactions. When a perturbation disrupts homeostasis, it triggers a sequence of afferent and efferent signal transmissions. These signals are processed by the control center, or signal integration center, which coordinates the appropriate response. The system demonstrates both negative feedback loops, where deviations from the set point are corrected to restore stability, and positive feedback loops, where responses are amplified to restore homeostasis. Together, these feedback mechanisms play essential roles in maintaining or altering physiological balance in biological systems

Feedback disruptions, particularly in diseases like Parkinson's and Huntington's, reveal the crucial role of these systems in coordinated motor and sensory processing [157, 162, 215]. After SCI, similar feedback control failures lead to various physiological impairments, from dysregulated BP and muscle tone to aberrant pain signaling and thermoregulation.

Besides internal homeostasis, living organisms need mechanisms to interact with their environment through non-conscious processes (e.g., thermoregulation), conscious decisions, and voluntary activity. Voluntary activities such as walking require multiple hierarchical feedback controls [137]. Central to these interactions are complex signaling networks that enable organisms to sense and respond to a wide range of stimuli. Feedback control regulates these networks through neural structures and neurotransmitter-molecular interactions and is also associated with response memory to increase system efficiency [27].

Historically, concepts of feedback control were explored in both engineering and physiology. Early examples include James Watt's flyball governor and Claude Bernard's concept of a self-regulating internal environment, "milieu intérieur." In biology, Walter Cannon expanded this to *adaptive homeostasis*, describing physiological responses, such as "fight or flight," coordinated by the sympathetic and parasympathetic systems [26]. These principles highlight the feedback loops that counteract or amplify physiological changes as needed—illustrated by processes such as blood glucose regulation (negative feedback) and oxytocin release during childbirth (positive feedback).

The nervous system is based on dynamic electrochemical neural communication. Spinal cord injuries (SCI) can significantly disrupt feedback control mechanisms. The spinal cord is a crucial conduit for signals between the brain and the rest of the body and for local signal processing to regulate sensory, motor, and autonomic functions. Insight into disrupted feedback loops is essential in developing therapeutics. Knowledge of feedback control concepts is applied in advanced medical technologies. For example, artificial prosthetic feedback systems can enhance functionality and user experience by providing real-time sensory feedback, mimicking natural limb movements [180].

19.3 Sensory, Motor, Autonomic, and Inhibitory Circuits of the Spinal Cord

The spinal cord transmits and processes sensory, motor, and autonomic signals between the body and the brain through electrochemical communication along afferent and efferent axonal pathways. These pathways regulate body functions by enabling motor outputs, sensory inputs, and autonomic control. The spinal cord consists of afferent and efferent nerve roots, regulatory circuits in gray matter, intersegmental pathways, and axonal tracts. Together, they manage body functions through ascending sensory, descending motor, and autonomic signals, and descending inhibitory axons. Neuroplasticity, which entails structural changes in neural circuits, often occurs after SCI. This process modifies communication pathways by altering neurotransmitter signaling across synapses [32] and promoting the growth of new neurite processes after SCI deafferentation [161].

19.3.1 Afferent Signals

Sensory axons of the afferent nervous system convey data from peripheral sensors in skin, muscles, and organs to the central nervous system (CNS). The axons arise from peripheral ganglia and synapse within circuits that convey peripheral sensory information to the spinal cord, brainstem, and cerebellum. Few, if any, primary afferents synapse directly in the cortex [25, 134]. Sensory modalities include conscious perceptions, touch, pressure, position, and pain, as well as non-conscious inputs like temperature, chemogenomic signals, and mechanical-baroreceptor inputs. Sensory receptors transduce stimuli into temporal action potential sequences. Peripheral ganglia neural cell bodies are pseudo-unipolar, with both a peripheral and a central projection branch. The T-junction between branches provides the first afferent filtering site before spinal cord entry [79]. Afferents either synapse on specific dorsal horn neurons or ascend as tract axons. Some sensory circuits, such as baroreceptors, travel directly to the brainstem via cranial nerves and are spared after SCI. Local sensorimotor integration for rapid feedback also occurs [54].

The spinal cord sensory circuits are primarily organized into three major ascending tracts: the dorsal column, spinothalamic tracts, and spinocerebellar tracts. The dorsal column conveys conscious proprioceptive information, including fine touch, two-point discrimination, and vibration. Sensory axons enter the spinal cord via dorsal roots and ascend without synapsing ipsilaterally to the lower medulla, where they synapse in the cuneate and gracile nuclei. Second-order neurons decussate and project to the thalamus. Third-order neurons project to the cortices, where conscious perception is created.

The anterolateral spinothalamic tract carries pain, temperature, and crude touch signals. Sensory axons enter from dorsal rootlets into the short ascending tract of Lissauer and synapse primarily in lamina II. Second-order neurons cross to the contralateral side and ascend to the thalamus, projecting to the sensory cortex. The spinothalamic synapses within the spinal cord dorsal horn can be highly affected by post-SCI neuroplasticity [60]. There are also ascending nociceptive pathways directly connected to the hypothalamus (limbic system) and the striatum [67].

Spinocerebellar tracts convey unconscious proprioceptive information from muscle spindles and Golgi tendon organs. Afferents terminate in intraspinal nuclei (such as Clarke's nucleus and spinal border cells), whose secondary axons ascend to the cerebellum to coordinate movement and maintain balance. Following SCI, the loss of ascending axons may cause cerebellar atrophy [107]. The spino-olivary tract connects to the inferior olivary nucleus, which sends climbing fibers to the cerebellar Purkinje cells. Deafferentation causes changes in Purkinje cell synapses [197].

19.3.2 Efferent Signals

Motor outputs from the spinal cord are conveyed in the ventral roots. Those to striated muscles originate in ventral horn motor neurons with direct muscle connections, whereas preganglionic axons to smooth muscles, such as those in the bowel, travel to a secondary ganglion to synapse on a postganglionic motor neuron that then innervates the organ. Smooth muscle innervation is generally considered part of the autonomic nervous system (ANS). The enteric nervous system contains both excitatory and inhibitory motor neurons that underlie its peristaltic movements [177]. Bladder motor control includes both voluntary and parasympathetic motor circuits.

For voluntary movements, the intention is transmitted from the brain to synapse on combinations of spinal effector motor inter-neurons to coordinate actions such as walking or grasping, which is simultaneously feedback-regulated by local and ascending sensory circuits. Anatomical descriptions of tracts tend to create false conceptual isolation, but as a generalization, the two main descending motor pathways are the pyramidal–corticospinal tract and the extrapyramidal system. The corticospinal tract originates in the motor cortex. Axons descend through the brainstem, decussate in the medullary pyramids, and descend in the lateral corticospinal tract to synapse with motor neurons in the anterior horn of the spinal cord, which directly innervate skeletal muscles. Additionally, the corticospinal tract extends multi-segmental collaterals and has extensive connections with regulatory interneurons [194].

The "extrapyramidal system" consists of brainstem motor pathways that modulate human muscle tone, posture, reflexes, gait, and balance mainly via the reticulospinal and vestibulospinal pathways. These tracts synapse with interneurons and gamma motor neurons in the spinal cord [123]. Humans have a limited rubrospinal tract [140]. Extrapyramidal motor outputs require constant sensory modulation through proprioceptive feedback loops [43], providing the basis for both voluntary movements and postural adjustments.

19.3.3 Descending Inhibitory Systems

Circuit modulation through inhibitory signaling is critical in the CNS. It includes local spinal cord neurons and descending systems [88] that arise from the midbrain and brainstem [101], including the monoaminergic, noradrenergic, and serotonergic systems [145]. The human spinal cord dorsal horn receives noradrenergic projections primarily from the locus coeruleus, which is a sympathetic nervous system component [12]. These fibers can block noxious pain signaling through presynaptic inhibition (α2a receptors), volume conduction, and activation of GABA-releasing inhibitory interneurons. Descending pain inhibition is also mediated by the cerulean and periaqueductal grey-rostroventral medulla systems. The rostroventral medulla is a component of the reticulospinal system that sends serotoninergic fibers to the spinal cord, activating inhibitory 5-HT receptors for pain modulation [86]. Monoaminergic systems also regulate function by varying gain control in motor neurons [172, 207].

19.3.4 Autonomic Nervous System

The spinal cord critically regulates unconscious physiological functions via the ANS neurons that are regulated by the descending hypothalamic and brainstem systems. The ANS has sympathetic and parasympathetic branches that regulate heart rate, BP, digestion, bladder control, and thermoregulation.

Sympathetic preganglionic neurons are primarily located in the thoracolumbar spinal cord's "intermediate" column, from T1 to L2. They project via ventral roots to paraspinal sympathetic ganglia, synapsing with postganglionic neurons that innervate organs and tissues, including the heart, blood vessels, and sweat glands. Sympathetic activation can prepare the body for "fight or flight" responses, increasing HR and BP and redirecting blood flow to essential organs and muscles. Parasympathetic preganglionic neurons are found in the craniosacral regions, primarily sacral segments S2 to S4. The parasympathetic ANS promotes "rest and digest" functions, decreasing heart rate, promoting digestion, and aiding energy conservation. Its vagal neural component is usually spared after SCI.

Following SCI, the disruption of these autonomic pathways leads to dysregulation of cardiovascular, respiratory, gut, and thermoregulatory functions, significantly impacting an individual's quality of life.

19.4 Phases of Spinal Cord Injury and Impact of Neuroplasticity

Traumatic SCI causes a sudden disruption in the transmission of axonal potential information, leading to functional paralysis across multiple systems, followed by variable degrees of recovery. Acutely, there may be severe neurogenic shock and bradycardia driven by the loss of sympathetically mediated vascular tone and cardiac output, along with unopposed vagal activity. There is also a transient loss of all detectable tendon reflex activity below the level of injury [47]. Unopposed parasympathetic activity from S2 to S4 may be associated with acute priapism [188]. Reflex activity gradually recovers, but spasticity, neuropathic pain, and autonomic dysfunction may emerge [85] (Fig. 19.2).

"Neuroplasticity" is a broad term for changes in the function of the nervous system that may be either adaptive or harmful [37, 198]. SCI leads to extensive deafferentation, prompting neuroplastic changes via synaptic modulation and the sprouting of local neurite processes, which alter circuit activity. Typically, there is competition for access to synaptic sites and the massive denervation of local neuronal dendrites after SCI allows for wide-ranging unstructured neuroplasticity from local neurons [14].

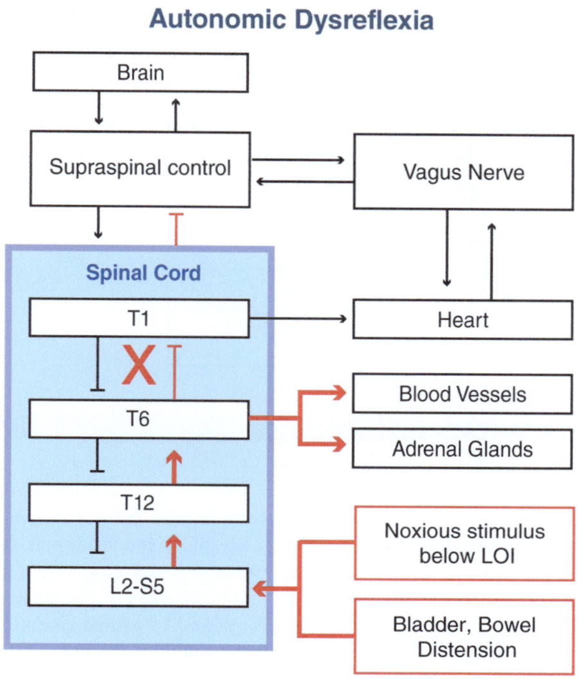

Fig. 19.2 Pathophysiology of autonomic dysreflexia (AD), a condition that can occur in individuals with spinal cord injuries at and above T6 level. In AD, a noxious afferent stimulus, such as bladder distention or bowel irritation, activates an exaggerated peripheral sympathetic response below the level of injury, leading to widespread vasoconstriction, mobilization of splanchnic venous blood into the circulation, and a sudden rise in blood pressure. The afferents from the bladder and bowel undergo post-injury plasticity in response to the deafferentation, resulting in significant circuit changes that amplify their signals and the circuit gain

19.5 Disordered Cardiovascular Function and Blood Pressure Regulation

SCI disruption of descending autonomic pathways affects multiple organ systems. Injuries at the cervical to mid-thoracic (T6) levels lead to loss of regulation of sympathetic neurons that innervate the heart and blood vessels. The clinical effects on the cardiovascular system are established acutely and can persist throughout an individual's lifetime [76, 149] (Fig. 19.3). Individuals with such injuries typically experience persistent hypotension as well as orthostatic hypotension due to loss of vasomotor tone, unstable BP, AD, and bradycardia [91, 205]. During the chronic phase, the cardiovascular system undergoes long-term adaptations due to altered hemodynamics and decreased physical activity [61]. Impaired function and

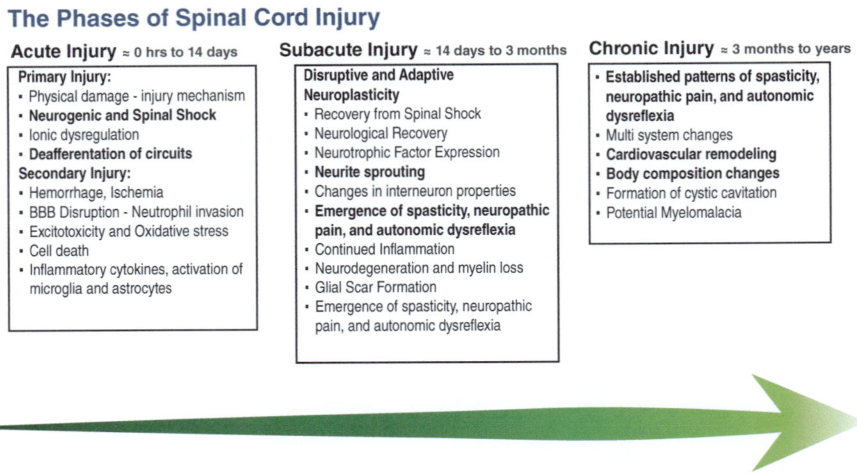

Fig. 19.3 The three phases of SCI and their key physiological and pathological processes that occur during each phase. The acute phase begins after the injury and lasts approximately 2 weeks. It is characterized by a shock state, massive deafferentation, and progressive secondary injury processes such as inflammation and neuronal death. This is followed by the subacute phase, which spans from 2 weeks to approximately 3 months and is marked by axonal sprouting, glial scar formation, multiple changes in body systems, and some neurological recovery. Finally, the chronic phase extends beyond 3 months and can persist for the patient's lifetime, involving long-term circuit remodeling and potential complications such as spasticity and chronic pain

sensitivity of arterial baroreceptors lead to dysregulated feedback control after severe SCI [131, 150, 152]. Vascular effects such as increased stiffness [87], together with metabolic dysfunction can increase the risk of cardiovascular disease, resulting in increased morbidity and mortality in SCI patients [64].

Orthostatic hypotension is common after SCI at or above the T6 level. It is defined as a drop in BP of 20 mm Hg systolic and 10 mm Hg diastolic that persists for 3 min after transitioning from a supine to a vertical tilt or upright position [185]. It can significantly interfere with activities of daily living and rehabilitation, and its symptoms can worsen during transfers or after meals [89]. Orthostatic hypotension can also reduce cognitive performance and is associated with fatigue. When using a tilt table, verticalized individuals with symptoms experience a decrease in cerebral blood flow velocity [69, 203], and the dynamic autoregulation of cerebral blood flow is impaired [151, 163]. The expected release of epinephrine and norepinephrine is reduced compared to control subjects and those with lower thoracic injuries. The sympathetic skin reflex test is usually absent in those with significant orthostatic hypotension [33, 209], and heart rate variability in response to a Valsalva maneuver is reduced [16]. International standards for documenting autonomic function following SCI (ISAFSCI) have been established and are recommended for use [206].

19.6 Autonomic Dysreflexia

AD arises from impaired negative feedback mechanisms in the ANS, aberrant neuroplasticity, and pathological gain in the input-output circuits. It is characterized by sudden hypertensive episodes that can rapidly shift significant blood volumes from the splanchnic circulation [40]. AD occurs when a noxious stimulus below the level of injury triggers a massive sympathetic response, leading to uncontrolled hypertension [75, 93, 114, 115, 142]. Due to the disruption in descending inhibitory pathways, the body cannot regulate this sympathetic outflow (Fig. 19.4).

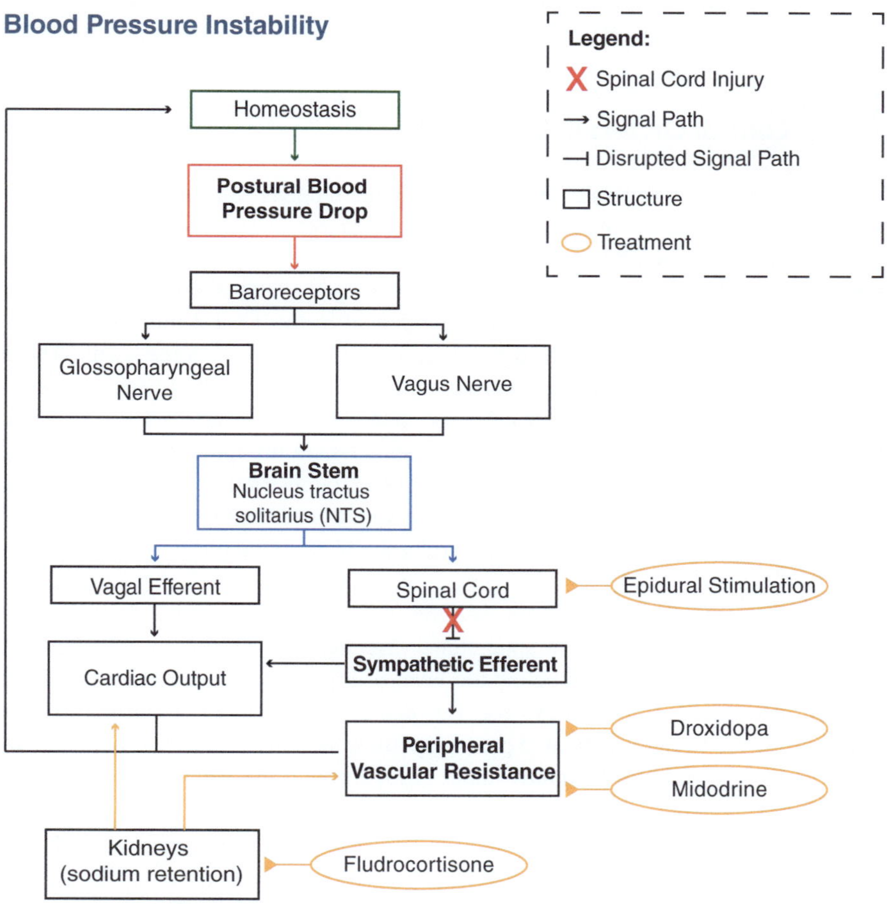

Fig. 19.4 Loss of BP control in SCI. In an intact system, baroreceptors detect BP changes and signal the brainstem, which activates both sympathetic and parasympathetic responses to re-establish homeostasis (adequate tissue blood flow). In SCI, disruption of sympathetic pathways impairs BP regulation, while unopposed parasympathetic vagal activity contributes to imbalance. BP may be labile and may decrease significantly in the sitting (or standing) position. Treatment targets include the peripheral vascular system, cardiac output, blood volume increases, and epidural spinal cord stimulation to enhance sympathetic efferent activity

AD significantly contributes to BP instability, and individuals may not realize they are having multiple daily episodes [91]. Bladder or bowel distention is the most common trigger, responsible for 75–85% of episodes [173]. Other nociceptive inputs, such as skin injuries, can also initiate AD. Symptoms include headaches, nasal congestion, blurred vision, and sweating above the injury level, often accompanied by piloerection and skin pallor below the injury [36, 63]. It is a potentially life-threatening condition for individuals with SCI above the T6 level. The acute hypertension, if severe may lead to stroke, myocardial infarction, or intracranial hemorrhage [55], increasing overall stroke and mortality risks [199]. Complete SCI is more likely to result in AD than incomplete injury [45]. AD can be prevented by careful mitigation of triggering factors. Treatment with acutely BP-lowering medications may be needed for severe episodes.

19.6.1 Control Circuits Related to AD

The lower brainstem regulates BP, specifically the nucleus solitarius, gigantocellular area, and the rostral ventrolateral medulla, which send axons into the spinal cord [39, 211]. Arterial stretch baroreceptors provide essential feedback control of BP to the brainstem. Cardiac, endocrine, and renal feedback systems also play important roles. Sympathetic preganglionic neurons, located in the T1–L2 intermediolateral column of the spinal cord, extend autonomic axons into the ventral roots. These neurons are responsible for the primary neural regulation of BP by releasing acetylcholine at synapses with postganglionic adrenergic neurons [34, 119, 139]. Postganglionic neurons extend to blood vessels, where norepinephrine is released and binds to alpha-1 receptors, causing excess vasoconstriction and BP elevation. Sympathetic preganglionic neurons also innervate the adrenal medulla, where cholinergic synapses [112] stimulate the release of norepinephrine and epinephrine [170].

The celiac ganglia (T12-L1) are essential nodes that regulate BP through their vasomotor nerve innervation of splanchnic vascular tone. During an AD episode, excessive sensory stimulation below the level of injury causes increased BP and a reduced heart rate [75, 100]. Baroreceptors detect this rise in BP and trigger reflex bradycardia due to vagal-mediated parasympathetic activity [3, 187], as parasympathetic control of the heart remains intact [100] through the vagus nerve from the medulla [17].

19.6.2 Neuroplastic Changes Underlying AD Development

Several neuroplastic changes occur following SCI that increase the likelihood of AD in response to triggering stimuli. Structural changes in sympathetic preganglionic neurons following SCI are associated with AD progression [98]. In rodent models, the soma and dendritic arbors of sympathetic preganglionic neurons shrink within the first week post-injury due to the loss of synaptic input from supraspinal axons [95]. However, these structures recover in size after a few weeks, which coincides with the development of AD [95, 98]. This recovery is likely driven by new synaptic connections from primary afferent fibers below the level of injury, increasing intraspinal reflex strength and AD severity [99].

Biological drivers of neuroplasticity contributing to AD have been identified in animal SCI models. Tissue levels of nerve growth factor (NGF), essential for sensory and sympathetic neuron survival, increase after SCI [24] and are associated with the sprouting of small-diameter afferent fibers and dendritic arbor expansion in the dorsal horn [71, 99, 192, 193]. This correlates with the sprouting of sensory afferents that express the high-affinity NGF receptor trkA [9, 97] into the dorsal horns of lumbar segments in rats after SCI [97], coinciding with the development of AD [93, 114]. Bladder distention, which is a major trigger of AD, activates visceral-vascular reflexes [30] that undergo neuroplastic changes after SCI. Amplified sensory input enhances spinal reflex responses [92, 168], leading to a stronger uninhibited sympathetic response due to loss of descending inhibition.

Neuroinflammatory cytokines, including TNF-α, interleukin-6 (IL-6) and interleukin-1 beta (IL-1β), can also potentiate the development of AD [10, 82, 126, 178] through release from activated astrocytes and microglia [82, 182]. IL-6 and IL-1β increase NGF levels, promoting sensory afferent sprouting [99], while TNFα inhibition decreases such sprouting [126, 127].

Extracellular matrix glycoproteins known as thrombospondins promote the formation of excitatory synapses by interacting with the calcium channel subunit α2δ-1 (referred to as the gabapentin receptor) [31, 56, 159]. After SCI, levels of both TNFα and thrombospondin increase in cord tissue [48, 126]. Gabapentin blocks the binding of thrombospondin to α2δ, which reduces excitatory synaptogenesis and sympathetic circuit excitability [56, 159].

After T3-level SCI in rats, neurons in the lumbar spinal dorsal root ganglia upregulate the transient receptor potential (TRP) channel TRPV1 (capsaicin receptor) and undergo hypertrophy that is associated with experimental AD [155]. TRPV1 is also upregulated on bladder-afferent C-fibers [214].

Connections between lumbosacral afferents and thoracic preganglionic neurons play a crucial role in integrating sensory and autonomic regulation of vascular tone for standing and locomotion. V2 and V3 class glutamatergic interneurons of the lumbosacral and thoracic spinal cord contribute to the regulation of movement and BP and are strongly implicated in AD after SCI [28].

After SCI, calcitonin gene-related peptide sensory afferents sprout into the deeper lamina of the sacral segment dorsal horns, forming synapses on V3 glutamatergic lumbar interneurons that connect with thoracic sympathetic preganglionic neurons [28]. Lumbosacral Vglut2 neurons develop new processes onto local thoracic glutamatergic interneurons that synapse on the sympathetic preganglionic neurons, enhancing their excitation during bladder distention [176]. The local plasticity of thoracic VGluT2(+) neurons is also implicated in AD development [136], and tonic GABAergic inhibition of sympathetic preganglionic neurons is impaired after experimental SCI [201]. In peripheral circuits downstream of the spinal cord, cholinergic and noradrenergic collaterals in the stellate ganglion may undergo cross-talk after SCI, amplifying the incoming sympathetic preganglionic neuron signals to increase postganglionic neuron transmission [1, 34]. Thus, several neuroplastic circuit changes underlie AD development.

Genetic predisposition may also contribute to AD vulnerability, as shown in studies where Wistar but not Sprague-Dawley rats developed AD after SCI [104]. AD also causes post-SCI immune depression syndrome in animal models [130, 216].

19.7 Spasticity

19.7.1 Introduction to Spasticity Following SCI

After SCI, signals from the brain to motor neurons and interneurons below the injury site are disrupted. This initially causes a phase of flaccid paralysis and reflex loss, known as spinal shock. Over time, however, exaggerated reflexes, increased muscle tone, and involuntary spasms gradually emerge. These are hallmarks of spasticity [41].

Spasticity is the most prominent manifestation of disrupted sensorimotor control after SCI. It is a complex, multi-mechanistic condition, often challenging to define and treat due to its varied presentations (Fig. 19.5). Critical contributors to spasticity include neuroplastic changes in neuronal connectivity and function, impaired feedback control at both segmental and supraspinal levels, and intrinsic muscle changes exacerbated by immobilization after SCI [110, 138]. Spasticity affects both paraplegic and tetraplegic individuals, with high prevalence rates: 93% of those with complete (AIS A) cervical SCI and 78% with incomplete (AIS B-D) injuries report symptoms [108, 124].

Spasticity can significantly impact quality of life by limiting daily activities, impairing mobility and self-care, increasing pain and fatigue, disrupting sleep, and increasing the risk of contractures, pressure ulcers, infections, and rehabilitation difficulties [1]. Despite these adverse effects, some individuals report that spasticity can provide functional benefits, such as increased stability in sitting and standing, enhanced muscle bulk, and improved venous return. Spasticity is also a significant clinical issue in other neurological disorders, such as stroke and cerebral palsy.

19.7.2 Understanding the Physiology of Spasticity

At rest, muscles are typically EMG silent, with tone maintained by myofascial properties [116]. Reflexes, essential for posture and efficient movement, operate through segmental and multi-segmental arcs. SCI disrupts these systems, particularly through altered proprioceptive feedback and reflex regulation.

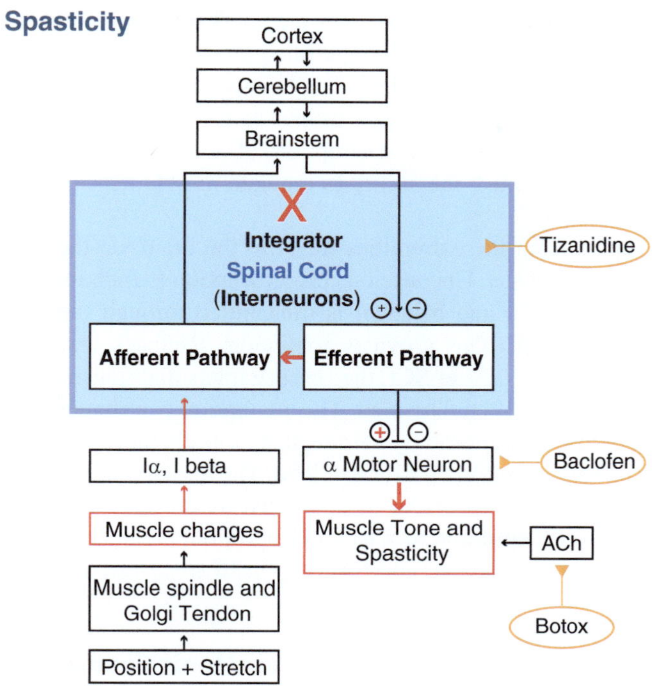

Fig. 19.5 Circuits involved in spasticity and treatment targets. The external input source is the stretch of muscle fibers, generating afferent impulses that travel to the spinal cord via 1α and 1β sensory fibers. There is local integration in the associated spinal segments. In an intact system, sensory impulses ascend to the cortex, cerebellum, and brainstem for processing. Motor responses descend for local segmental integration, motor neuron output, and muscle activation. In SCI, afferent impulses are amplified due to the loss of descending inhibition and alterations in interneuron function, leading to heightened and disorganized segmental motor outputs. Therapeutic interventions target different levels of the spasticity circuit. Peripherally, botulinum toxin can act at the neuromuscular junction to reduce muscle activation. Baclofen can modulate GABA B receptor-mediated ionic currents at alpha motor neurons to reduce spasticity. Tizanidine can modulate glutamatergic synaptic transmission at interneurons to decrease muscle tone

19.7.3 Proprioceptive Feedback Disruption

The terminology of proprioception can be confusing, so it is important to distinguish between proprioceptors, propriospinal neurons, propriospinal tracts, and the sense of proprioception. Proprioceptors, including muscle spindles and Golgi tendon organs, relay feedback from the muscles and joints about position and movement to the spinal cord and higher centers [154]. Propriospinal neurons in the spinal cord normally integrate sensory information with descending motor commands [102]. Conscious proprioception is essential for the brain to create a sense of position in space and to plan and execute movement.

Muscle spindles detect muscle length and stretch rates to regulate muscle contractions. Their afferent signals are transmitted through Ia and II afferent fibers, which help control reflex arcs. Reflex arcs mediate essential involuntary responses to sensory stimuli, such as the Ia-mediated stretch reflex. After SCI, muscle spindle feedback may become dysregulated, leading to excessive reflex activity and spasticity. Golgi tendon organs sense changes in muscle tension and usually work to prevent excessive force generation. Disruption of Golgi tendon organ feedback following SCI can diminish the ability to regulate muscle tension, contributing to ongoing spasticity.

Sensory inputs from the extremities travel to the brain via the dorsal column-medial lemniscus pathway. Unconscious proprioception (which involves automatic regulation of movement and balance) is transmitted through the spinocerebellar tracts to the cerebellum. This provides continuous feedback that helps modulate muscle tone and reflexes. After SCI, the sensory tracts that transmit proprioceptive signals to the brain are often disrupted. This disruption contributes to a breakdown in the feedback loops that normally help regulate muscle tone, leading to an inability to adjust to changes in body position or load. The loss of proprioceptive feedback can contribute to the development of spasticity, as muscles may become overly active or excessively tense due to a lack of appropriate regulatory inhibition. The balanced activity of the reticular and corticospinal tracts is also disrupted [167].

19.7.4 Changes in Excitation Balance and Ionic Channels

Normally, the supraspinal centers provide inhibitory modulation over reflexes to prevent exaggerated muscle contraction. SCI may result in a loss of descending inhibitory control from the brain, causing exaggerated reflex responses to muscle stretch or other stimuli that can lead to involuntary muscle contractions and stiffness. A delicate balance between excitatory and inhibitory inputs in the spinal cord is necessary to regulate muscle tone and movement smoothly.

Inhibitory interneurons in the spinal cord, such as Renshaw cells and Ia inhibitory interneurons, play a critical role in modulating motor neuron activity. After SCI, the function of these inhibitory interneurons may be compromised. For example, damage to the descending pathways that influence interneuron activity can reduce their inhibitory connections. This imbalance makes motor neurons more excitable, contributing to the sustained muscle contractions seen in spasticity.

The loss of inhibitory interneuron activity also disrupts the normal feedback mechanisms that regulate reflexes, leading to exaggerated muscle responses. Interneuronal properties may also change, contributing to spasticity. Many interneurons have inhibitory functions, releasing GABA or glycine; however, their inhibitory phenotype changes after SCI through alterations in ion channels and signaling. These include the downregulation of glutamic acid decarboxylase and the potassium chloride cotransporter KCC2 [18]. Reduced KCC2 channel activity decreases chloride currents, making neurons more excitable [23]. Motor neuron excitability may increase due to persistent inward currents of sodium and calcium (65- [83]). SCI shifts the excitation-inhibition balance due to the loss of inhibitory inputs, resulting in hyperexcitability of spinal motor circuits and leading to increased muscle tone and involuntary muscle contractions. The overactivity of excitatory pathways and reduced inhibitory control create a feedback loop that perpetuates and exacerbates spasticity. As described for AD, deafferentation can also lead to afferent sprouting after SCI as a source of aberrant circuits underlying spasticity [96, 118].

19.7.5 Defining and Characterizing Spasticity

The increased muscle tone following SCI results from denervation hypersensitivity, changes in muscle properties that include fibrosis and atrophy, and alterations in elastic properties, contributing to increased passive tension. While precisely defining spasticity can be challenging, definitions can provide a mechanistic focus since the afferent receptors are well known. Lance defined spasticity as "a motor disorder characterized by a velocity-dependent increase in tonic stretch reflexes (muscle tone) with exaggerated tendon jerks, resulting from hyperexcitability of the stretch reflex, as one component of the upper motor neuron syndrome [103]." However, this definition does not account for clonus, involuntary spasms, and primarily increased muscle tone, defining features of post-SCI muscle hyperactivity. Decq proposed a modified definition dividing spasticity into three components: (1) intrinsic tonic spasticity, characterized by an exaggeration of the tonic component of the stretch reflex, resulting in increased muscle tone; (2) intrinsic phasic spasticity, marked by an exaggeration of the phasic component of the stretch reflex, leading to symptoms such as tendon hyperreflexia and clonus; and (3) extrinsic spasticity, which involves exaggerated globalized flexion or extension spinal reflexes [44].

Intrinsic tonic spasticity refers to a *continuous*, prolonged increase in muscle tone characterized by sustained, involuntary muscle contractions and resistance to passive movement. Patients often describe this as "stiffness." Tonic spasticity is associated with persistent hyperexcitability of motor neurons and a loss of inhibitory control [191]. This type of spasticity is velocity-dependent, meaning that faster stretching results in greater reflex activity [186].

On the other hand, intrinsic phasic spasticity refers to *intermittent*, rapid muscle contractions or "spasms" in response to stimuli, such as quick stretching of the muscle or sudden movement. It is observed as exaggerated rhythmic stretch reflexes due to heightened sensitivity of the muscle spindle reflex. It includes symptoms such as tendon hyperreflexia and clonus, both resulting from the exaggeration of the phasic component of the stretch reflex. Tendon tap hyperreflexia likely arises from reduced presynaptic inhibition of Ia fibers. Clonus is characterized by involuntary, rhythmic muscle contractions, usually at the ankle, due to recurrent activation of stretch reflexes or a central oscillator in the spinal cord. Tonic and phasic spasticity differ in their underlying mechanisms and are both part of post-SCI disordered motor control, which also includes excessive co-contraction of muscles [117].

Extrinsic spasticity refers to involuntary flexor muscle spasms triggered by noxious stimuli originating from outside the muscle, such as skin, muscle, and joint receptors, or even a full bladder or bowel [1]. These spasms are mediated by polysynaptic reflexes within the multisegmental internuncial integrative interneuron system [20, 166], which normally provides inter-joint protective responses. SCI can disrupt the normal inhibition of these reflexes by supraspinal pathways, leading to hyperexcitability and lower thresholds for reflex activation.

19.7.6 Measurement of Spasticity

The diverse definitions of spasticity make its assessment challenging. The Ashworth and modified Ashworth scales are the most commonly used tools [22]. The results of spasticity assessments can differ significantly depending on the clinical context and individual factors. This has led to recommendations for using a combination of assessment methods that incorporate clinical, neurophysiological, and biomechanical techniques. However, there is often a limited correlation between clinical scales, decreases in spasticity, measures, and improved function [62].

19.8 Neuropathic Pain

Normally, pain serves protective functions to limit injury. Post-SCI neuropathic pain, however, is a significant and challenging complication. It is the only consciously experienced secondary condition discussed in this chapter. Defined as "pain caused by a lesion or disease of the somatosensory nervous system," neuropathic pain represents a sensory processing disorder. It can arise from injury to nerves, the spinal cord, and brain centers, including the thalamus [13] (Fig. 19.6). Like AD and spasticity, neuropathic pain arises from the loss of circuit inhibition and aberrant neuroplasticity [160]. Several neuroplastic mechanisms contribute to neuropathic pain [59], especially within the dorsal horn [77, 120] where, descending monoaminergic axons normally provide feedback-regulated inhibition [11, 84]. Anatomically, pain-processing synapses are typically compartmentalized in the lamina II substantia gelatinosa.

19.8.1 Molecular Mechanisms of Neuropathic Pain

Several molecular changes contribute to neuropathic pain, including loss of inhibition, neuroinflammation, central sensitization, alterations in receptors and ion channels, modifications in second messenger systems, and long-term potentiation.

Loss of Inhibitory Control Normally, GABA and glycine neurotransmitters regulate neuronal excitability in the dorsal horn. However, in neuropathic pain, there is often a reduction in GABAergic and glycinergic inhibition due to decreased synthesis, release, or receptor function [109]. This loss of inhibitory control contributes to unopposed excitatory signaling and the maintenance of central pain sensitization.

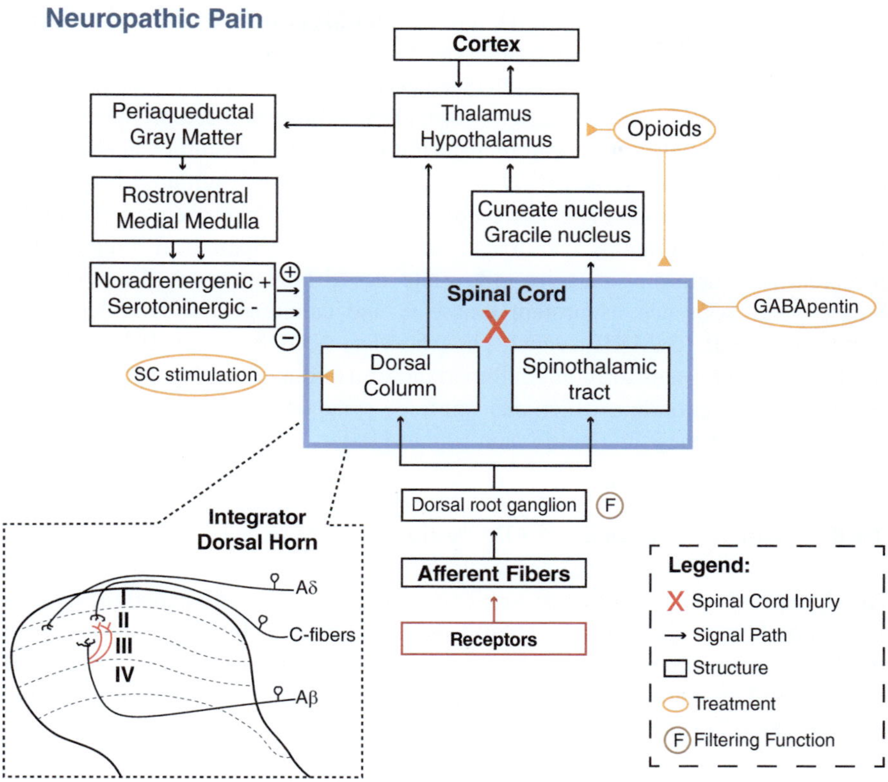

Fig. 19.6 Neuropathic pain arises after peripheral nerve root injury and disruption of ascending pathways due to SCI, leading to abnormal signal transmission and the development of chronic neuropathic pain that is difficult to manage. Nociceptor function may be amplified, and neuroplastic changes occur within the dorsal horn and other circuit regions. Different combinations of therapies are often employed to target neuropathic pain. Gabapentin and opioids are commonly used to alleviate neuropathic pain by modulating pain signals and reducing neuronal hyperexcitability. Some epidural spinal cord stimulation paradigms have efficacy

Role of Neuroinflammatory Mediators Locally, after SCI, activated microglia and astrocytes release pro-inflammatory cytokines, including TNFα, IL-1β, IL-6, and chemokines, contributing to the maintenance of central sensitization. Inflammatory mediators also promote the production of prostaglandins and nitric oxide, which can enhance the excitability of dorsal horn neurons and further promote pain hypersensitivity.

Central Sensitization Increased responsiveness (hyperexcitability) to normal or subthreshold afferent input may develop in CNS neurons, particularly in the dorsal horn of the spinal cord, with resultant amplification of signals. Central sensitization is caused by enhanced synaptic transmission, increased excitability of dorsal horn neurons, and reduced inhibitory signaling, which often persist into the chronic injury phase [113].

Changes in Receptor, Ion Channel, and Second Messenger Systems Following SCI, changes occur in the expression and function of ion channels, such as the upregulation of voltage-gated sodium channels (e.g., Nav1.7, Nav1.8) [78] and calcium channels, resulting in increased neuronal excitability and ectopic spontaneous neuronal firing. Glutamate, the primary excitatory neurotransmitter in the dorsal horn, binds to NMDA (N-methyl-D-aspartate) and AMPA (α-amino-3-hydroxy-5-methyl-4-isoxazolepropionic acid) receptors. Persistent or high-frequency stimulation of nociceptive afferents leads to excessive glutamate release, activating NMDA receptors and increasing calcium influx into dorsal horn neurons. This activates kinase pathways, such as protein kinase C and calcium/calmodulin-dependent protein kinase II (CaMKII), which phosphorylate NMDA and AMPA receptors, reinforcing central sensitization. An important form of dorsal horn synaptic plasticity is long-term potentiation, which can reinforce synaptic connections and enhance neuron responsiveness to amplify pain signals [164].

19.8.2 Anatomical Basis of Allodynia

Allodynia, a classic type of neuropathic pain, is characterized by experiencing pain from stimuli that are not usually painful such contact with clothing. It occurs when mechanoreceptor fibers sprout from their normal termination sites in laminae III and IV into Lamina II, resulting in the transduction of an innocuous sensation into pain [51, 175, 212].

19.8.3 Pain Signal Blockade

The brain contains a network of structures that work together to block pain, including the periaqueductal gray, locus coeruleus, and nuclei of the rostroventral medulla (specifically, the raphe magnus and nucleus reticularis gigantocellularis) [15]. The descending periaqueductal gray-locus coeruleus pain suppression pathway inhibits pain by releasing norepinephrine, which binds to presynaptic alpha-2 receptors in the dorsal horn. Additionally, periaqueductal gray-rostroventral medulla axons release serotonin that binds to 5-HT receptors. Local interneurons releasing enkephalin provide presynaptic inhibition by binding to opiate receptors. Additionally, the hypothalamus and pituitary gland release endorphins in response to pain or stress, which relieve pain and create a general feeling of well-being.

19.8.4 Genetic and Epigenetic Modifications

Chronic pain is associated with gene expression changes in dorsal horn neurons, which lead to the upregulation of pain-related receptors, ion channels, and signaling molecules. Epigenetic changes, including DNA methylation and histone modification, can sustain the expression of genes involved in central sensitization, perpetuating neuropathic pain [46].

19.8.5 Clinical Implications

Understanding these mechanisms is crucial for developing therapies that reduce central sensitization. Potential targets include NMDA receptors, ion channels, inflammatory mediators, and pathways that increase inhibitory neurotransmission.

19.9 Thermoregulation

Normal body core temperature is regulated at 37±0.6 C. Individuals with SCI experience reduced sensory input to the thermoregulatory center, resulting in a loss of sweating capacity and vasomotor control below the SCI level. The severity of thermoregulatory impairment is proportional to the level and completeness of injury, with athletes with SCI being particularly at risk [70] for abnormally high body temperatures in a hot environment or during exercise [72]. In addition, many individuals with tetraplegia report feeling cold even in ambient temperatures not regarded as cold by those without injury. Impaired thermoregulation has been associated with an increased risk of developing pressure ulcers due to impaired skin vasoregulation and sweating [196], and it can complicate the interpretation of fever in individuals with SCI [169]. At extremes, thermoregulatory impairment can affect essential physiological processes, including enzyme efficiency and cellular energetic stability [129].

19.9.1 Thermoregulatory Mechanisms

Thermoregulation is a crucial feedback-regulated homeostatic function involving heat production and dissipation control through the ANS. The hypothalamus controls thermoregulation by maintaining a set core temperature and integrating sensory inputs related to temperature changes [171]. Cold sensors, primarily located in the epidermis but also present within the midbrain and spinal cord, and warm temperature sensors in the preoptic anterior hypothalamus convey afferent signals. Heat-sensitive neurons also synapse with higher cortical regions to motivate corrective behavior [171].

Central mechanisms are usually triggered when ambient temperatures fall below ≈ 27 °C or rise above ≈ 33 °C [128, 147]. Temperatures outside this ambient range may drive core temperature fluctuation and influence vasomotor tone, metabolism, and cortical signaling, prompting the need for environmental adjustments [171]. Cold temperatures usually lead to vasoconstriction, which reduces peripheral heat loss, increases catecholamine release, boosts metabolism, and triggers shivering, a process regulated by the posterior hypothalamus that can boost heat production by a factor of 4–5 [171]. In contrast, elevated body temperatures resulting from external ambient heat or exercise prompt vasodilation, allowing heat dissipation through the skin. Sympathetic mechanisms mediate this vasodilation, including nitric oxide release, cholinergic activation of muscarinic receptors, and beta-2 adrenergic receptor activation [147]. Sweating, a sudomotor response, is another potent mechanism for reducing body temperature [171].

19.9.2 Impact of Temperature Changes on Arousal and Alertness

Temperature fluctuations can trigger increased arousal, alertness, and stress, prompting corrective actions. After SCI, this supraspinal output to levels below the injury is impaired, disrupting thermoregulatory efferent output and amplifying the effects of environmental temperature or exercise. This disruption can lead to partial poikilothermia, resulting in hypothermia or hyperthermia [4, 8, 122, 189].

19.9.3 Spinal Cord Injury and Thermoregulation

Following SCI, vascular changes contribute to thermoregulatory dysfunction [42, 208]. Post-SCI exercise intolerance is observed as reduced cardiac output hinders cardiovascular responses to increased demand during physical activity [42, 129, 184]. Normal skin perfusion is further disrupted due to oscillations in arterial diameter, exacerbating the difficulty in maintaining a stable body temperature [42, 132, 141]. Increased subcutaneous fat mass and body fat percentage following injury raise thermal resistance between the skin and internal structures, further impairing thermal regulation following core temperature changes [174, 179].

Vasomotor tone changes, regulated by spinal segments T1-L2, are retained above the injury level in people with paraplegia but are less effective in complete tetraplegia with loss of supraspinal input [156, 171]. People with paraplegia retain some ability to increase metabolism using residual muscle innervation, but those with complete cervical injuries lose efferent output and the ability to shiver below the injury level [49, 50, 171]. SCI diminishes supraspinal descending output, reducing sudomotor ability and further contributing to exercise intolerance [65, 144, 213]. Individuals with incomplete tetraplegia have a 50%–76% reduction in sweating compared to uninjured controls [144, 213], while complete cervical injury causes loss of all sudomotor ability below the lesion [190].

Education is essential to guide individuals with SCI in managing extreme temperatures when normal feedback mechanisms are impaired. Proactive regulation of body temperature is necessary, and wearable or peripheral devices like cell phones can help track environmental and skin temperatures. Individuals can learn new physiological cues, such as excessive sweating above the injury level, the onset of AD, and muscle stiffness or skin color changes. In cold temperatures, early decisions to move to warmer locations, wear increased clothing, use heaters, or ingest warm liquids can help raise the core temperature [171]. In hot conditions, fans and other cooling measures can aid in maintaining a safe body temperature.

19.9.4 Clinical Relevance

Thermoregulatory dysfunction in SCI can have significant effects. Extreme temperature fluctuations can impact organ function, immune response, and fluid balance and exacerbate neurologic impairment. Hypothermia may lead to bradycardia and potentially harmful hypotension, while hyperthermia may induce cardiovascular strain and promote AD [74]. Thermal monitoring and environmental management are essential to prevent further complications within the SCI population. In emergencies, treatments include surface rewarming or cooling, warmed or chilled intravenous fluids, antipyretics and inotropic agents, and even gastric lavage [195].

19.10 Treatment Targets and Therapy for Disrupted Feedback Regulation

We have approached SCI from the perspective of dysregulated feedback. In this manner, one can consider the sites of action of therapeutics to be within the afferent, integrative, efferent, and end-organ sites, as illustrated in Figs. 19.1, 19.2, 19.3, 19.4, 19.5 and 19.6. Physical therapy, drugs, and electrical neuromodulation are commonly used to target post-SCI complications arising from loss of feedback control (Table 19.1).

Effective post-SCI neuroprotection, which is an area of significant effort in the SCI field [73], could mitigate the complications we have discussed. Human MRI evidence supports the importance of tissue preservation, with even modest amounts of spared tissues associated with better recovery [148]. Early spinal cord decompression, tissue hypothermia, and drug and biologics therapies have been studied for neuroprotection [58].

An example of effective neuroprotection reducing autonomic complications was an inverse relationship between white matter sparing and the occurrence/severity of AD in a rat SCI model [202]. In this experiment, treatment with a monoclonal antibody targeting CD11d/CD18 integrin receptors reduced inflammation and white matter loss, preserving supraspinal control and reducing AD frequency [202].

Neuromodulation using drugs and electrical stimulation is an approach to mitigate the severity of complications in the chronic SCI state. An important neuromodulatory strategy is modifying ion channel activity. Baclofen is a $GABA^B$ channel agonist used for spasticity that can be delivered continuously by an infusion pump. Gabapentinoids (gabapentin, pregabalin) modulate the α-2-δ-1 subunit of voltage-gated calcium channels to alleviate neuropathic pain. Epidural stimulation (ES) was initially proposed to treat neuropathic pain based on the gate control theory [121]. Numerous trials have studied its effects on several forms of chronic pain [90, 146] with designs that include placebo/sham stimulation, which is essential due to placebo effects in pain studies [52]. The efficacy of ES is greater with new burst modes of stimulation, which at high frequencies do not result in paresthesias. An early application of ES was to treat spasticity [158], and recently, ES approaches have been developed to treat orthostatic hypotension [81], as discussed below.

Table 19.1 Therapeutics

Treatment	Target condition	Method of action	Feedback loop role
Baclofen	Spasticity	$GABA^B$ receptor agonist; enhances inhibitory signaling in the spinal cord to reduce muscle tone and spasms	Spinal segmental integration modulator
Epidural stimulation	Neuropathic pain, orthostatic hypotension	Modulates spinal circuits to enhance signal processing and autonomic function	Spinal segmental and tract modulator
Gabapentinoids (gabapentin, pregabalin)	Neuropathic pain	Modulates the α-2-δ subunit of voltage-gated Ca+ channels to reduce excitability and pain transmission	Spinal segmental downstream modulator
Botulinum toxin (botox)	Spasticity	Blocks acetylcholine release at neuromuscular junctions, reducing overactive muscle contractions	End organ neurotransmission blocker
Midodrine	Orthostatic hypotension	α-1 receptor agonist, vasoconstriction to increase BP	End organ effector
Droxidopa	Orthostatic hypotension	Synthetic norepinephrine; enhances adrenergic receptor activation to maintain BP	End organ effector
Fludrocortisone	Orthostatic hypotension	Increases blood volume by promoting Na retention and enhances vascular response to norepinephrine	Alters cardiovascular volume
Botox (bladder control)	Bladder spasticity	Injected into bladder muscles to reduce involuntary contractions by inhibiting neurotransmitter release	End organ
Sacral neuromodulation	Bladder and bowel dysfunction	Electrical stimulation of sacral nerves to restore sensory and motor feedback	Spinal segment modulator
Physical therapy	Spasticity, orthostatic tolerance	Stretching and strengthening exercises to improve joint mobility and tone control	Multifactorial effects
Capsaicin/ resiniferatoxin	Autonomic dysreflexia (bladder)	Desensitizes C-fiber afferents by binding to TRPV1 receptors, reducing overactivity	Afferent fiber blocker
Anticholinergic	Bladder spasticity	Competitive antagonist at muscarinic receptors, reducing involuntary muscle spasms	End organ
Biofeedback training	General autonomic control	Real-time monitoring (e.g., BP, HR) to train conscious control over autonomic functions	Primarily mediated by vagal circuits

(continued)

Table 19.1 (continued)

Treatment	Target condition	Method of action	Feedback loop role
Stem cell therapy (experimental)	Neuropathic pain, spasticity	Aims to repair damaged circuits and restore inhibitory control by transplanting GABAergic neurons	Spinal segmental function restoration
Tizanidine	Spasticity	α2-adrenergic receptor agonist; reduces excitatory neurotransmitter	Spinal segmental modulator

19.10.1 Treatment of Orthostatic Hypotension

Many therapies have been tested for orthostatic hypotension, including rehabilitation and functional electrical stimulation of the legs. However, substantial and persistent BP improvements are difficult to achieve. Garments that compress the legs and abdomen are commonly worn to reduce venous pooling. Pharmacotherapy for orthostatic hypotension often includes fludrocortisone and midodrine. Midodrine provides a *downstream* approach for feedback regulation. Midodrine is a prodrug whose derivative, desglymidrodine, is an A1 receptor agonist, the same receptor to which noradrenaline binds, causing direct vasoconstriction. Midodrine may cause supine hypertension. Droxidopa can also raise BP without causing supine hypertension [204]. Droxidopa is a synthetic precursor to noradrenaline that can cross the blood-brain barrier and has agonist activity at α and β adrenergic receptors. Fludrocortisone increases blood volume by promoting sodium retention, thus increasing intravascular volume. It also sensitizes blood vessels to the effects of norepinephrine [125], improving BP regulation in patients with low BP.

Neuromodulation

Epidural and transcutaneous spinal cord stimulation are reported to improve BP stability [2, 7, 81, 153] by directly regulating thoracic sympathetic preganglionic neuron output. The location of the stimulation is controversial, and thoracic afferent stimulation may be safer and more effective than lumbar stimulation (Courtine et al. accepted 2024).

Physical Therapy Approaches have targeted enhancing baroreceptor sensitivity to improve BP control. Extensive stand and respiratory training can improve orthostatic tolerance [6, 81, 80].

Biofeedback Techniques Real-time monitoring (e.g., BP and heart rate) trains individuals to influence autonomic responses consciously through cognitive strategies.

Stem Cell Therapy Experimental studies are investigating whether stem cells can repair damaged circuits involved in autonomic control, such as restoring the inhibitory regulation of pain signaling by transplanted GABA-expressing neuronal cells [53].

19.10.2 Treatment of Autonomic Dysreflexia

BP measurement is crucial for diagnosing AD. It is essential to compare the BP to the patient's baseline values [36]. SCI patients typically have a supine systolic BP between 90 and 110 mm Hg [94], so a hypertensive BP in the moderate range for non-SCI patients may indicate the presence of AD in those with SCI. Generally, a systolic BP over 150 mm Hg or a BP value >40 mm Hg above baseline represents a severe episode for which treatment should be initiated.

The first step in managing AD is to identify and remove the noxious stimulus, such as a full bladder or bowel distention. If this is unsuccessful, fast-acting medications like sublingual nifedipine or nitroglycerin paste may be applied to acutely lower BP. Alpha-blockers (e.g., prazosin) block the effects of norepinephrine, reducing BP spikes during AD. Nitroglycerin and nitrates act as vasodilators to lower BP during AD episodes.

Bladder and Bowel Feedback Regulation The bladder is a significant source of afferent impulses that can provoke AD episodes. SCI often results in neurogenic bladder and bowel dysfunction, leading to incontinence, retention, or abnormal reflexes. Normal feedback control over bladder and bowel emptying is disrupted. Conducting urodynamic studies, which can replicate bladder-filling/bladder-sphincter dyssynergia, can trigger AD [66].

Reduction of Bladder Afferent Signaling Capsaicin or resiniferatoxin can be instilled into the bladder to desensitize C-fibers by binding to the TRPV1 receptor, leading to reduced bladder reactivity [29].

Reduction of Efferent Signaling Botulinum toxin can be injected into the bladder or bowel muscles to reduce spasticity and improve control over bladder and bowel reflexes.

Drugs to Relax the Bladder Oxybutynin is an anticholinergic medication whose active metabolite N-desethyloxybutynin is a competitive antagonist of the postganglionic muscarinic M1 and M3 receptors of smooth muscle endplates. Tolterodine is more selective for the M2 and M3 receptors.

Sacral Neuromodulation Implantable devices stimulate the sacral nerves to restore bladder and bowel function, improving sensory feedback and motor control. Implants as well as rhizotomy of the sacral dorsal rootlets have been associated with significantly reduced AD [38].

19.10.3 Treatment of Spasticity

Assessment The diverse definitions of spasticity complicate its assessment. The Ashworth and modified Ashworth scales are the most commonly used tools [22].

The outcomes of spasticity assessments can vary significantly depending on the clinical context and individual factors. This has led to recommendations for a battery of assessment tools incorporating clinical, neurophysiological, and biomechanical techniques. However, there is generally a poor correlation among clinical scales, and reductions in spasticity do not necessarily translate to improved function [19].

A wide range of therapies has been applied to spasticity due to its multiple etiologies, including stroke, cerebral palsy, and SCI. Treatment approaches include physical therapy, pharmacotherapy, and neuromodulation.

Physical Therapy Stretching is the most common method to modify spasticity by increasing joint range of motion, soft tissue extensibility, and the reflex state by inducing adaptation of muscle spindles to a stretched position. In general, the effects are transitory [68]. Tendon and muscle vibration have also been shown to improve walking speed in those individuals with incomplete SCI [135]. Vibration is believed to exert its effects at the level of muscle spindles by enhancing inhibitory feedback to control excessive muscle contractions. This effect has been documented by observation of reduced H reflexes [133].

Another direct muscle-focused therapy is botulinum toxin. Although this has been mentioned above, it is discussed here for use in skeletal muscles. Botulinum toxin injections reduce local muscle overactivity by blocking the release of acetylcholine at motor end plates, with robust effects lasting for a few months [183]. A primary mechanism of action is the cleavage of critical presynaptic endocytic proteins [21].

Drugs The most commonly used anti-spasticity drug is baclofen, a GABA-B receptor agonist that enhances inhibitory signaling in the spinal cord, thereby reducing spasticity because of decreased calcium conductance in presynaptic neurons and increased potassium conductance at post-synaptic sites, resulting in hyperpolarization [200]. Intrathecal baclofen delivery can deliver increased therapeutic efficacy by pump-mediated delivery to the spinal fluid, allowing for more targeted control of spasticity [143].

Spinal Stimulation Neuromodulation approaches for spasticity, including epidural and transcutaneous stimulation, have shown promising effects. However, few adequately powered studies have been conducted [165, 181].

19.10.4 Treatment of Neuropathic Pain

Neuropathic pain following SCI results from disrupted feedback in sensory pathways, where abnormal signals are generated in response to non-painful stimuli (allodynia) or exaggerated pain responses (hyperalgesia). It is the most subjective of the post-SCI complications discussed in this chapter. Numerous therapeutic approaches target multiple loci in the involved pathways, from the skin surface to thalamocortical function.

Drugs The most commonly prescribed medications for neuropathic pain are anticonvulsants, antidepressants, and cannabinoids. Gabapentin and pregabalin modulate overactive pain signals by targeting calcium channels in neurons. Antidepressants (e.g., amitriptyline and duloxetine) modify pain pathways by increasing serotonin and norepinephrine levels. The role of cannabinoids in modulating pain pathways is being investigated to provide relief from neuropathic pain [210].

Neurostimulation Multiple types of electrical neuromodulation have been tested for neuropathic pain. These include nerve and dorsal root ganglion stimulation, epidural stimulation, repetitive transcranial magnetic stimulation, direct current stimulation, and deep brain stimulation [106]. This range of approaches underscores the greater complexity of neuropathic pain as compared to orthostatic hypotension, AD, and spasticity.

19.10.5 Treatment of Altered Thermoregulation

Currently, there are no drug or device treatments to restore thermoregulation. Experimental methods for specific optogenetic stimulation of hypothalamic targets can regulate body temperature [217]. Non-thermoregulatory reflex sweating and hyperhidrosis can occur after SCI [57]. Beta-blockers may be a therapeutic option.

19.11 Summary

We have reviewed several post-SCI problems caused by impaired feedback control and aberrant neuroplasticity. By understanding the involved feedback systems, we can identify potentially effective intervention points. However, circuits are altered by the neuroplastic changes following SCI deafferentation, and the alterations in interneuronal segmental signaling are only partially understood. Some approaches downstream of regulatory mechanisms are useful, such as using midodrine to elevate BP. However, a lack of feedback controls limits their efficacy and safety. Modulatory drugs like baclofen and gabapentin act within the control circuits. Electrical neuromodulation for hemodynamic fluctuations, spasticity, and pain is rapidly reversible and adjustable, and in some applications, closed-loop control could be restored. Post-SCI deafferentation neural sprouting and novel circuit formation are significant issues, and early treatments to better regulate these need to be developed before the changes are established. Inducing new regenerative process growth in residual descending systems is one approach that will remain for the future. Post-SCI neuroprotective treatments are essential to retain sufficient regulatory circuits and should remain a primary focus in the SCI field.

Acknowledgments James Guest, Neil Datta, and Pedro Saravia gratefully acknowledge the support from the Miami Project to Cure Paralysis. Josh Ceisler is a first-year PhD student in the Program in Biomedical Sciences at the University of Miami.

References

1. Adams MM, Hicks AL. Spasticity after spinal cord injury. Spinal Cord. 2005;43:577–86.
2. Ahuja CS, Wilson JR, Nori S, Kotter MRN, Druschel C, Curt A, Fehlings MG. Traumatic spinal cord injury. Nat Rev Dis Primers. 2017;3(1). https://doi.org/10.1038/nrdp.2017.18.
3. Alexander N, Decuir M. Role of aortic and Vagus nerves in arterial Baroreflex bradycardia in rabbits. Am J Phys. 1963;205:775–80.
4. Altus P, Hickman JW, Nord HJ. accidental hypothermia in a healthy quadriplegic patient. Neurology. 1985;35(3):427–8.
5. Anderson CR, Mclachlan EM, Srb-Christie O. Distribution of sympathetic preganglionic neurons and monoaminergic nerve terminals in the spinal cord of the rat. J Comp Neurol. 1989;283:269–84.
6. Aslan SC, Randall DC, Krassioukov AV, Phillips A, Ovechkin AV. Respiratory training improves blood pressure regulation in individuals with chronic spinal cord injury. Arch Phys Med Rehabil. 2016;97:964–73.
7. Aslan SC, Legg Ditterline BE, Park MC, Angeli CA, Rejc E, Chen Y, Ovechkin AV, Krassioukov A, Harkema SJ. Epidural spinal cord stimulation of lumbosacral networks modulates arterial blood pressure in individuals with spinal cord injury-induced cardiovascular deficits. Front Physiol. 2018;9:565.
8. Attia M, Engel P. thermoregulatory set point in patients with spinal-cord injuries (spinal man). Paraplegia. 1983;21(4):233–48.
9. Averill S, Mcmahon BS, Clary OD, Reichardt FL, Priestley VJ. Immunocytochemical localization of trkA receptors in chemically identified subgroups of adult rat sensory neurons. Eur J Neurosci. 1995;7:1484–94.
10. Bandtlow CE, Meyer M, Lindholm D, Spranger M, Heumann R, Thoenen H. Regional and cellular codistribution of interleukin 1 beta and nerve growth factor mRNA in the adult rat brain: possible relationship to the regulation of nerve growth factor synthesis. J Cell Biol. 1990;111:1701–11.
11. Bannister K, Dickenson AH. What do monoamines do in pain modulation? Curr Opin Support Palliat Care. 2016;10:143–8.
12. Bannister K, Bee LA, Dickenson AH. Preclinical and early clinical investigations related to monoaminergic pain modulation. Neurotherapeutics. 2009;6:703–12.
13. Baron R, Binder A, Wasner G. Neuropathic pain: diagnosis, pathophysiological mechanisms, and treatment. Lancet Neurol. 2010;9:807–19.
14. Beauparlant J, Van Den Brand R, Barraud Q, Friedli L, Musienko P, Dietz V, Courtine G. Undirected compensatory plasticity contributes to neuronal dysfunction after severe spinal cord injury. Brain. 2013;136:3347–61.
15. Benarroch EE. Descending monoaminergic pain modulation: bidirectional control and clinical relevance. Neurology. 2008;71:217–21.
16. Berger MJ, Kimpinski K, Currie KD, Nouraei H, Sadeghi M, Krassioukov AV. Multi-domain assessment of autonomic function in spinal cord injury using a modified autonomic reflex screen. J Neurotrauma. 2017;34:2624–33.
17. Berthoud HR, Neuhuber WL. Functional and chemical anatomy of the afferent vagal system. Auton Neurosci. 2000;85:1–17.
18. Bhagwani A, Chopra M, Kumar H. Spinal cord injury provoked neuropathic pain and spasticity, and their Gabaergic connection. Neurospine. 2022;19:646–68.
19. Biering-Sorensen F, Nielsen JB, Klinge K. Spasticity-assessment: a review. Spinal Cord. 2006;44:708–22.
20. Biraben A, Roby-Brami A, Azouvi P, Tougeron A, Bussel B. Physiopathology of spasticity and flexion spasms. Therapie. 1990;45:259–62.
21. Blasi J, Chapman ER, Link E, Binz T, Yamasaki S, De Camilli P, Südhof TC, Niemann H, Jahn R. Botulinum neurotoxin A selectively cleaves the synaptic protein SNAP-25. Nature. 1993;365:160–3.

22. Bohannon RW, Smith MB. Interrater reliability of a modified Ashworth scale of muscle spasticity. Phys Ther. 1987;67:206–7.
23. Boulenguez P, Liabeuf S, Bos R, Bras H, Jean-Xavier C, Brocard C, Stil A, Darbon P, Cattaert D, Delpire E, Marsala M, Vinay L. Down-regulation of the potassium-chloride cotransporter KCC2 contributes to spasticity after spinal cord injury. Nat Med. 2010;16:302–U97.
24. Brown A, Ricci MJ, Weaver LC. NGF message and protein distribution in the injured rat spinal cord. Exp Neurol. 2004;188:115–27.
25. Cai B, Wu D, Xie H, Chen Y, Wang H, Jin S, Song Y, Li A, Huang S, Wang S, Lu Y, Bao L, Xu F, Gong H, Li C, Zhang X. A direct spino-cortical circuit bypassing the thalamus modulates nociception. Cell Res. 2023;33:775–89.
26. Cannon WB. Organization for physiological homeostasis. Physiol Rev. 1929;9:399–431.
27. Carew T, Castellucci VF, Kandel ER. Sensitization in Aplysia: restoration of transmission in synapses inactivated by long-term habituation. Science. 1979;205:417–9.
28. Chacon C, Nwachukwu CV, Shahsavani N, Cowley KC, Chopek JW. Lumbar V3 interneurons provide direct excitatory synaptic input onto thoracic sympathetic preganglionic neurons, linking locomotor, and autonomic spinal systems. Front Neural Circuits. 2023;17
29. Chancellor MB, De Groat WC. Intravesical capsaicin and Resiniferatoxin therapy: spicing up the ways to treat the overactive bladder. J Urol. 1999;162:3–11.
30. Chuang Y-C, Fraser MO, Yu Y, Beckel JM, Seki S, Nakanishi Y, Yokoyama H, Chancellor MB, Yoshimura N, De Groat WC. Analysis of the afferent limb of the vesicovascular reflex using neurotoxins, resiniferatoxin and capsaicin. Am J Phys Regul Integr Comp Phys. 2001;281:R1302–10.
31. Christopherson KS, Ullian EM, Stokes CCA, Mullowney CE, Hell JW, Agah A, et al. Thrombospondins are astrocyte-secreted proteins that promote CNS synaptogenesis. Cell. 2005;120(3):421–33.
32. Citri A, Malenka RC. Synaptic plasticity: multiple forms, functions, and mechanisms. Neuropsychopharmacology. 2008;33:18–41.
33. Claydon VE, Krassioukov AV. Orthostatic hypotension and autonomic pathways after spinal cord injury. J Neurotrauma. 2006;23:1713–25.
34. Clyburn C, Li MH, Ingram SL, Andresen MC, Habecker BA. Cholinergic collaterals arising from noradrenergic sympathetic neurons in mice. J Physiol. 2023;601:1247–64.
35. Connelly WM, Laing M, Errington AC, Crunelli V. The thalamus as a low pass filter: filtering at the cellular level does not equate with filtering at the network level. Frontiers in Neural Circuits. 2016;9
36. Cowan H, Lakra C, Desai M. Autonomic dysreflexia in spinal cord injury. BMJ. 2020;371:m3596.
37. Cramer SC, Sur M, Dobkin BH, O'brien C, Sanger TD, Trojanowski JQ, Rumsey JM, Hicks R, Cameron J, Chen D, Chen WG, Cohen LG, Decharms C, Duffy CJ, Eden GF, Fetz EE, Filart R, Freund M, Grant SJ, Haber S, Kalivas PW, Kolb B, Kramer AF, Lynch M, Mayberg HS, Mcquillen PS, Nitkin R, Pascual-Leone A, Reuter-Lorenz P, Schiff N, Sharma A, Shekim L, Stryker M, Sullivan EV, Vinogradov S. Harnessing neuroplasticity for clinical applications. Brain. 2011;134:1591–609.
38. Creasey GH, Grill JH, Korsten M, Hoi Sang U, Betz R, Anderson R, Walter J, Implanted Neuroprosthesis Research, G. An implantable neuroprosthesis for restoring bladder and bowel control to patients with spinal cord injuries: a multicenter trial. Arch Phys Med Rehabil. 2001;82:1512–9.
39. Crill W, Reis D. Distribution of carotid sinus and depressor nerves in cat brain stem. Am J Physiol-Legacy Content. 1968;214:269–76.
40. Curt A, Nitsche B, Rodic B, Schurch B, Dietz V. Assessment of autonomic dysreflexia in patients with spinal cord injury. J Neurol Neurosurg Psychiatry. 1997;62:473–7.
41. D'amico JM, Condliffe EG, Martins KJB, Bennett DJ, Gorassini MA. Recovery of neuronal and network excitability after spinal cord injury and implications for spasticity. Front Integr Neurosci. 2014;8

42. de Groot PC, Bleeker MW, van Kuppevelt DH, van der Woude LH, Hopman MT. Rapid and extensive arterial adaptations after spinal cord injury. Archives of Physical Medicine and Rehabilitation. 2006;87(5):688–96.
43. Dean JC. Proprioceptive feedback and preferred patterns of human movement. Exerc Sport Sci Rev. 2013;41:36–43.
44. Decq P. Pathophysiology of spasticity. Neuro-chirurgie. 2003;49:163–84.
45. Del Fabro AS, Mejia M, Nemunaitis G. An investigation of the relationship between autonomic dysreflexia and intrathecal baclofen in patients with spinal cord injury. J Spinal Cord Med. 2018;41:102–5.
46. Descalzi G, Ikegami D, Ushijima T, Nestler EJ, Zachariou V, Narita M. Epigenetic mechanisms of chronic pain. Trends Neurosci. 2015;38:237–46.
47. Ditunno JF, Little JW, Tessler A, Burns AS. Spinal shock revisited: a four-phase model. Spinal Cord. 2004;42:383–95.
48. Donnelly DJ, Popovich PG. Inflammation and its role in neuroprotection, axonal regeneration and functional recovery after spinal cord injury. Exp Neurol. 2008;209:378–88.
49. Downey JA, Chiodi HP, Darling RC. central temperature regulation in spinal man. Journal of Applied Physiology. 1967;22(1):91–94.
50. Downey JA, Miller JM, Darling RC. thermoregulatory responses to deep and superficial cooling in spinal man. Journal of Applied Physiology. 1969;27(2):209-213.1
51. Duan B, Cheng L, Bourane S, Britz O, Padilla C, Garcia-Campmany L, Krashes M, Knowlton W, Velasquez T, Ren X, Ross SE, Lowell BB, Wang Y, Goulding M, Ma Q. Identification of spinal circuits transmitting and gating mechanical pain. Cell. 2014;159:1417–32.
52. Duarte RV, Nevitt S, Mcnicol E, Taylor RS, Buchser E, North RB, Eldabe S. Systematic review and meta-analysis of placebo/sham controlled randomised trials of spinal cord stimulation for neuropathic pain. Pain. 2020;161:24–35.
53. Eaton MJ, Plunkett JA, Martinez MA, Lopez T, Karmally S, Cejas P, Whittemore SR. Article commentary: transplants of neuronal cells bioengineered to synthesize GABA alleviate chronic neuropathic pain. Cell Transplant. 1999;8:87–101.
54. Edwards LL, King EM, Buetefisch CM, Borich MR. Putting the "Sensory" into sensorimotor control: the role of sensorimotor integration in goal-directed hand movements after stroke. Front Integr Neurosci. 2019;13:16.
55. Eltorai I, Kim R, Vulpe M, Kasravi H, Ho W. Fatal cerebral hemorrhage due to autonomic dysreflexia in a tetraplegic patient: case report and review. Paraplegia. 1992;30:355–60.
56. Eroglu Ç, Allen NJ, Susman MW, O'Rourke NA, Park CY, Özkan E, et al. Gabapentin Receptor α2δ-1 Is a Neuronal Thrombospondin Receptor Responsible for Excitatory CNS Synaptogenesis. Cell. 2009;139(2):380–92.
57. Fast A. Reflex sweating in patients with spinal cord injury: a review. Arch Phys Med Rehabil. 1977;58:435–7.
58. Fehlings MG, Moghaddamjou A, Harrop JS, Stanford R, Ball J, Aarabi B, Freeman BJC, Arnold PM, Guest JD, Kurpad SN, Schuster JM, Nassr A, Schmitt KM, Wilson JR, Brodke DS, Ahmad FU, Yee A, Ray WZ, Brooks NP, Wilson J, Chow DS, Toups EG, Kopjar B. Safety and efficacy of Riluzole in acute spinal cord injury study (RISCIS): A multi-center, randomized, placebo-controlled, double-blinded trial. J Neurotrauma. 2023;40:1878–88.
59. Finnerup NB, Kuner R, Jensen TS. Neuropathic pain: from mechanisms to treatment. Physiol Rev. 2021;101:259–301.
60. Fisher KM, Garner JP, Darian-Smith C. Chronic adaptations in the dorsal horn following a cervical spinal cord injury in primates. J Neurosci. 2024;44:e0877232023.
61. Fossey MPM, Balthazaar SJT, Squair JW, Williams AM, Poormasjedi-Meibod M-S, Nightingale TE, Erskine E, Hayes B, Ahmadian M, Jackson GS, Hunter DV, Currie KD, Tsang TSM, Walter M, Little JP, Ramer MS, Krassioukov AV, West CR. Spinal cord injury impairs cardiac function due to impaired bulbospinal sympathetic control. Nat Commun. 2022;13:1382.

62. Francis HP, Wade DT, Turner-Stokes L, Kingswell RS, Dott CS, Coxon EA. Does reducing spasticity translate into functional benefit? An exploratory meta-analysis. J Neurol Neurosurg Psychiatry. 2004;75:1547–51.
63. Furlan JC. Headache attributed to autonomic dysreflexia: an underrecognized clinical entity. Neurology. 2011;77(8):792–8.
64. Garshick E, Kelley A, Cohen SA, Garrison A, Tun CG, Gagnon D, Brown R. A prospective assessment of mortality in chronic spinal cord injury. Spinal Cord. 2005;43:408–16.
65. Gerner HJ, Engel P, Gass GC, Gass EM, Hannich T, Feldmann G. The effects of sauna on tetraplegic and paraplegic subjects. Paraplegia. 1992;30(6):410–9.1.
66. Giannantoni A, Di Stasi SM, Scivoletto G, Mollo A, Silecchia A, Fuoco U, Vespasiani G. Autonomic dysreflexia during urodynamics. Spinal Cord. 1998;36:756–60.
67. Giesler GJ Jr, Katter JT, Dado RJ. Direct spinal pathways to the limbic system for nociceptive information. Trends Neurosci. 1994;17:244–50.
68. Gomez-Cuaresma L, Lucena-Anton D, Gonzalez-Medina G, Martin-Vega FJ, Galan-Mercant A, Luque-Moreno C. Effectiveness of stretching in post-stroke spasticity and range of motion: systematic review and meta-analysis. J Pers Med. 2021;11:1074.
69. Gonzalez F, Chang JY, Banovac K, Messina D, Martinez-Arizala A, Kelley RE. Autoregulation of cerebral blood flow in patients with orthostatic hypotension after spinal cord injury. Paraplegia. 1991;29:1–7.
70. Griggs KE, Price MJ, Goosey-Tolfrey VL. Cooling athletes with a spinal cord injury. Sports Med. 2015;45:9–21.
71. Grill RJ, Blesch A, Tuszynski MH. Robust growth of chronically injured spinal cord axons induced by grafts of genetically modified NGF-secreting cells. Exp Neurol. 1997;148:444–52.
72. Grossmann F, Perret C, Roelands B, Meeusen R, Flueck JL. Fluid balance and thermoregulatory responses during wheelchair basketball games in hot vs. temperate conditions. Nutrients. 2022;14
73. Guest J, Datta N, Jimsheleishvili G, Gater DR Jr. Pathophysiology, classification and comorbidities after traumatic spinal cord injury. J Pers Med. 2022;12
74. Gunduz H, Binak DF. Autonomic dysreflexia: An important cardiovascular complication in spinal cord injury patients. Cardiology Journal. 2012;19(2):215–9.
75. Guttmann L, Whitteridge D. Effects of bladder distension on autonomic mechanisms after spinal cord injuries. Brain. 1947;70:361–404.
76. Hagen EM, Rekand T, Gronning M, Faerestrand S. Cardiovascular complications of spinal cord injury. Tidsskr Nor Laegeforen. 2012;132:1115–20.
77. Hains BC, Klein JP, Saab CY, Craner MJ, Black JA, Waxman SG. Upregulation of sodium channel Nav1.3 and functional involvement in neuronal hyperexcitability associated with central neuropathic pain after spinal cord injury. J Neurosci. 2003;23:8881–92.
78. Hameed S. Na(v)1.7 and Na(v)1.8: role in the pathophysiology of pain. Mol Pain. 2019;15:1744806919858801.
79. Hao H, Ramli R, Wang C, Liu C, Shah S, Mullen P, Lall V, Jones F, Shao J, Zhang H, Jaffe DB, Gamper N, Du X. Dorsal root ganglia control nociceptive input to the central nervous system. PLoS Biol. 2023;21:e3001958.
80. Harkema SJ, Ferreira CK, Van Den Brand RJ, Krassioukov AV. Improvements in orthostatic instability with stand locomotor training in individuals with spinal cord injury. J Neurotrauma. 2008;25:1467–75.
81. Harkema SJ, Legg Ditterline B, Wang S, Aslan S, Angeli CA, Ovechkin A, Hirsch GA. Epidural spinal cord stimulation training and sustained recovery of cardiovascular function in individuals with chronic cervical spinal cord injury. JAMA Neurol. 2018;75:1569–71.
82. Hayashi M, Ueyama T, Nemoto K, Tamaki T, Senba E. Sequential mRNA expression for immediate early genes, cytokines, and neurotrophins in spinal cord injury. Journal of Neurotrauma. 2000;17(3):203–18.
83. Heckman CJ, Gorassini MA, Bennett DJ. Persistent inward currents in motoneuron dendrites: implications for motor output. Muscle Nerve. 2005;31:135–56.

84. Heinricher MM, Tavares I, Leith JL, Lumb BM. Descending control of nociception: specificity, recruitment and plasticity. Brain Res Rev. 2009;60:214–25.
85. Hiersemenzel LP, Curt A, Dietz V. From spinal shock to spasticity: neuronal adaptations to a spinal cord injury. Neurology. 2000;54:1574–82.
86. Hornung JP. The human raphe nuclei and the serotonergic system. J Chem Neuroanat. 2003;26:331–43.
87. Huang SC, May-Kuen Wong A, Lien HY, Fuk-Tan Tang S, Fu TC, Lin Y, Wang JS. Systemic vascular resistance is increased and associated with accelerated arterial stiffening change in patients with chronic cervical spinal cord injury. Eur J Phys Rehabil Med. 2013;49:41–9.
88. Hughes DI, Todd AJ. Central nervous system targets: inhibitory interneurons in the spinal cord. Neurotherapeutics. 2020;17:874–85.
89. Illman A, Stiller K, Williams M. The prevalence of orthostatic hypotension during physiotherapy treatment in patients with an acute spinal cord injury. Spinal Cord. 2000;38:741–7.
90. Joosten EA, Franken G. Spinal cord stimulation in chronic neuropathic pain: mechanisms of action, new locations, new paradigms. Pain. 2020;161:S104.
91. Katzelnick CG, Weir JP, Jones A, Galea M, Dyson-Hudson TA, Kirshblum SC, Wecht JM. Blood pressure instability in persons with SCI: evidence from a 30-day home monitoring observation. Am J Hypertens. 2019;32:938–44.
92. Koizumi K, Collin R, Kaufman A, Brooks cmc. contribution of unmyelinated afferent excitation to sympathetic reflexes. Brain Research. 1970;20(1):99–&.
93. Krassioukov AV, Weaver LC. Episodic hypertension due to autonomic dysreflexia in acute and chronic spinal cord-injured rats. Am J Phys. 1995;268:H2077–83.
94. Krassioukov A, Linsenmeyer TA, Beck LA, Elliott S, Gorman P, Kirshblum S, et al. Evaluation and Man-agement of Autonomic Dysreflexia and Other Autonomic Dysfunctions: Preventing the Highs and Lows: Management of Blood Pressure, Sweating, and Temperature Dysfunction. Top Spinal Cord Inj Rehabil. 2021;27(2):225–90.
95. Krassioukov AV, Weaver LC. Morphological changes in sympathetic preganglionic neurons after spinal cord injury in rats. Neuroscience. 1996;70:211–25.
96. Krenz NR, Weaver LC. Sprouting of primary afferent fibers after spinal cord transection in the rat. Neuroscience. 1998a;85:443–58.
97. Krenz NR, Weaver LC. Sprouting of primary afferent fibers after spinal cord transection in the rat. Neuroscience. 1998b;85:443–58.
98. Krenz RN, Weaver CL. Changes in the morphology of sympathetic preganglionic neurons parallel the development of autonomic dysreflexia after spinal cord injury in rats. Neurosci Lett. 1998c;243:61–4.
99. Krenz NR, Meakin SO, Krassioukov AV, Weaver LC. Neutralizing intraspinal nerve growth factor blocks autonomic dysreflexia caused by spinal cord injury. J Neurosci. 1999;19:7405–14.
100. Krum H, Howes LG, Brown DJ, Louis WJ. Blood pressure variability in tetraplegic patients with autonomic hyperreflexia. Paraplegia. 1989;27:284–8.
101. Kwon M, Altin M, Duenas H, Alev L. The role of descending inhibitory pathways on chronic pain modulation and clinical implications. Pain Pract. 2014;14:656–67.
102. Laliberte AM, Goltash S, Lalonde NR, Bui TV. Propriospinal neurons: essential elements of locomotor control in the intact and possibly the injured spinal cord. Front Cell Neurosci. 2019;13
103. Lance JW. The control of muscle tone, reflexes, and movement: Robert Wartenberg Lecture. Neurology. 1980;30:1303–13.
104. Landrum LM, Thompson GM, Blair RW. Does postsynaptic alpha 1-adrenergic receptor supersensitivity contribute to autonomic dysreflexia? Am J Phys. 1998;274:H1090–8.
105. Langley JN. On the union of cranial autonomic (visceral) Fibres with the nerve cells of the superior cervical ganglion. J Physiol. 1898;23:240–70.

106. Lefaucheur JP, Aleman A, Baeken C, Benninger DH, Brunelin J, Di Lazzaro V, Filipovic SR, Grefkes C, Hasan A, Hummel FC, Jääskeläinen SK, Langguth B, Leocani L, Londero A, Nardone R, Nguyen JP, Nyffeler T, Oliveira-Maia AJ, Oliviero A, Padberg F, Palm U, Paulus W, Poulet E, Quartarone A, Rachid F, Rektorová I, Rossi S, Sahlsten H, Schecklmann M, Szekely D, Ziemann U. Evidence-based guidelines on the therapeutic use of repetitive transcranial magnetic stimulation (rTMS): an update (2014-2018). Clin Neurophysiol. 2020;131:474–528.
107. Lei Y, Perez MA. Cerebellar contribution to sensorimotor adaptation deficits in humans with spinal cord injury. Sci Rep. 2021;11:2507.
108. Li YR, Gorassini MA, Bennett DJ. Role of persistent sodium and calcium currents in motoneuron firing and spasticity in chronic spinal rats. J Neurophysiol. 2004;91:767–83.
109. Li C, Lei Y, Tian Y, Xu S, Shen X, Wu H, Bao S, Wang F. The etiological contribution of Gabaergic plasticity to the pathogenesis of neuropathic pain. Mol Pain. 2019;15:1744806919847366.
110. Lieber RL, Steinman S, Barash IA, Chambers H. Structural and functional changes in spastic skeletal muscle. Muscle Nerve. 2004;29:615–27.
111. Lu Y, Doroshenko M, Lauzadis J, Kanjiya MP, Rebecchi MJ, Kaczocha M, Puopolo M. Presynaptic inhibition of primary nociceptive signals to dorsal horn lamina I neurons by dopamine. J Neurosci. 2018;38:8809–21.
112. Lumb R, Tata M, Xu XJ, Joyce A, Marchant C, Harvey N, et al. Neuropilins guide preganglionic sympa-thetic axons and chromaffin cell precursors to establish the adrenal medulla. Development. 2018;145(21).
113. Lütolf R, Rosner J, Curt A, Hubli M. Indicators of central sensitization in chronic neuropathic pain after spinal cord injury. Eur J Pain. 2022;26:2162–75.
114. Maiorov DN, Weaver LC, Krassioukov AV. Relationship between sympathetic activity and arterial pressure in conscious spinal rats. Am J Phys. 1997;272:H625–31.
115. Maiorov DN, Fehlings MG, Krassioukov AV. Relationship between severity of spinal cord injury and abnormalities in neurogenic cardiovascular control in conscious rats. J Neurotrauma. 1998;15:365–74.
116. Masi AT, Hannon JC. Human resting muscle tone (HRMT): narrative introduction and modern concepts. J Bodyw Mov Ther. 2008;12:320–32.
117. Mayo M, Deforest BA, Castellanos M, Thomas CK. Characterization of involuntary contractions after spinal cord injury reveals associations between physiological and self-reported measures of spasticity. Front Integr Neurosci. 2017;11
118. Mccouch GP, Austin GM, Liu CN, Liu CY. Sprouting as A cause of spasticity. J Neurophysiol. 1958;21:205–16.
119. McLachlan EM, Oldfield BJ. Some observations on the catecholaminergic innervation of the intermediate zone of the thoracolumbar spinal cord of the cat. J Comp Neurol. 1981;200:529–44.
120. Meisner JG, Marsh AD, Marsh DR. Loss of GABAergic interneurons in laminae I-III of the spinal cord dorsal horn contributes to reduced GABAergic tone and neuropathic pain after spinal cord injury. J Neurotrauma. 2010;27:729–37.
121. Melzack R, Wall PD. Pain mechanisms: a new theory. Science. 1965;150:971–9.
122. Menard MR, Hahn G. acute and chronic hypothermia in a man with spinal-cord injury -environmental and pharmacological causes. Archives of Physical Medicine and Rehabilita-tion. 1991;72(6):421–4.
123. Miall RC. Systems descending from the brainstem: basic principles. In: Pfaff DW, editor. Neuroscience in the 21st century: from basic to clinical. New York: Springer New York; 2013.
124. Milligan J, Ryan K, Lee J. Demystifying spasticity in primary care. Can Fam Physician. 2019;65:697–703.

125. Mion D Jr, Rea RF, Anderson EA, Kahn D, Sinkey CA, Mark AL. Effects of fludrocortisone on sympathetic nerve activity in humans. Hypertension. 1994;23:123–30.
126. Mironets E, Osei-Owusu P, Bracchi-Ricard V, Fischer R, Owens EA, Ricard J, Wu D, Saltos T, Collyer E, Hou S, Bethea JR, Tom VJ. Soluble TNFalpha signaling within the spinal cord contributes to the development of autonomic Dysreflexia and ensuing vascular and immune dysfunction after spinal cord injury. J Neurosci. 2018;38:4146–62.
127. Mironets E, Fischer R, Bracchi-Ricard V, Saltos TM, Truglio TS, O'Reilly ML, et al. Attenuating Neurogen-ic Sympathetic Hyperreflexia Robustly Improves Antibacterial Immunity After Chronic Spinal Cord Injury. Journal of Neuroscience. 2020;40(2):478–92.
128. Mitchell D, Laburn HP. Pathophysiology of temperature regulation. Physiologist. 1985;28:507–17.
129. Mneimneh F, Moussalem C, Ghaddar N, Aboughali K, Omeis I. Influence of cervical spinal cord injury on thermoregulatory and cardiovascular responses in the human body: literature review. J Clin Neurosci. 2019;69:7–14.
130. Moura MM, Monteiro A, Salgado AJ, Silva NA, Monteiro S. Disrupted autonomic pathways in spinal cord injury: implications for the immune regulation. Neurobiol Dis. 2024;195:106500.
131. Munakata M, Kameyama J, Nunokawa T, Ito N, Yoshinaga K. Altered Mayer wave and baroreflex profiles in high spinal cord injury. Am J Hypertens. 2001;14:141–8.
132. Muraki S, Yamasaki M, Ishii K, Kikuchi K, Seki K. Relationship core temperature and skin blood flux in lower limbs during prolonged arm exercise in persons with spinal cord injury. European Journal of Ap-plied Physiology and Occupational Physiology. 1996;72(4):330–4.1.
133. Murillo N, Valls-Sole J, Vidal J, Opisso E, Medina J, Kumru H. Focal vibration in neurorehabilitation. Eur J Phys Rehabil Med. 2014;50:231–42.
134. Nathan PW, Smith MC. Spino-cortical fibres in man. J Neurol Neurosurg Psychiatry. 1955;18:181–90.
135. Ness LL, Field-Fote EC. Whole-body vibration improves walking function in individuals with spinal cord injury: a pilot study. Gait Posture. 2009;30:436–40.
136. Noble BT, Brennan FH, Wang Y, Guan Z, Mo X, Schwab JM, Popovich PG. Thoracic VGluT2(+) spinal interneurons regulate structural and functional plasticity of sympathetic networks after high-level spinal cord injury. J Neurosci. 2022;42:3659–75.
137. Noga BR, Opris I, Lebedev MA, Mitchell GS. Editorial: Neuromodulatory control of brainstem function in health and disease. Front Neurosci. 2020;14:86.
138. O'dwyer NJ, Ada L. Reflex hyperexcitability and muscle contracture in relation to spastic hypertonia. Curr Opin Neurol. 1996;9:451–5.
139. Oldfield BJ, McLachlan EM. An analysis of the sympathetic preganglionic neurons projecting from the upper thoracic spinal roots of the cat. Journal of Comparative Neurol-ogy. 1981;196(2):329–45
140. Olivares-Moreno R, Rodriguez-Moreno P, Lopez-Virgen V, Macías M, Altamira-Camacho M, Rojas-Piloni G. Corticospinal vs Rubrospinal revisited: an evolutionary perspective for sensorimotor integration. Front Neurosci. 2021;15:686481.
141. Olive JL, McCully K, Dudley GA. Blood flow response in individuals with incomplete spinal cord injuries. Spinal Cord. 2002;40(12):639–45.
142. Osborn JW, Taylor RF, Schramm LP. Chronic cervical spinal cord injury and autonomic hyperreflexia in rats. Am J Phys. 1990;258:R169–74.
143. Penn RD, Savoy SM, Corcos D, Latash M, Gottlieb G, Parke B, Kroin JS. Intrathecal baclofen for severe spinal spasticity. N Engl J Med. 1989;320:1517–21.
144. Petrofsky JS, Stacy R. The effect of training on endurance and the cardiovascular-responses of individuals with paraplegia during dynamic exercise induced by functional electrical-stimulation. European Journal of Applied Physiology. 1992;64(6):487–92.
145. Pertovaara A, Almeida A. Chapter 13: Descending inhibitory systems. Handb Clin Neurol. 2006;81:179–92.

146. Petersen EA, Stauss TG, Scowcroft JA, Brooks ES, White JL, Sills SM, Amirdelfan K, Guirguis MN, Xu J, Yu C, Nairizi A, Patterson DG, Tsoulfas KC, Creamer MJ, Galan V, Bundschu RH, Paul CA, Mehta ND, Choi H, Sayed D, Lad SP, Dibenedetto DJ, Sethi KA, Goree JH, Bennett MT, Harrison NJ, Israel AF, Chang P, Wu PW, Gekht G, Argoff CE, Nasr CE, Taylor RS, Subbaroyan J, Gliner BE, Caraway DL, Mekhail NA. Effect of high-frequency (10-kHz) spinal cord stimulation in patients with painful diabetic neuropathy: A randomized clinical trial. JAMA Neurol. 2021;78:687–98.
147. Petrofsky JS. Control of skin blood flow. In: Farage MA, Miller KW, Maibach HI, editors. Textbook of aging skin. Berlin/Heidelberg: Springer Berlin Heidelberg; 2017.
148. Pfyffer D, Smith AC, Weber KA 2nd, Grillhoesl A, Mach O, Draganich C, Berliner JC, Tefertiller C, Leister I, Maier D, Schwab JM, Thompson A, Curt A, Freund P. Prognostic value of tissue bridges in cervical spinal cord injury: a longitudinal, multicentre, retrospective cohort study. Lancet Neurol. 2024;23:816–25.
149. Phillips AA, Krassioukov AV. Contemporary cardiovascular concerns after spinal cord injury: mechanisms, Maladaptations, and management. J Neurotrauma. 2015;32:1927–42.
150. Phillips AA, Krassioukov AV, Ainslie PN, Warburton DE. Baroreflex function after spinal cord injury. J Neurotrauma. 2012;29:2431–45.
151. Phillips AA, Ainslie PN, Krassioukov AV, Warburton DE. Regulation of cerebral blood flow after spinal cord injury. J Neurotrauma. 2013;30:1551–63.
152. Phillips AA, Krassioukov AV, Ainslie PN, Cote AT, Warburton DE. Increased central arterial stiffness explains baroreflex dysfunction in spinal cord injury. J Neurotrauma. 2014;31:1122–8.
153. Phillips AA, Squair JW, Sayenko DG, Edgerton VR, Gerasimenko Y, Krassioukov AV. An autonomic Neuroprosthesis: noninvasive electrical spinal cord stimulation restores autonomic cardiovascular function in individuals with spinal cord injury. J Neurotrauma. 2018;35:446–51.
154. Proske U. The role of muscle proprioceptors in human limb position sense: a hypothesis. J Anat. 2015;227:178–83.
155. Ramer LM, Van Stolk AP, Inskip JA, Ramer MS, Krassioukov AV. Plasticity of TRPV1-expressing sensory neurons mediating autonomic Dysreflexia following spinal cord injury. Front Physiol. 2012;3
156. Randall WC, Wurster RD, Lewin RJ. Responses of patients with high spinal transection to high ambient temperatures. J Appl Physiol. 1966;21(3):985–93.
157. Reiner A, Deng YP. Disrupted striatal neuron inputs and outputs in Huntington's disease. CNS Neurosci Ther. 2018;24:250–80.
158. Reynolds AF, Oakley JC. High frequency cervical epidural stimulation for spasticity. Appl Neurophysiol. 1982;45:93–7.
159. Risher WC, Kim N, Koh S, Choi JE, Mitev P, Spence EF, et al. Thrombospondin receptor α2δ-1 pro-motes synaptogenesis and spinogenesis via postsynaptic Rac1. Journal of Cell Biology. 2018;217(10):3747-65.1.1.
160. Roberts LA, Beyer C, Komisaruk BR. Nociceptive responses to altered GABAergic activity at the spinal cord. Life Sci. 1986;39:1667–74.
161. Rosenzweig ES, Courtine G, Jindrich DL, Brock JH, Ferguson AR, Strand SC, Nout YS, Roy RR, Miller DM, Beattie MS, Havton LA, Bresnahan JC, Edgerton VR, Tuszynski MH. Extensive spontaneous plasticity of corticospinal projections after primate spinal cord injury. Nat Neurosci. 2010;13:1505–10.
162. Sabino-Carvalho JL, Falquetto B, Takakura AC, Vianna LC. Baroreflex dysfunction in Parkinson's disease: integration of central and peripheral mechanisms. J Neurophysiol. 2021;125:1425–39.
163. Sahota IS, Ravensbergen HR, Mcgrath MS, Claydon VE. Cerebrovascular responses to orthostatic stress after spinal cord injury. J Neurotrauma. 2012;29:2446–56.
164. Sandkühler J. Understanding LTP in pain pathways. Mol Pain. 2007;3:9.

165. Sandler EB, Condon K, Field-Fote EC. Efficacy of transcutaneous spinal stimulation versus whole body vibration for spasticity reduction in persons with spinal cord injury. J Clin Med. 2021;10
166. Sandrini G, Serrao M, Rossi P, Romaniello A, Cruccu G, Willer JC. The lower limb flexion reflex in humans. Prog Neurobiol. 2005;77:353–95.
167. Sangari S, Perez MA. Imbalanced corticospinal and Reticulospinal contributions to spasticity in humans with spinal cord injury. J Neurosci. 2019;39:7872–81.
168. Sato A, Schmidt RF. somatosympathetic reflexes - afferent fibers, central path-ways, discharge characteristics. Physiological Reviews. 1973;53(4):916–47.
169. Savage KE, Oleson CV, Schroeder GD, Sidhu GS, Vaccaro AR. Neurogenic fever after acute traumatic spinal cord injury: A qualitative systematic review. Global Spine J. 2016;6:607–14.
170. Scheurink AJW, Steffens AB, Bouritius H, Dreteler GH, Bruntink R, Remie R, et al. Adrenal and sympathetic catecholamines in exercising rats. American Journal of Physiology. 1989;256(1):R155–R60.
171. Schmidt DK, Chan WC. Thermoregulation and fever in Normal persons and in those with spinal cord injuries. Mayo Clin Proc. 1992;67:469–75.
172. Sharples SA, Koblinger K, Humphreys JM, Whelan PJ. Dopamine: a parallel pathway for the modulation of spinal locomotor networks. Front Neural Circuits. 2014;8
173. Shergill IS, Arya M, Hamid R, Khastgir J, Patel HR, Shah PJ. The importance of autonomic dysreflexia to the urologist. BJU Int. 2004;93(7):923–6.
174. Singh R, Rohilla RK, Saini G, Kaur K. Longitudinal study of body composition in spinal cord injury pa-tients. Indian Journal of Orthopaedics. 2014;48(2):168–77.
175. Sliwinski C, Heutehaus L, Taberner FJ, Weiss L, Kampanis V, Tolou-Dabbaghian B, Cheng X, Motsch M, Heppenstall PA, Kuner R, Franz S, Lechner SG, Weidner N, Puttagunta R. Contribution of mechanoreceptors to spinal cord injury–induced mechanical allodynia. Pain. 2024;165:1336.
176. Soriano JE, Hudelle R, Mahe L, Gautier M, Teo YY, Skinnider MA, Laskaratos A, Ceto S, Kathe C, Hutson T, Charbonneau R, Girgis F, Casha S, Rimok J, Tso M, Larkin-Kaiser K, Hankov N, Gandhi AP, Amir S, Kang X, Vyza Y, Martin-Moraud E, Lacour S, Demesmaeker R, Asboth L, Barraud Q, Anderson MA, Bloch J, Squair JW, Phillips AA, Courtine G. The neuronal architecture of autonomic dysreflexia. bioRxiv. 2024:2024.05.06.592781.
177. Spencer NJ, Hu H. Enteric nervous system: sensory transduction, neural circuits and gastrointestinal motility. Nat Rev Gastroenterol Hepatol. 2020;17:338–51.
178. Spranger M, Lindholm D, Bandtlow C, Heumann R, Gnahn H, Naher-Noe M, Thoenen H. Regulation of nerve growth factor (NGF) synthesis in the rat central nervous system: comparison between the effects of Interleukin-1 and various growth factors in astrocyte cultures and in vivo. Eur J Neurosci. 1990;2:69–76.
179. Spungen AM, Adkins RH, Stewart CA, Wang J, Pierson RN, Waters RL, et al. Factors influencing body composition in persons with spinal cord injury: a cross-sectional study. Journal of Applied Physiology. 2003;95(6):2398–407.
180. Srinivasan SS, Tuckute G, Zou J, Gutierrez-Arango S, Song H, Barry RL, Herr HM. Agonist-antagonist myoneural interface amputation preserves proprioceptive sensorimotor neurophysiology in lower limbs. Sci Transl Med. 2020;12:eabc5926.
181. Stampas A, Hook M, Korupolu R, Jethani L, Kaner MT, Pemberton E, Li S, Francisco GE. Evidence of treating spasticity before it develops: a systematic review of spasticity outcomes in acute spinal cord injury interventional trials. Ther Adv Neurol Disord. 2022;15:17562864211070657.
182. Streit WJ, Semple-Rowland SL, Hurley SD, Miller RC, Popovich PG, Stokes BT. Cytokine mRNA profiles in contused spinal cord and axotomized facial nucleus suggest a beneficial role for inflammation and gliosis. Experimental Neurology. 1998;152(1):74–87.
183. Sumsuzzman DM, Khan ZA, Nila IS, Moran VMV, Rajesh M, Yang WJ, Hong Y. Effects of botulinum toxin-A for spasticity and nociceptive pain in individuals with spinal cord injury: A systematic review and meta-analysis. Ann Rehabil Med. 2024;48:192–202.

184. Takahashi M, Sakaguchi A, Matsukawa K, Komine H, Kawaguchi K, Onari K. Cardiovascular control during voluntary static exercise in humans with tetraplegia. J Appl Physiol. 2004;1985(97):2077–82.
185. The Consensus Committee of the American Autonomic Society and the American Academy of Neurology. Consensus statement on the definition of orthostatic hypotension, pure autonomic failure, and multiple system atrophy. Neurology. 1996;46:1470.
186. Thilmann AF, Fellows SJ, Garms E. The mechanism of spastic muscle hypertonus – variation in reflex gain over the time course of spasticity. Brain. 1991;114:233–44.
187. Thompson GW, Levett JM, Miller SM, Hill MR, Meffert WG, Kolata RJ, Clem MF, Murphy DA, Armour JA. Bradycardia induced by intravascular versus direct stimulation of the vagus nerve. Ann Thorac Surg. 1998;65:637–42.
188. Todd NV. Priapism in acute spinal cord injury. Spinal Cord. 2011;49:1033–5.
189. Tomoda Y, Kagawa S, Kurata S, Tanaka K. Hyperthermia due to heat retention in chronic spinal cord inju-ry: A case report. J Gen Fam Med. 2019;20(3):111–3.1.
190. Trbovich M, Ford A, Wu Y, Koek W, Wecht J, Kellogg D, Jr. Correlation of neurological level and sweat-ing level of injury in persons with spinal cord injury. J Spinal Cord Med. 2021;44(6):902–9.
191. Trompetto C, Marinelli L, Mori L, Pelosin E, Currà A, Molfetta L, Abbruzzese G. Pathophysiology of spasticity: implications for neurorehabilitation. Biomed Res Int. 2014;2014:354906.
192. Tuszynski MH, Peterson DA, Ray J, Baird A, Nakahara Y, Gage FH. Fibroblasts genetically modified to produce nerve growth factor induce robust neuritic ingrowth after grafting to the spinal cord. Exp Neurol. 1994;126:1–14.
193. Tuszynski MH, Gabriel K, Gage FH, Suhr S, Meyer S, Rosetti A. Nerve growth factor delivery by gene transfer induces differential outgrowth of sensory, motor, and noradrenergic neurites after adult spinal cord injury. Exp Neurol. 1996;137:157–73.
194. Ueno M, Nakamura Y, Li J, Gu Z, Niehaus J, Maezawa M, Crone SA, Goulding M, Baccei ML, Yoshida Y. Corticospinal circuits from the sensory and motor cortices differentially regulate skilled movements through distinct spinal interneurons. Cell Rep. 2018;23:1286–1300.e7.
195. Ulger F, Dilek A, Karakaya D, Senel A, Sarihasan B. Fatal Fever of Unknown Origin in Acute Cervical Spinal Cord Injury: Five Cases. Journal of Spinal Cord Medicine. 2009;32(3):343–8.
196. Vecin NM, Gater DR. Pressure injuries and management after spinal cord injury. J Pers Med. 2022;12
197. Visavadiya NP, Springer JE. Altered cerebellar circuitry following thoracic spinal cord injury in adult rats. Neural Plast. 2016;2016:8181393.
198. Voss P, Thomas ME, Cisneros-Franco JM, De Villers-Sidani É. Dynamic brains and the changing rules of neuroplasticity: implications for learning and recovery. Front Psychol. 2017;8:1657.
199. Wan D, Krassioukov AV. Life-threatening outcomes associated with autonomic dysreflexia: a clinical re-view. J Spinal Cord Med. 2014;37(1):2–10.
200. Wang X, Lambert NA. GABA(B) receptors couple to potassium and calcium channels on identified lateral perforant pathway projection neurons. J Neurophysiol. 2000;83:1073–8.
201. Wang L, Spary E, Deuchars J, Deuchars SA. Tonic Gabaergic inhibition of sympathetic preganglionic neurons: a novel substrate for sympathetic control. J Neurosci. 2008;28:12445–52.
202. Weaver LC, Marsh DR, Gris D, Brown A, Dekaban GA. Autonomic dysreflexia after spinal cord injury: central mechanisms and strategies for prevention. In: Weaver LC, Polosa C, editors. Autonomic Dysfunc-tion after Spinal Cord Injury. Progress in Brain Research. 1522006. p. 245–63.
203. Wecht JM, Rosado-Rivera D, Handrakis JP, Radulovic M, Bauman WA. Effects of midodrine hydrochloride on blood pressure and cerebral blood flow during orthostasis in persons with chronic tetraplegia. Arch Phys Med Rehabil. 2010;91:1429–35.

204. Wecht JM, Rosado-Rivera D, Weir JP, Ivan A, Yen C, Bauman WA. Hemodynamic effects of L-threo-3,4-dihydroxyphenylserine (Droxidopa) in hypotensive individuals with spinal cord injury. Arch Phys Med Rehabil. 2013;94:2006–12.
205. Wecht JM, Harel NY, Guest J, Kirshblum SC, Forrest GF, Bloom O, Ovechkin AV, Harkema S. Cardiovascular autonomic dysfunction in spinal cord injury: epidemiology, diagnosis, and management. Semin Neurol. 2020;40:550–9.
206. Wecht JM, Krassioukov AV, Alexander M, Handrakis JP, Mckenna SL, Kennelly M, Trbovich M, Biering-Sorensen F, Burns S, Elliott SL, Graves D, Hamer J, Krogh K, Linsenmeyer TA, Liu N, Hagen EM, Phillips AA, Previnaire JG, Rodriguez GM, Slocum C, Wilson JR. International standards to document autonomic function following SCI (ISAFSCI): second edition. Top Spinal Cord Inj Rehabil. 2021;27:23–49.
207. Wei K, Glaser JI, Deng L, Thompson CK, Stevenson IH, Wang Q, Hornby TG, Heckman CJ, Kording KP. Serotonin affects movement gain control in the spinal cord. J Neurosci. 2014;34:12690–700.
208. West CR, AlYahya A, Laher I, Krassioukov A. Peripheral vascular function in spinal cord injury: a system-atic review. Spinal Cord. 2013;51(1):10–9.
209. West CR, Wong SC, Krassioukov AV. Autonomic cardiovascular control in Paralympic athletes with spinal cord injury. Med Sci Sports Exerc. 2014;46:60–8.
210. Whiting PF, Wolff RF, Deshpande S, Di Nisio M, Duffy S, Hernandez AV, Keurentjes JC, Lang S, Misso K, Ryder S, Schmidlkofer S, Westwood M, Kleijnen J. Cannabinoids for medical use A systematic review and meta-analysis. JAMA. 2015;313:2456–73.
211. Willette RN, Barcas PP, Krieger AJ, Sapru HN. Vasopressor and depressor areas in the rat medulla. Neuropharmacology. 1983;22:1071–9.
212. Woolf CJ, Shortland P, Coggeshall RE. Peripheral nerve injury triggers central sprouting of myelinated afferents. Nature. 1992;355:75–8.
213. Yaggie JA, Niemi TJ, Buono MJ. Adaptive sweat gland response after spinal cord injury. Archives of Physical Medicine and Rehabilitation. 2002;83(6):802–5.
214. Yoshizawa T, Kadekawa K, Tyagi P, Yoshikawa S, Takahashi R, Takahashi S, Yoshimura N. Mechanisms inducing autonomic dysreflexia during urinary bladder distention in rats with spinal cord injury. Spinal Cord. 2015;53:190–4.
215. Zesiewicz TA, Baker MJ, Wahba M, Hauser RA. Autonomic nervous system dysfunction in Parkinson's disease. Curr Treat Options Neurol. 2003;5:149–60.
216. Zhang Y, Guan Z, Reader B, Shawler T, Mandrekar-Colucci S, Huang K, Weil Z, Bratasz A, Wells J, Powell ND, Sheridan JF, Whitacre CC, Rabchevsky AG, Nash MS, Popovich PG. Autonomic dysreflexia causes chronic immune suppression after spinal cord injury. J Neurosci. 2013;33:12970–81.
217. Zhao Z-D, Yang WZ, Gao C, Fu X, Zhang W, Zhou Q, Chen W, Ni X, Lin J-K, Yang J, Xu X-H, Shen WL. A hypothalamic circuit that controls body temperature. Proc Natl Acad Sci. 2017;114:2042–7.

Part IV

Neurorehabilitation and Long Term-Prognosis

20 Neural Repair and Regeneration After Spinal Cord Injury

Anant Naik, Abhigyan Datta, Shivaniben Chaudhary, Jacob Weiner, and Ann M. Parr

20.1 Introduction

The spinal cord is a vital component of the central nervous system (CNS) which enables signal transmission from the brain to the body and vice versa, enabling execution of motor activities and perception of sensory inputs. Injury to the spinal cord significantly impacts life expectancy and quality of life. Some reports suggest a global incidence of nearly one million per year, and over 20 million individuals are living with spinal cord injury (SCI). The total years lived with disability are calculated to be 6.2 million in a study by Ding et al. [1]. Unfortunately, SCI rates increased significantly from 1990 to 2019 [2], and overall incidence and prevalence of SCI are higher in developing countries, mainly because of a higher incidence of road traffic accidents and an increase in the size of the overall population at risk.

Given the immense burden on patients, their families, and communities, significant efforts have been made to develop new treatments for SCI. Importantly, SCIs are not all the same, and therapies that might be helpful in acute SCI may not be successful in chronic SCI. In general, neuroprotective therapies are more likely to show benefit in acute or subacute SCI, whereas regenerative therapies are likely needed to benefit patients with chronic injuries. The caveat to this is the potential role of chronic inflammation in chronic SCI, which is understudied and poorly understood. This overview seeks to review the pathophysiology of SCI from the lens of both neuroprotective and neuroregenerative efforts, to summarize the advances made to date, and to chart a trajectory for the future of this field.

A. Naik · S. Chaudhary · J. Weiner · A. M. Parr (✉)
Department of Neurosurgery, University of Minnesota, Minneapolis, MN, USA
e-mail: amparr@umn.edu

A. Datta
Department of Neurology, University of Minnesota, Minneapolis, MN, USA

E. Brogi et al. (eds.), *Traumatic Spinal Cord Injury*, Hot Topics in Acute Care Surgery and Trauma, https://doi.org/10.1007/978-3-031-99890-4_20

20.2 Pathophysiology of Spinal Cord Injury

The pathophysiology of SCI involves a complex interplay of distinct cellular processes that extend beyond the initial injury site. A cascade of biochemical and cellular events coupled with profound neuro-architectural alterations leads to substantial CNS dysfunction. Both primary and secondary injury mechanisms occur, contributing to acute and chronic alterations in spinal cord structure and function. Primary injury mechanisms occur within seconds to minutes of the initial trauma, while secondary mechanisms unfold over the subsequent hours, days, and weeks.

20.2.1 Primary Injury Mechanisms

Primary injury refers to the immediate mechanical damage to the spinal cord, most commonly caused by contusion and compression, with transection being much less likely [3–5]. This initial trauma disrupts axons, blood vessels, and cell membranes, leading to hemorrhage and cell death. The vertebral column and supporting spinal ligaments are often compromised [3, 4, 6]. This severe irreversible damage limits capacity for intrinsic cellular recovery, a problem which only worsens with time. These initial injury mechanisms result in a cascade of secondary injury processes that further perturb the already-damaged nervous system.

20.2.2 Secondary Injury Mechanisms

20.2.2.1 Ischemia, Vascular Disruption, and Inflammation

This injury phase is further subdivided into three distinct categories: acute, subacute, and chronic. The acute phase follows the primary injury, involving the disruption of the blood-spinal cord barrier, resulting in ischemia and hypoxia [7–9]. This compromise of blood and oxygen supply aggravates neuronal and glial cell death, which may contribute to the development of additional neural deficits [9–11]. A key aspect of secondary injury is the body's inflammatory response, which is characterized by infiltration of immune cells, particularly neutrophils, macrophages, and lymphocytes. These immune cells release pro-inflammatory cytokines (such as TNF-α and IL-6), further damaging neural tissue via leukocyte and lymphocyte activity and often leading to eventual scar formation via fibrosis [10–12].

20.2.2.2 Oxidative Stress, Excitotoxicity, and Apoptosis

The excessive production of reactive oxygen species and reactive nitrogen species leads to widespread cellular damage, including lipid peroxidation, protein oxidation, and DNA damage [12–14]. This oxidative stress disrupts essential cellular processes, including enzymatic and metabolic processes crucial for neuronal survival and function. The inflammatory cascade triggered by SCI involves the release of cytokines, free radicals, and other inflammatory molecules that exacerbate tissue damage [8, 10, 11, 13]. Concurrently, excessive glutamate release induces excitotoxicity, causing an influx of calcium and other ions into neurons. This unregulated ionic imbalance triggers various cell death mechanisms, including irreversible apoptosis and necrosis, which are defining facets of the secondary injury phase. The activation of initiator and executioner caspases, key components of the internal and external apoptotic pathways, results in the systematic disassembly of cellular components, organelles, and cytoarchitectural filaments necessary for physiological processes. Neurons are not impacted in isolation; glial and endothelial cells, which are essential for regulatory and support functions, are also degraded and lost over time. Thus, crucial cellular components necessary for maintaining spinal cord integrity and functionality are significantly altered from the pre-injury state [10, 11].

20.2.2.3 Cellular and Molecular Responses

The final phase of secondary injury is the chronic stage, characterized by glial scar formation and astrocyte activation, which can exacerbate such responses as axonal retraction and degeneration and thereby worsen prognosis. Over time, gliosis can result in additional scar tissue formation, further disrupting neurocircuitry above and below the injury site. This scarring typically surrounds a cystic cavity, which may expand as a syrinx (thought to be caused by resultant arachnoiditis) and cause further spinal cord compression. The severity of these outcomes is influenced by such factors as age, sex, injury location, and overall severity, potentially resulting in greater neurological deficits in certain patients. Individualized therapeutic strategies are crucial to mitigate SCI pathophysiology [8, 10, 11, 13].

20.2.2.4 Cellular and Molecular Mechanisms in Repair

Repair in the nervous system takes place through neuronal sprouting and regeneration. Sprouting occurs when an uninjured neuron forms new synapses and connections. This typically occurs locally at the site of injury and does not result in long-distance regeneration. Various proteins are involved in the sprouting response, including L1, c-Jun, and c-Fos (cytoskeleton proteins) and GAP-43 (growth-associated proteins), whose production is upregulated and potentially contributes to neuroplasticity [15]. On the other hand, regeneration may result from the proximal segment of an injured neuron, either from the tip or from the shaft, and would ideally traverse the site of injury to reach the next targeted relay neuron.

20.2.2.5 Role of Glial Cells

Various cells are recruited to help facilitate regeneration after neuronal injury in the spinal cord. The perilesional areas are rich in reactive astrocytes and other cells like macrophages and microglia. Processes of these cells form an inhibitory mesh-like array at the site of the lesion. Astrocytes and microglia have also been found to release inhibitory extracellular matrix proteins such as chondroitin sulfate proteoglycans, tenascin, and NG2 proteoglycan (also known as chondroitin sulfate proteoglycan 4). Cells and secreted proteins together form the glial scar. Pericytes have also been found in perilesional areas, where they proliferate and secrete extracellular matrix proteins that also contribute to inhibition of the growth cone from injured axons [16]. However, the glial scar also plays a role in restraining the cytotoxic cells and inflammatory markers from damaging perilesional spinal cord axons. Interestingly, despite the dogma of the glial scar being inhibitory, a complete lack of astrocytes has been shown to be detrimental in experimental rodent models [17, 18]. This apparent dual role of astrocytes remains controversial and requires further research [19].

20.2.2.6 Neurotrophic Factors

Neurotrophic factors play a crucial role in neuronal survival, growth, and regeneration following SCI. Brain-derived neurotrophic factor (BDNF), first identified by Yves Barde and Hans Thoenen in 1982, was found to be influential for growth and maintenance of dopaminergic, cholinergic, GABAergic, and serotonergic neurons in the CNS [20, 21]. BDNF exerts neuroprotective effects by decreasing the activation of caspase-3-like enzymes involved in glutamate-mediated apoptotic cell death and by increasing the expression of anti-apoptotic proteins such as B-cell lymphoma 2 (Bcl-2) [22]. In studies examining peripheral nerve injury, BDNF was found to be upregulated by Schwann cells, inhibiting retrograde atrophy of the proximal ends of injured axons, degrading growth inhibitors, and activating intrinsic growth programs at the injury site. This facilitated rapid regeneration in these models. Administration of BDNF and neurotrophin-3 (NT-3) has been shown to enhance neuronal survival and promote sprouting at the injury site [23–25]. However, their role in promoting regeneration beyond the lesion site is limited. Another group of factors includes fibroblast growth factors (FGFs), which are a family of polypeptides with 22 structurally similar members. FGFs facilitate determination of neuronal cell fate, migration, and differentiation [26]. In some studies using peripheral nerve grafts, FGF treatment has led to regrowth of cholinergic fibers in spinal cord neurons in rats [27]. Other factors include glial-derived neurotrophic factor, nerve growth factor, and ciliary neurotrophic factor.

20.3 Strategies for Neural Repair and Regeneration

20.3.1 Pharmacologic Interventions

20.3.1.1 Neuroprotective Agents

Several pharmacological agents have been investigated as potential neuroprotective agents after SCI. Methylprednisolone sodium succinate (MPSS) is postulated to act by reducing inflammation, edema, and lipid peroxidation of cell membranes during the secondary injury phase. While the NASCIS II and III trials showed short-term motor improvements when MPSS was administered within eight hours of injury, more recent analyses have highlighted no long-term benefits [28, 29]. Furthermore, a new case-matched analysis [30] that used data from the NASCIS II and Sygen trials but excluded patients who would not meet contemporary diagnostic criteria (such as injury levels T10 to caudal, or ASIA motor scores >4–5), revealed no neurological improvement from MPSS 26 weeks after SCI, suggesting that prior positive findings may have been due to randomization imbalances. A meta-analysis of eight guidelines on MPSS use found divided opinions: three recommended its use, three advised against it, and two remained neutral. Overall, given doubts about its efficacy, MPSS is now rarely used as a neuroprotective agent after SCI [31].

Minocycline is an antibiotic that has been studied in SCI for its anti-inflammatory and anti-apoptotic effects (reduction in caspase 3 and TNF alpha activity), in addition to its protective effects against NMDA-mediated glutamate excitotoxicity. Rat studies [32] have also shown minocycline to reduce the severity of autonomic dysreflexia, which is a significant concern in patients with SCI. However, clinical trials have not shown this benefit. A phase II trial [33] showed modest motor improvements in patients receiving minocycline. A recent study comparing MPSS alone with a combination of MPSS and minocycline demonstrated significantly better neurological recovery with the combined treatment [34].

Riluzole acts by blocking sodium channels (preventing cellular swelling and death) and reducing glutamate excitotoxicity, which is a key factor in secondary injury following SCI. Preclinical studies as well as a phase I trial [35] showed improved motor scores in patients with cervical SCI. More recently, although the Riluzole in Spinal Cord Injury Study (RISCIS*)* did not meet its primary endpoint, it demonstrated promise in complete injuries [36]. Clinical trials are also underway to determine the effects of riluzole on spasticity in SCI.

As enthusiasm for MPSS decreased, intravenous immune globulin (IVIG) attracted interest due to its immunomodulatory effects (neutralization of antibodies, complement inhibition, cytokine suppression) [37] and a possible neuroprotective effect thought to be mediated through improved myelin preservation (mechanism unclear) [38, 39]. Preclinical studies have been promising, and a phase I/II trial is currently underway to evaluate its clinical efficacy in SCI. The tyrosine kinase inhibitor imatinib has shown promise in reducing intramedullary hemorrhage and inflammation and improving hindlimb locomotor function in rat models by inhibition of c-kit-triggered cytokine production [40]. A phase II trial is evaluating its safety and benefit in patients with cervical SCI (NCT02363361) [41].

20.3.1.2 Neural Regenerative Agents

Whereas neuroprotective therapies aim to preserve function in existing neurons, neural regenerative agents seek to restore function in dysfunctional neurons or to replace them entirely. Nogo-A is a protein that inhibits axonal growth, and blocking its activity has been proposed as a strategy to enhance neural regeneration. In a phase I trial [42], anti-Nogo-A treatment was found to be safe, but paraplegic patients did not demonstrate significant motor recovery. However, tetraplegic patients showed modest improvement, leading to an ongoing phase II trial that should soon be nearing completion.

Repulsive guidance molecule A (RGMa) is another inhibitor of neurite growth that is upregulated around the SCI lesion site [43]. Elezanumab, an anti-RGMa monoclonal antibody, has shown promise in preclinical studies by promoting neuroplasticity and motor recovery, and a phase II clinical trial is currently ongoing. Another example is in the pathway of the Rho-associated coiled-coil protein kinase

(Rho-ROCK). This is a downstream effector of Rho, which limits axonal regrowth following SCI. VX-210 (Cethrin), a recombinant C3 transferase that inhibits Rho-ROCK, showed encouraging motor improvements in a phase I/IIa trial [44]. However, a phase IIb/III trial was terminated early and did not show benefit [44]. Finally, magnesium [45, 46] and lithium [47] have been studied in SCI, but the existing evidence for both is currently ambiguous.

Various growth factors have been investigated for their capacity to improve regeneration in SCI. Known for its hematopoietic properties, erythropoietin has also shown neuroprotective effects in SCI. Animal studies demonstrated motor improvements [48, 49], but human trials investigating individual as well as combined effects of recombinant human EPO [50, 51] have not replicated these benefits, and concerns remain regarding the risk for thrombosis. Granulocyte colony stimulating factor (G-CSF) is known for its ability to mobilize stem cells and enhance neural regeneration. Although preclinical studies showed positive outcomes, a phase 3 clinical trial [52] failed to show changes in American Spinal Injury Association (ASIA) motor scores. Another example is hepatocyte growth factor (HGF), which has demonstrated significant neuroprotective effects in SCI [53] through anti-apoptotic mechanisms and promotion of angiogenesis. A phase I/II trial [54] using recombinant HGF (KP-100) showed improved motor recovery in patients, making HGF a promising therapeutic agent. Fibroblast growth factor (FGF), particularly basic FGF, enhances neural precursor cell survival and responsiveness to other growth signals [55], supporting its role in neural cell proliferation. Preclinical studies further demonstrated FGF-mediated axonal regeneration in SCI models [26, 27]. Clinically, the FGF-mimetic SUN13837 was evaluated for neurological recovery after SCI. Although preclinical data suggested neuroprotection despite limited penetration of the blood–spinal cord barrier, subsequent clinical testing (ASCENT-ASCI) failed to show significant benefits [56].

20.3.2 Stem Cell Therapies

Stem cell therapies in SCI offer a promising regenerative approach by potentially replacing damaged cells, modulating immune responses, and promoting tissue repair [57, 58]. Various cell types, including neural stem cells (NSCs), mesenchymal stem cells (MSCs), oligodendrocyte progenitor cells (OPCs), olfactory ensheathing cells (OECs), and Schwann cells (SCs), have all been explored for their potential to enhance recovery and restore function in SCI patients [29, 57].

20.3.2.1 Neural Stem Cells

NSC therapy presents a promising regenerative treatment for spinal cord injury (SCI) through replacement of damaged neurons and glial cells [59, 60]. Although the adult spinal cord contains endogenous neural precursor cells (NPCs), their limited number and ability to generate new neurons and oligodendrocytes (favoring astrocytes that contribute to glial scar formation) render endogenous repair inadequate, especially in the SCI environment [61–63]. Thus, exogenous NPC transplantation has emerged as a more effective method for SCI repair, promoting cell replacement, neuroprotection, axonal regeneration, and remyelination [64].

NPCs can be sourced from adult and fetal CNS tissue, embryonic stem cells (ESCs), or induced pluripotent stem cells (iPSCs) [65]. ESCs offer robust neural induction potential through modulation of signaling pathways such as BMP/SMAD1 and FGF/Erk, but they are controversial because of ethical concerns and tumorigenicity risks [65–68]. iPSCs derived from reprogrammed somatic cells avoid these ethical dilemmas and enable autologous transplantation, which reduces rejection risks [69, 70]. However, iPSCs still have tumor formation risks and high costs, though research is ongoing to mitigate these issues by inhibiting pathways like NOTCH [71]. Direct transdifferentiation of NPCs from adult somatic cells, bypassing pluripotency, is a newer approach that holds potential [65]. Despite NPC therapies showing significant promise, clinical trials have reported only modest outcomes, primarily due to poor graft survival and limited integration within the spinal cord [59, 72–75].

Given the significant impact of the SCI microenvironment on NPC efficacy, combinatorial strategies represent a logical therapeutic approach [59]. These include enhancement of the microenvironment with specific growth factors, co-transplantation with other cell types, molecular-based approaches, and incorporation of NPCs into biomaterials [76–78]. Evidence suggests that such strategies are essential to improve the survival, cell replacement capacity, and overall therapeutic outcomes of NPC transplantation in SCI [59].

20.3.2.2 Mesenchymal Stem Cells

MSCs may be derived from bone marrow, adipose tissue, or the umbilical cord and show potential in treating SCI because of their ability to differentiate into multiple cell types [79–81]. Their relative accessibility and low immunogenicity make MSCs well-suited for clinical study [82, 83]. In SCI, MSCs have been shown to promote angiogenesis and modulate immune responses [83, 84]. MSCs transplanted directly into the spinal cord can modulate macrophage activation and improve tissue preservation [85]. Although preclinical trials have shown variable outcomes, with some reporting significant functional improvements and others showing limited benefits, a recent Mayo Clinic phase I trial of intrathecal delivery of adipose-derived MSCs in traumatic SCI demonstrated that seven out of ten patients with ASIA Impairment Scale (AIS) grade A or B injuries improved in AIS grade, meeting the primary endpoint [86]. Ongoing research aims to enhance MSC therapeutic effects through genetic engineering, including IGF-1 overexpression, TNF-alpha inhibition, and microRNA-124 modification.

20.3.2.3 Other Cells

OPCs are capable of remyelinating axons and promoting motor recovery by preserving white matter and modulating immune responses. A recent phase I/IIa clinical trial demonstrated promising results, with clinical improvement of at least one AIS grade in 96% of patients, along with MRI evidence of regeneration and functional improvements [87]. OECs support axonal regeneration by clearing debris and secreting neurotrophic factors. Although early clinical trials demonstrated safety, results for efficacy have been inconsistent, warranting further investigation [88]. SCs are essential for peripheral nervous system repair and provide structural scaffolds for axonal growth and remyelination. A recent phase 1 safety trial of autologous SC transplants in eight patients with SCI demonstrated safety in all patients, and one patient demonstrated sustained minor improvement in level of injury [89].

20.3.3 Gene Therapy

Gene therapy holds promise for enhancement of neural repair and functional recovery after SCI [90]. Technologies like CRISPR/Cas9 and application of adeno-associated viruses (AAV) enable precise gene delivery with minimal off-target effects [91]. Two main approaches are in vivo gene delivery directly to the spinal cord and ex vivo transduction of cells, which are then transplanted. Among these, in vivo delivery using AAV vectors (unlike other vectors such as lentiviral vectors) allows sustained episomal expression of therapeutic genes to target various aspects of injury repair, such as promoting pro-regenerative factors, modulating neural circuits, suppressing inhibitory molecules, and degrading the glial scar [92].

A key focus of gene therapy is enhancing pro-regenerative factors like KLF7 and SOX11, which boost axonal growth [93, 94]. Combining multiple growth-promoting genes like insulin-like growth factor, FGF2, and neurotrophic factors like ciliary neurotrophic factor and BDNF further accelerates axon regeneration [95]. Circuit modulation is another promising area of investigation. Dormant but preserved neural tissue around SCI lesions can be reactivated in a sustained manner using neuroplasticity-based strategies [96, 97]. For example, AAV-mediated overexpression of KCC2 improves neural function and recovery by maintaining sustained synaptic inhibition, whereas pharmacological KCC2 agonists would require daily administration to maintain therapeutic benefits [97]. Similarly, using gene therapy as a delivery tool for enzymes like chondroitin ABC, which can degrade chondroitin sulfate proteoglycans (a component of the glial scar and a barrier to regeneration), avoids the need for multiple repeated spinal cord infusions of the enzyme [98–101].

Other avenues of research include using gene therapy to promote NCAM (neural cell adhesion molecule) expression (which has been shown to improve locomotor recovery and reduce apoptosis), counteract inhibitory factors (such as silencing the tumor suppressor PTEN through short-hairpin RNA constructs to boost axonal regrowth by activating the mTOR pathway), and development of chemogenetic tools such as DREADDs (Designer Receptors Exclusively Activated by Designer Drugs), which may offer precise control over neuronal activity by using synthetic ligands to modulate specific circuits, such as pain circuits [101–105].

Other than AAV vectors, CRISPR-Cas9 has emerged as an additional powerful tool for genome editing, enabling precise modulation of gene expression in SCI research [106]. Preclinical studies have shown that CRISPR-based gene therapy can be effective in many ways, including silencing growth inhibitors, inducing the expression of axonal growth promoters, and delivering targeted immunotherapy [106, 107]. Other novel tools are being explored to enhance other forms of therapy, such as use of optogenetics to integrate new neurons produced by NSC-based therapies into pre-existing functional neuronal networks [108].

Despite its potential, gene therapy faces such challenges as optimizing delivery vectors, addressing immunogenicity, and ensuring safety [109]. However, with ongoing advancements in viral vector technology and the ability to fine-tune gene expression, gene therapy holds great promise as a personalized treatment for SCI, offering hope for better recovery and improved quality of life.

20.3.4 Biomaterials and Scaffolds

Scaffolds and hydrogels are increasingly being utilized in SCI treatment to enhance stem cell therapy by providing a supportive structure that facilitates cell survival, differentiation, and integration into the host tissue [110]. These biomaterials aim to bridge lesion cavities, replace damaged extracellular matrices, and create a conducive environment for neural regeneration.

Hydrogels are particularly valuable due to their soft, three-dimensional network structure that mimics the natural extracellular matrix, providing a supportive microenvironment for stem cells [90]. Laminin-coated hydrogels, for example, have been shown to enhance the viability of induced pluripotent stem cell-derived neural progenitors, promote host axonal growth, and stimulate astrocyte migration to the injury site, thereby improving functional recovery. Additionally, self-assembling peptides that form nanofibers within hydrogels can act as scaffolding to promote synaptic connectivity while reducing inflammation and the formation of cystic cavities, as demonstrated in animal models of cervical SCI.

Scaffolds made from materials such as collagen, fibrin, and silk fibroin, often combined with neurotrophic factors, also play a crucial role in supporting neural regeneration [111–113]. These scaffolds not only promote the survival and differentiation of transplanted cells, but also inhibit inflammation and astrogliosis, which are key barriers to axonal regrowth. For instance, N-cadherin-modified collagen scaffolds have been shown to enhance the migration and differentiation of endogenous neural progenitor cells, significantly improving motor recovery in SCI models. Furthermore, combining stem cell therapies with biodegradable scaffolds, such as chitin conduits and fibrin matrices, has shown promise in improving outcomes [114]. These scaffolds help prevent scar formation, promote angiogenesis, and create a microenvironment favorable to MSC survival and function, as demonstrated by improved tissue retention and structural recovery after SCI.

20.3.5 Neuromodulation

Neuromodulation-based approaches also stand at the forefront of neural regenerative efforts. These interventions aim to reactivate neural circuits and enhance neuroplasticity and thereby augment neural repair and functional recovery. Some studies have demonstrated that electrical stimulation increases neuronal excitability, which amplifies low-amplitude inputs and helps translate these into voluntary motor function that helps to induce plasticity [115]. Repeated stimulation allows for the strengthening of synapses and facilitates sprouting by increasing the probability of firing events in a Hebbian framework [116].

Epidural spinal cord stimulation (eSCS) is a promising therapy for restoring volitional movement and autonomic function in SCI individuals. Animal research has shown that eSCS can promote motor functional recovery after SCI by enhancing oligodendrocyte survival and differentiation along with myelin preservation, suggesting a potential mechanism for improved neural connectivity and function. Preliminary clinical studies suggest that eSCS can enhance motor control and cardiovascular function in individuals with chronic SCI, although the precise mechanisms of action remain under investigation [117]. For example, the Epidural Stimulation After Neurological Damage (ESTAND) clinical trial is evaluating the effects of eSCS on volitional movement and autonomic outcomes, with a focus on optimizing epidural stimulation parameters [118]. Promising results from the trial demonstrate that eSCS may afford additional autonomic benefits over time (such as restoration of sexual function) along with improvement in functional volitional movement [119]. Transcutaneous electrical stimulation utilizes similar principles but thus far has predominantly been used for pain relief rather than facilitation of neural regeneration.

20.4 Conclusion

Spinal cord regeneration is a multifaceted and highly complex process that presents many potential therapeutic targets. Ongoing clinical and preclinical studies seek to uncover the complex molecular and cellular dynamics underlying neuronal regeneration. Future treatments will leverage these mechanisms to improve patient outcomes.

References

1. Ding W, Hu S, Wang P, et al. Spinal cord injury: the global incidence, prevalence, and disability from the global burden of disease study 2019. Spine (Phila Pa 1976). 2022;47(21):1532–40. https://doi.org/10.1097/BRS.0000000000004417.
2. Safdarian M, Trinka E, Rahimi-Movaghar V, Thomschewski A, Aali A, Abady GG, et al. Global, regional, and national burden of spinal cord injury, 1990–2019: a systematic analysis for the Global Burden of Disease Study 2019. Lancet Neurol. 2023;22(11):1026–47.
3. Anjum A, Yazid MD, Fauzi Daud M, Idris J, Ng AMH, Selvi Naicker A, Ismail OHR, Athi Kumar RK, Lokanathan Y. Spinal cord injury: pathophysiology, multimolecular interactions, and underlying recovery mechanisms. Int J Mol Sci. 2020;21(20):7533. https://doi.org/10.3390/ijms21207533. PMID: 33066029; PMCID: PMC7589539.
4. Alizadeh A, Dyck SM, Karimi-Abdolrezaee S. Traumatic spinal cord injury: an overview of pathophysiology, models and acute injury mechanisms. Front Neurol. 2019;10:282. https://doi.org/10.3389/fneur.2019.00282. PMID: 30967837; PMCID: PMC6439316.

5. Cheriyan T, Ryan DJ, Weinreb JH, Cheriyan J, Paul JC, Lafage V, Kirsch T, Errico TJ. Spinal cord injury models: a review. Spinal Cord. 2014;52(8):588–95. https://doi.org/10.1038/sc.2014.91. Epub 2014 Jun 10. PMID: 24912546.
6. Ahuja CS, Wilson JR, Nori S, Kotter MRN, Druschel C, Curt A, Fehlings MG. Traumatic spinal cord injury. Nat Rev Dis Primers. 2017;3:17018. https://doi.org/10.1038/nrdp.2017.18. PMID: 28447605.
7. Oyinbo CA. Secondary injury mechanisms in traumatic spinal cord injury: a nugget of this multiply cascade. Acta Neurobiol Exp (Wars). 2011;71(2):281–99. https://doi.org/10.55782/ane-2011-1848. PMID: 21731081.
8. Fatima G, Sharma VP, Das SK, Mahdi AA. Oxidative stress and antioxidative parameters in patients with spinal cord injury: implications in the pathogenesis of disease. Spinal Cord. 2015;53(1):3–6. https://doi.org/10.1038/sc.2014.178. Epub 2014 Nov 4. PMID: 25366528.
9. Zhang N, Yin Y, Xu SJ, Wu YP, Chen WS. Inflammation & apoptosis in spinal cord injury. Indian J Med Res. 2012;135(3):287–96. PMID: 22561613; PMCID: PMC3361863.
10. Salvador AFM, Dykstra T, Rustenhoven J, Gao W, Blackburn SM, Bhasiin K, Dong MQ, Guimarães RM, Gonuguntla S, Smirnov I, Kipnis J, Herz J. Age-dependent immune and lymphatic responses after spinal cord injury. Neuron. 2023;111(14):2155–2169.e9. https://doi.org/10.1016/j.neuron.2023.04.011. Epub 2023 May 5. PMID: 37148871; PMCID: PMC10523880.
11. Sutherland TC, Mathews KJ, Mao Y, Nguyen T, Gorrie CA. Differences in the cellular response to acute spinal cord injury between developing and mature rats highlights the potential significance of the inflammatory response. Front Cell Neurosci. 2017;10:310. https://doi.org/10.3389/fncel.2016.00310. PMID: 28133446; PMCID: PMC5233684.
12. Hu X, Xu W, Ren Y, Wang Z, He X, Huang R, Ma B, Zhao J, Zhu R, Cheng L. Spinal cord injury: molecular mechanisms and therapeutic interventions. Signal Transduct Target Ther. 2023;8(1):245. https://doi.org/10.1038/s41392-023-01477-6. PMID: 37357239; PMCID: PMC10291001.
13. Yu B, Yao C, Wang Y, Mao S, Wang Y, Wu R, Feng W, Chen Y, Yang J, Xue C, Liu D, Ding F, Gu X. The landscape of gene expression and molecular regulation following spinal cord hemisection in rats. Front Mol Neurosci. 2019;12:287. https://doi.org/10.3389/fnmol.2019.00287. PMID: 31824262; PMCID: PMC6883948.
14. Li C, Wu Z, Zhou L, Shao J, Hu X, Xu W, Ren Y, Zhu X, Ge W, Zhang K, Liu J, Huang R, Yu J, Luo D, Yang X, Zhu W, Zhu R, Zheng C, Sun YE, Cheng L. Correction to: temporal and spatial cellular and molecular pathological alterations with single-cell resolution in the adult spinal cord after injury. Signal Transduct Target Ther. 2022;7(1):154. https://doi.org/10.1038/s41392-022-01012-z. Erratum for: Signal Transduct Target Ther. 2022 Mar 2;7(1):65. doi: 10.1038/s41392-022-00885-4. PMID: 35538055; PMCID: PMC9091229.
15. Maier IC, Schwab ME. Sprouting, regeneration and circuit formation in the injured spinal cord: factors and activity. Philos Trans R Soc Lond Ser B Biol Sci. 2006;361(1473):1611–34. https://doi.org/10.1098/rstb.2006.1890.
16. Cregg JM, DePaul MA, Filous AR, Lang BT, Tran A, Silver J. Functional regeneration beyond the glial scar. Exp Neurol. 2014;253:197–207.
17. Rolls A, Shechter R, Schwartz M. The bright side of the glial scar in CNS repair. Nat Rev Neurosci. 2009;10(3):235–41.
18. Anderson MA, Burda JE, Ren Y, Ao Y, O'Shea TM, Kawaguchi R, et al. Astrocyte scar formation aids central nervous system axon regeneration. Nature. 2016;532(7598):195–200.
19. Ahuja C, Wilson J, Nori S, et al. Traumatic spinal cord injury. Nat Rev Dis Primers. 2017;3:17018.
20. Barde YA, Edgar D, Thoenen H. Purification of a new neurotrophic factor from mammalian brain. EMBO J. 1982;1(5):549–53.
21. Pillai A. Brain-derived neurotropic factor/TrkB signaling in the pathogenesis and novel pharmacotherapy of schizophrenia. Neurosignals. 2008;16(2–3):183–93.
22. Almeida RD, Manadas BJ, Melo CV, Gomes JR, Mendes CS, Graos MM, et al. Neuroprotection by BDNF against glutamate-induced apoptotic cell death is mediated by ERK and PI3-kinase pathways. Cell Death Differ. 2005;12(10):1329–43.

23. Lu P, Tuszynski MH. Growth factors and combinatorial therapies for CNS regeneration. Exp Neurol. 2008;209(2):313–20.
24. Hammond EN, Tetzlaff W, Mestres P, Giehl KM. BDNF, but not NT-3, promotes long-term survival of axotomized adult rat corticospinal neurons in vivo. Neuroreport. 1999;10(12):2671–5.
25. Liu Y, Kim D, Himes BT, Chow SY, Schallert T, Murray M, et al. Transplants of fibroblasts genetically modified to express BDNF promote regeneration of adult rat rubrospinal axons and recovery of forelimb function. J Neurosci. 1999;19(11):4370–87.
26. Zhou Y, Wang Z, Li J, Li X, Xiao J. Fibroblast growth factors in the management of spinal cord injury. J Cell Mol Med. 2018;22(1):25–37. https://doi.org/10.1111/jcmm.13353.
27. Kuo HS, Tsai MJ, Huang MC, et al. The combination of peripheral nerve grafts and acidic fibroblast growth factor enhances arginase I and polyamine spermine expression in transected rat spinal cords. Biochem Biophys Res Commun. 2007;357(1):1–7. https://doi.org/10.1016/j.bbrc.2007.02.167.
28. Evaniew N, Belley-Côté EP, Fallah N, Noonan VK, Rivers CS, Dvorak MF. Methylprednisolone for the treatment of patients with acute spinal cord injuries: a systematic review and meta-analysis. J Neurotrauma. 2016;33(5):468–81. https://doi.org/10.1089/neu.2015.4192.
29. Liu Z, Yang Y, He L, et al. High-dose methylprednisolone for acute traumatic spinal cord injury: a meta-analysis. Neurology. 2019;93(9) https://doi.org/10.1212/WNL.0000000000007998.
30. Geisler FH, Moghaddamjou A, Wilson JRF, Fehlings MG. Methylprednisolone in acute traumatic spinal cord injury: case-matched outcomes from the NASCIS2 and Sygen historical spinal cord injury studies with contemporary statistical analysis. J Neurosurg Spine Published online January 1, 2023:1–12. https://doi.org/10.3171/2022.12.SPINE22713, 38.
31. Guan B, Fan Y, Zheng R, et al. A critical appraisal of clinical practice guidelines on pharmacological treatments for spinal cord injury. Spine J. 2023;23(3):392–402. https://doi.org/10.1016/j.spinee.2022.09.009.
32. Squair JW, Ruiz I, Phillips AA, et al. Minocycline reduces the severity of autonomic Dysreflexia after experimental spinal cord injury. J Neurotrauma. 2018;35(24):2861–71. https://doi.org/10.1089/neu.2018.5703.
33. Casha S, Zygun D, McGowan MD, Bains I, Yong VW, John Hurlbert R. Results of a phase II placebo-controlled randomized trial of minocycline in acute spinal cord injury. Brain. 2012;135(4):1224–36. https://doi.org/10.1093/brain/aws072.
34. Meshkini A, Dabbagh Ohadi MA, Mirghaderi P, Mirzaei F, Rafiei E, Allahyari N, et al. Combined treatment with minocycline and methylprednisolone in acute traumatic spinal cord injury: a pilot study. Interdiscip Neurosurg. 2024;36:101883. https://doi.org/10.1016/j.inat.2023.101883.
35. Grossman RG, Fehlings MG, Frankowski RF, et al. A prospective, multicenter, phase I matched-comparison group trial of safety, pharmacokinetics, and preliminary efficacy of Riluzole in patients with traumatic spinal cord injury. J Neurotrauma. 2014;31(3):239–55. https://doi.org/10.1089/neu.2013.2969.
36. Fehlings MG, Moghaddamjou A, Harrop JS, et al. Safety and efficacy of Riluzole in acute spinal cord injury study (RISCIS): a multi-center, randomized, placebo-controlled. Double-blinded trial. J Neurotrauma. 2023;40(17–18):1878–88. https://doi.org/10.1089/neu.2023.0163.
37. Brennan FH, Kurniawan ND, Vukovic J, Bartlett PF, Käsermann F, Arumugam TV, et al. IVIg attenuates complement and improves spinal cord injury outcomes in mice. Ann Clin Transl Neurol. 2016;3(7):495–511. https://doi.org/10.1002/acn3.318.
38. Gillespie ER, Ruitenberg MJ. Neuroinflammation after SCI: current insights and therapeutic potential of intravenous immunoglobulin. J Neurotrauma. 2022;39(3–4):320–32. https://doi.org/10.1089/neu.2019.6952.
39. Nimmerjahn F, Ravetch JV. Anti-inflammatory actions of intravenous immunoglobulin. Annu Rev Immunol. 2008;26(1):513–33. https://doi.org/10.1146/annurev.immunol.26.021607.090232.

40. Abrams MB, Nilsson I, Lewandowski SA, et al. Imatinib enhances functional outcome after spinal cord injury. Harvey AR, ed. PLoS ONE. 2012;7(6):e38760. https://doi.org/10.1371/journal.pone.0038760.
41. Treatment of Cervical Spinal Cord Injury With Imatinib - a Safety and Feasibility Study (NCT02363361). https://clinicaltrials.gov/study/NCT02363361?term=NCT02363361&rank=1
42. Kucher K, Johns D, Maier D, et al. First-in-man intrathecal application of neurite growth-promoting anti-Nogo-a antibodies in acute spinal cord injury. Neurorehabil Neural Repair. 2018;32(6–7):578–89. https://doi.org/10.1177/1545968318776371.
43. Schwab JM, Monnier PP, Schluesener HJ, et al. Central nervous system injury-induced repulsive guidance molecule expression in the adult human brain. Arch Neurol. 2005;62(10):1561–8. https://doi.org/10.1001/archneur.62.10.1561.
44. Fehlings MG, Theodore N, Harrop J, et al. A phase I/IIa clinical trial of a recombinant rho protein antagonist in acute spinal cord injury. J Neurotrauma. 2011;28(5):787–96. https://doi.org/10.1089/neu.2011.1765.
45. Temkin NR, Anderson GD, Winn HR, et al. Magnesium sulfate for neuroprotection after traumatic brain injury: a randomised controlled trial. Lancet Neurol. 2007;6(1):29–38. https://doi.org/10.1016/S1474-4422(06)70630-5.
46. Sperl A, Heller RA, Biglari B, et al. The role of magnesium in the secondary phase after traumatic spinal cord injury. A prospective clinical observer study. Antioxidants. 2019;8(11):509. https://doi.org/10.3390/antiox8110509.
47. Yang ML, Li JJ, So KF, et al. Efficacy and safety of lithium carbonate treatment of chronic spinal cord injuries: a double-blind, randomized, placebo-controlled clinical trial. Spinal Cord. 2012;50(2):141–6. https://doi.org/10.1038/sc.2011.126.
48. Boran BO, Colak A, Kutlay M. Erythropoietin enhances neurological recovery after experimental spinal cord injury. Restor Neurol Neurosci. 2005;23(5–6):341–5.
49. Cerri G, Montagna M, Madaschi L, et al. Erythropoietin effect on sensorimotor recovery after contusive spinal cord injury: an electrophysiological study in rats. Neuroscience. 2012;219:290–301. https://doi.org/10.1016/j.neuroscience.2012.05.041.
50. Alibai EA, Baghban F, Farrokhi MR, Mohebali N, Ashraf MH. Effects of human erythropoietin on functional outcome of patients with traumatic cervical cord injury; a pilot randomized clinical trial. Bull Emerg Trauma. 2015;3(3):79–85.
51. Ganjeifar B, Rezaee H, Keykhosravi E, et al. The effect of combination therapy with erythropoietin and methylprednisolone in patients with traumatic cervical spinal cord injury: a pilot randomized controlled trial. Spinal Cord. 2021;59(3):347–53. https://doi.org/10.1038/s41393-020-00604-2.
52. Koda M, Hanaoka H, Fujii Y, et al. Randomized trial of granulocyte colony-stimulating factor for spinal cord injury. Brain J Neurol. 2021;144(3):789–99. https://doi.org/10.1093/brain/awaa466.
53. Yamane K, Misawa H, Takigawa T, Ito Y, Ozaki T, Matsukawa A. Multipotent neurotrophic effects of hepatocyte growth factor in spinal cord injury. Int J Mol Sci. 2019;20(23):6078. https://doi.org/10.3390/ijms20236078.
54. Nagoshi N, Tsuji O, Kitamura K, et al. Phase I/II study of intrathecal administration of recombinant human hepatocyte growth factor in patients with acute spinal cord injury: a double-blind, randomized clinical trial of safety and efficacy. J Neurotrauma. 2020;37(15):1752–8. https://doi.org/10.1089/neu.2019.6854.
55. Santa-Olalla J, Covarrubias L. Basic fibroblast growth factor promotes epidermal growth factor responsiveness and survival of mesencephalic neural precursor cells. J Neurobiol. 1999;40(1):14–27. https://doi.org/10.1002/(SICI)1097-4695(199907)40:1<14::AID-NEU2>3.0.CO;2-U.
56. Levinson B. SUN13837 in treatment of acute spinal cord injury, the ASCENT-ASCI study. Clin Neurol Neurosci. 2018;2(1):1. https://doi.org/10.11648/j.cnn.20180201.11.
57. Takahashi K, Yamanaka S. Induction of pluripotent stem cells from mouse embryonic and adult fibroblast cultures by defined factors. Cell. 2006;126(4):663–76. https://doi.org/10.1016/j.cell.2006.07.024. Epub 2006 Aug 10. PMID: 16904174.

58. Okubo T, Nagoshi N, Kohyama J, Tsuji O, Shinozaki M, Shibata S, Kase Y, Matsumoto M, Nakamura M, Okano H. Treatment with a Gamma-Secretase Inhibitor Promotes Functional Recovery in Human iPSC-Derived Transplants for Chronic Spinal Cord Injury. Stem Cell Reports. 2018;11(6):1416-32. https://doi.org/10.1016/j.stemcr.2018.10.022.
59. Hosseini SM, Borys B, Karimi-Abdolrezaee S. Neural stem cell therapies for spinal cord injury repair: an update on recent preclinical and clinical advances. Brain. Published online November 17, 2023:awad392. https://doi.org/10.1093/brain/awad392.
60. Tetzlaff W, Okon EB, Karimi-Abdolrezaee S, et al. A systematic review of cellular transplantation therapies for spinal cord injury. J Neurotrauma. 2011;28(8):1611–82. https://doi.org/10.1089/neu.2009.1177.
61. Stenudd M, Sabelström H, Frisén J. Role of endogenous neural stem cells in spinal cord injury and repair. JAMA Neurol. 2015;72(2):235–7. https://doi.org/10.1001/jamaneurol.2014.2927.
62. Barnabé-Heider F, Göritz C, Sabelström H, et al. Origin of new glial cells in intact and injured adult spinal cord. Cell Stem Cell. 2010;7(4):470–82. https://doi.org/10.1016/j.stem.2010.07.014.
63. Llorens-Bobadilla E, Chell JM, Le Merre P, et al. A latent lineage potential in resident neural stem cells enables spinal cord repair. Science. 2020;370(6512):eabb8795. https://doi.org/10.1126/science.abb8795.
64. Zholudeva LV, Lane MA. Transplanting cells for spinal cord repair: who, what, when, where and why? Cell Transplant. 2019;28(4):388–99. https://doi.org/10.1177/0963689718824097.
65. Tang Y, Yu P, Cheng L. Current progress in the derivation and therapeutic application of neural stem cells. Cell Death Dis. 2017;8(10):e3108. https://doi.org/10.1038/cddis.2017.504.
66. Greber B, Coulon P, Zhang M, et al. FGF signalling inhibits neural induction in human embryonic stem cells. EMBO J. 2011;30(24):4874–84. https://doi.org/10.1038/emboj.2011.407.
67. Tomishima M. Neural induction - dual SMAD inhibition. StemBook Published online 2014. https://doi.org/10.3824/stembook.1.57.1.
68. Manzari-Tavakoli A, Babajani A, Farjoo MH, Hajinasrollah M, Bahrami S, Niknejad H. The cross-talks among bone morphogenetic protein (BMP) signaling and other prominent pathways involved in neural differentiation. Front Mol Neurosci. 2022;15:827275. https://doi.org/10.3389/fnmol.2022.827275.
69. Kolagar TA, Farzaneh M, Nikkar N, Khoshnam SE. Human pluripotent stem cells in neurodegenerative diseases: potentials, advances and limitations. Curr Stem Cell Res Ther. 2020;15(2):102–10. https://doi.org/10.2174/1574888X14666190823142911.
70. Takahashi K, Yamanaka S. Induction of pluripotent stem cells from mouse embryonic and adult fibroblast cultures by defined factors. Cell. 2006;126(4):663–76. https://doi.org/10.1016/j.cell.2006.07.024.
71. Okubo T, Nagoshi N, Kohyama J, et al. Treatment with a gamma-secretase inhibitor promotes functional recovery in human iPSC- derived transplants for chronic spinal cord injury. Stem Cell Rep. 2018;11(6):1416–32. https://doi.org/10.1016/j.stemcr.2018.10.022.
72. Curtis E, Martin JR, Gabel B, et al. A first-in-human, phase I study of neural stem cell transplantation for chronic spinal cord injury. Cell Stem Cell. 2018;22(6):941–950.e6. https://doi.org/10.1016/j.stem.2018.05.014.
73. Vaquero J, Zurita M, Rico MA, et al. Cell therapy with autologous mesenchymal stromal cells in post-traumatic syringomyelia. Cytotherapy. 2018;20(6):796–805. https://doi.org/10.1016/j.jcyt.2018.04.006.
74. Levi AD, Okonkwo DO, Park P, et al. Emerging safety of intramedullary transplantation of human neural stem cells in chronic cervical and thoracic spinal cord injury. Neurosurgery. 2018;82(4):562–75. https://doi.org/10.1093/neuros/nyx250.
75. Shin JC, Kim KN, Yoo J, et al. Clinical trial of human fetal brain-derived neural stem/progenitor cell transplantation in patients with traumatic cervical spinal cord injury. Neural Plast. 2015;2015:1–22. https://doi.org/10.1155/2015/630932.
76. Robinson J, Lu P. Optimization of trophic support for neural stem cell grafts in sites of spinal cord injury. Exp Neurol. 2017;291:87–97. https://doi.org/10.1016/j.expneurol.2017.02.007.

77. Hao M, Chen L, He J, et al. Multifunctional hydroxyapatite Nanobelt haystacks integrated neural stem cell spheroid for rapid spinal cord injury repair. Adv Funct Mater. 2023;33(23):2214869. https://doi.org/10.1002/adfm.202214869.
78. Wang Z, Zhao H, Tang X, et al. CNS organoid surpasses cell-laden microgel assembly to promote spinal cord injury repair. Research (Washington, DC). 2022;2022:9832128. https://doi.org/10.34133/2022/9832128.
79. Sasaki M, Radtke C, Tan AM, et al. BDNF-hypersecreting human mesenchymal stem cells promote functional recovery, axonal sprouting, and protection of corticospinal neurons after spinal cord injury. J Neurosci. 2009;29(47):14932–41. https://doi.org/10.1523/JNEUROSCI.2769-09.2009.
80. Ankeny DP, McTigue DM, Jakeman LB. Bone marrow transplants provide tissue protection and directional guidance for axons after contusive spinal cord injury in rats. Exp Neurol. 2004;190(1):17–31. https://doi.org/10.1016/j.expneurol.2004.05.045.
81. Hofstetter CP, Schwarz EJ, Hess D, et al. Marrow stromal cells form guiding strands in the injured spinal cord and promote recovery. Proc Natl Acad Sci. 2002;99(4):2199–204. https://doi.org/10.1073/pnas.042678299.
82. Dasari VR, Veeravalli KK, Dinh DH. Mesenchymal stem cells in the treatment of spinal cord injuries: a review. World J Stem Cells. 2014;6(2):120–33. https://doi.org/10.4252/wjsc.v6.i2.120.
83. Carrade DD, Affolter VK, Outerbridge CA, et al. Intradermal injections of equine allogeneic umbilical cord-derived mesenchymal stem cells are well tolerated and do not elicit immediate or delayed hypersensitivity reactions. Cytotherapy. 2011;13(10):1180–92. https://doi.org/10.3109/14653249.2011.602338.
84. Ulndreaj A, Chio JCT, Ahuja CS, Fehlings MG. Modulating the immune response in spinal cord injury. Expert Rev Neurother. 2016;16(10):1127–9. https://doi.org/10.1080/14737175.2016.1207532.
85. Nakajima H, Uchida K, Guerrero AR, et al. Transplantation of mesenchymal stem cells promotes an alternative pathway of macrophage activation and functional recovery after spinal cord injury. J Neurotrauma. 2012;29(8):1614–25. https://doi.org/10.1089/neu.2011.2109.
86. Bydon M, Qu W, Moinuddin FM, et al. Intrathecal delivery of adipose-derived mesenchymal stem cells in traumatic spinal cord injury: phase I trial. Nat Commun. 2024;15(1):2201. https://doi.org/10.1038/s41467-024-46259-y.
87. Fessler RG, Ehsanian R, Liu CY, et al. A phase 1/2a dose-escalation study of oligodendrocyte progenitor cells in individuals with subacute cervical spinal cord injury. J Neurosurg Spine. 2022;37(6):812–20. https://doi.org/10.3171/2022.5.SPINE22167.
88. Li L, Adnan H, Xu B, et al. Effects of transplantation of olfactory ensheathing cells in chronic spinal cord injury: a systematic review and meta-analysis. Eur Spine J. 2015;24(5):919–30. https://doi.org/10.1007/s00586-014-3416-6.
89. Gant KL, Guest JD, Palermo AE, et al. Phase 1 safety trial of autologous human Schwann cell transplantation in chronic spinal cord injury. J Neurotrauma. 2022;39(3–4):285–99. https://doi.org/10.1089/neu.2020.7590.
90. Zavvarian MM, Toossi A, Khazaei M, Hong J, Fehlings M. Novel innovations in cell and gene therapies for spinal cord injury. F1000Res. 2020;9:279. https://doi.org/10.12688/f1000research.21989.1.
91. Wang D, Tai PWL, Gao G. Adeno-associated virus vector as a platform for gene therapy delivery. Nat Rev Drug Discov. 2019;18(5):358–78. https://doi.org/10.1038/s41573-019-0012-9.
92. Stepankova K, Jendelova P, Machova UL. Planet of the AAVs: the spinal cord injury episode. Biomedicine. 2021;9(6):613. https://doi.org/10.3390/biomedicines9060613.
93. Wang Z, Reynolds A, Kirry A, Nienhaus C, Blackmore MG. Overexpression of Sox11 promotes corticospinal tract regeneration after spinal injury while interfering with functional recovery. J Neurosci. 2015;35(7):3139–45. https://doi.org/10.1523/JNEUROSCI.2832-14.2015.
94. Blackmore MG, Wang Z, Lerch JK, et al. Krüppel-like Factor 7 engineered for transcriptional activation promotes axon regeneration in the adult corticospinal tract. Proc Natl Acad Sci USA. 2012;109(19):7517–22. https://doi.org/10.1073/pnas.1120684109.

95. Anderson MA, O'Shea TM, Burda JE, et al. Required growth facilitators propel axon regeneration across complete spinal cord injury. Nature. 2018;561(7723):396–400. https://doi.org/10.1038/s41586-018-0467-6.
96. Richardson PM. Ciliary neurotrophic factor: a review. Pharmacol Ther. 1994;63(2):187–98. https://doi.org/10.1016/0163-7258(94)90045-0.
97. Zholudeva LV, Qiang L, Marchenko V, Dougherty KJ, Sakiyama-Elbert SE, Lane MA. The Neuroplastic and therapeutic potential of spinal interneurons in the injured spinal cord. Trends Neurosci. 2018;41(9):625–39. https://doi.org/10.1016/j.tins.2018.06.004.
98. Chen B, Li Y, Yu B, et al. Reactivation of dormant relay pathways in injured spinal cord by KCC2 manipulations. Cell. 2018;174(6):1599. https://doi.org/10.1016/j.cell.2018.08.050.
99. Burnside ER, De Winter F, Didangelos A, et al. Immune-evasive gene switch enables regulated delivery of chondroitinase after spinal cord injury. Brain. 2018;141(8):2362–81. https://doi.org/10.1093/brain/awy158.
100. Nori S, Khazaei M, Ahuja CS, et al. Human oligodendrogenic neural progenitor cells delivered with chondroitinase ABC facilitate functional repair of chronic spinal cord injury. Stem Cell Rep. 2018;11(6):1433–48. https://doi.org/10.1016/j.stemcr.2018.10.017.
101. Bradbury EJ, Moon LDF, Popat RJ, et al. Chondroitinase ABC promotes functional recovery after spinal cord injury. Nature. 2002;416(6881):636–40. https://doi.org/10.1038/416636a.
102. Danilov CA, Steward O. Conditional genetic deletion of PTEN after a spinal cord injury enhances regenerative growth of CST axons and motor function recovery in mice. Exp Neurol. 2015;266:147–60. https://doi.org/10.1016/j.expneurol.2015.02.012.
103. Liu K, Lu Y, Lee JK, et al. PTEN deletion enhances the regenerative ability of adult corticospinal neurons. Nat Neurosci. 2010;13(9):1075–81. https://doi.org/10.1038/nn.2603.
104. Saini V, Loers G, Kaur G, Schachner M, Jakovcevski I. Impact of neural cell adhesion molecule deletion on regeneration after mouse spinal cord injury. Kirik D, ed. Eur J Neurosci. 2016;44(1):1734–46. https://doi.org/10.1111/ejn.13271.
105. Grace PM, Wang X, Strand KA, et al. DREADDed microglia in pain: implications for spinal inflammatory signaling in male rats. Exp Neurol. 2018;304:125–31. https://doi.org/10.1016/j.expneurol.2018.03.005.
106. Paschon V, Correia FF, Morena BC, et al. CRISPR, prime editing, optogenetics, and DREADDs: new therapeutic approaches provided by emerging technologies in the treatment of spinal cord injury. Mol Neurobiol. 2020;57(4):2085–100. https://doi.org/10.1007/s12035-019-01861-w.
107. Wang B, Chang M, Zhang R, et al. Spinal cord injury target-immunotherapy with TNF-α autoregulated and feedback-controlled human umbilical cord mesenchymal stem cell derived exosomes remodelled by CRISPR/Cas9 plasmid. Biomater Adv. 2022;133:112624. https://doi.org/10.1016/j.msec.2021.112624.
108. Ahmad A, Ashraf S, Komai S. Optogenetics applications for treating spinal cord injury. Asian Spine J. 2015;9(2):299. https://doi.org/10.4184/asj.2015.9.2.299.
109. Hamilton BA, Wright JF. Challenges posed by immune responses to AAV vectors: addressing root causes. Front Immunol. 2021;12:675897. https://doi.org/10.3389/fimmu.2021.675897.
110. Assunção-Silva RC, Gomes ED, Sousa N, Silva NA, Salgado AJ. Hydrogels and cell based therapies in spinal cord injury regeneration. Stem Cells Int. 2015;2015:948040. https://doi.org/10.1155/2015/948040. Epub 2015 Jun 1. PMID: 26124844; PMCID: PMC4466497
111. King VR, Phillips JB, Hunt-Grubbe H, Brown R, Priestley JV. Characterization of non-neuronal elements within fibronectin mats implanted into the damaged adult rat spinal cord. Biomaterials. 2006;27(3):485–96.
112. Qu J, Wang D, Wang H, Dong Y, Zhang F, Zuo B, Zhang H. Electrospun silk fibroin nanofibers in different diameters support neurite outgrowth and promote astrocyte migration. J Biomed Mater Res A. 2013;101(9):2667–78.
113. Liu T, Houle JD, Xu J, Chan BP, Chew SY. Nanofibrous collagen nerve conduits for spinal cord repair. Tissue Eng A. 2012;18(9–10):1057–66.

114. Silva D, Sousa RA, Salgado AJ. Hydrogels as delivery systems for spinal cord injury regeneration. Mater Today Biol. 2021;9:100093. Published 2021 Jan 22. https://doi.org/10.1016/j.mtbio.2021.100093.
115. Grahn PJ, Lavrov IA, Sayenko DG, et al. Enabling task-specific volitional motor functions via spinal cord neuromodulation in a human with paraplegia. Mayo Clin Proc. 2017;92(4):544–54. https://doi.org/10.1016/j.mayocp.2017.02.014.
116. Rushton DN. Functional electrical stimulation and rehabilitation--an hypothesis. Med Eng Phys 2003;25(1):75–78. doi:https://doi.org/10.1016/s1350-4533(02)00040-1.
117. Chalif JI, Chavarro VS, Mensah E, et al. Epidural Spinal Cord Stimulation for Spinal Cord Injury in Humans: A Systematic Review. J Clin Med. 2024;13(4):1090. Published 2024 Feb 14. https://doi.org/10.3390/jcm13041090.
118. Darrow DP, Balser DY, Freeman D, et al. Effect of epidural spinal cord stimulation after chronic spinal cord injury on volitional movement and cardiovascular function: study protocol for the phase II open label controlled E-STAND trial. BMJ Open. 2022;12(7):e059126. Published 2022 Jul 18. https://doi.org/10.1136/bmjopen-2021-059126.
119. Darrow D, Balser D, Netoff TI, Krassioukov A, Phillips A, Parr A, et al. Epidural spinal cord stimulation facilitates immediate restoration of dormant motor and autonomic supraspinal pathways after chronic neurologically complete spinal cord injury. J Neurotrauma. 2019;36(15):2325–36. https://doi.org/10.1089/neu.2018.6006.

Prognostication, Long-Term Functional Trajectories, and Psychological Support for Patients and Families

21

Lauren M. Anderson, Fawaz Philip Tarzi, and Anaar E. Siletz

21.1 Prognostication at the Time of Injury

Prognostication after spinal cord injury (SCI) pertains to physiologic recovery such as motor and sensory function, bowel and bladder control, and the impact of the SCI on functionality and longevity. In addition to measures of physiologic function, it is important to assess the impact on patients' experiences and quality of life. Important considerations include the ability to live and work independently, the financial burdens SCI patients may experience, and the impact on social integration and relationships.

ASIA score, indicating the severity of functional deficits immediately after injury, remains the best predictor of outcome after SCI (Table 21.1) [1, 2]. Neurological level is also predictive of functional prognosis, with a higher likelihood of functional recovery with lower spinal cord injuries. The length of the spinal cord lesion on MRI or other imaging may also have some prognostic value, with better prognosis for shorter lesions [2]. Other clinical prediction tools have been evaluated with various degrees of reliability (Table 21.2).

L. M. Anderson
Drexel University College of Medicine, Philadelphia, PA, USA

F. P. Tarzi
Department of Neurology, University of Southern California, Keck school of Medicine, Los Angeles, CA, USA

A. E. Siletz (✉)
Department of Surgery, University of Southern California, Los Angeles, CA, USA

E. Brogi et al. (eds.), *Traumatic Spinal Cord Injury*, Hot Topics in Acute Care Surgery and Trauma, https://doi.org/10.1007/978-3-031-99890-4_21

Table 21.1 ASIA Impairment Scale (AIS)

ASIA impairment score	*Degree of impairment*	*Description*
A	Complete	No sensory or motor function in sacral segments S4-S5.
B	Sensory Incomplete	Sensory, but no motor function below the neurological level of injury and includes the sacral segments S4-S5, AND no motor function is preserved more than three levels below the motor level on either side of the body.
C	Motor Incomplete	Motor function preserved at the most caudal sacral segments for voluntary anal contraction OR the patient meets the criteria for sensory incomplete status (sensory function preserved at the most caudal sacral segments S4-5, and has some sparing of motor function more than three levels below the ipsilateral motor level on either side of the body. For AIS C, less than half of key muscle functions below the single NLI have a muscle grade ≥ 3.
D	Motor Incomplete	Motor incomplete status as defined above, with half or more key muscle functions below the neurologic level of injury having a muscle grade ≥ 3.
E	Normal	If sensation and motor function are graded as normal in all segments, and the patient had prior deficits, then the AIS grade is E. Someone without an initial SCI does not receive an AIS grade.
Sensory grading	*Score*	*Description*
	0	Absent
	1	Altered, either decreased/impaired sensation or hypersensitivity
	2	Normal
	NT	Not testable
	*	Non-SCI condition present
Motor function grading	*Score*	*Description*
	0	Total paralysis
	1	Palpable or visible contraction
	2	Active movement, full ROM with gravity eliminated
	3	Active movement, full ROM against gravity
	4	Active movement, full ROM against gravity and moderate resistance in a muscle specific position
	5	(Normal) Active movement, full ROM against gravity and full resistance in a muscle specific position expected from an otherwise unimpaired person
	NT	Not testable (i.e. due to immobilization, severe pain such that the patient cannot be graded, amputation of limb, or contracture of >50% of the range of motion
	NA	Non-SCI condition present

Source: Rupp et al. [21]
Abbreviations: *ROM* Range of motion

Table 21.2 Grading tools for assessing neurological function after spinal cord injury

Score	Definition	Citation
Dutch Clinical Prediction Rule (DCPR) [2]	Derived from EMSCI data set introduced in 2011 to aid in early prediction of independent ambulation among adult patients after SCI.	[2]
Functional Independence Measure (FIM) [22]	Assessment of functional outcome after SCI. Can be used on wide range of patients and is divided into motor subscale (self-care, sphincter management, transfers and locomotion) and a cognition subscale (communication and social cognition). Scores range from 1 (totally dependent) to 7 (device and helper- independent). Often performed at 1 year.	[22]
Lower Extremity Motor Score (LEMS) [21]	ASIA motor function grading of C5-T1	[21]
Upper Extremity Motor Scores (UEMS) [21]	ASIA motor function grading of L2-S1	[21]

Abbreviations: *EMSCI* European Multicenter Study About Spinal Cord Injury. *SCI* Spinal cord injury

21.2 Modifiable Prognostic Factors

21.2.1 Early Surgical Decompression

The evidence-based acute treatment of SCI, including indications for surgical decompression, is discussed elsewhere in this book. However, in patients for whom surgical decompression is indicated, earlier surgical decompression has been associated with improved functional outcomes. Decompression may allow greater blood flow to the affected spinal cord, decreasing the incidence of secondary injury. A secondary analysis of data from multiple clinical trials grouped patients into early (<24 h) and late (>24 h) surgical decompression groups, adjusting for injury characteristics [3]. The primary endpoint assessed was motor recovery at 1 year, for which there was 80% follow-up of 186 patients. In the early surgery group, there was significantly increased upper limb motor recovery compared to the late surgery group for ASIA grades A-C. However, there was no difference in lower limb recovery. Although a higher proportion of the early surgical group patients regained complete independence in functional activities as assessed by the Functional Independence Measure (FIM), none of the associations were statistically significant. When compared to surgical decompression after 7 days, earlier surgical decompression (within 7 days) also was associated with improved long-term outcomes in a retrospective study of cervical spine injury [4]. Both early and late surgical groups had significantly improved recovery compared to patients who opted out of surgery and underwent nonoperative management with mannitol and methylprednisolone.

21.2.2 Exercise and Rehabilitation

Exercise has many potential benefits as a therapeutic tool in SCI patient rehabilitation, due to its neuroprotective and regenerative potential. However, optimal duration, timing, and training type have yet to be determined [5]. SCI patients often are at a higher risk for musculoskeletal decline, bone demineralization, cardiovascular disease, dyslipidemia, and other autonomic comorbidities due to physical limitations resulting in a more sedentary lifestyle. Long-term consequences of physical deconditioning include bone and joint diseases, circulatory insufficiency, clotting disorders, and neuropathic pain. These conditions can be barriers to exercise therapy for SCI patients. Musculoskeletal changes following SCI include reductions in muscle fiber contractile protein, peak contractile forces, and fatigue resistance that can impede participation in not only exercise therapy but activities of daily life [6]. Considerations regarding exercise in SCI patients include reduced cardiac output and respiratory dysfunction in high spinal cord lesions, and functional motor changes limiting participation. Patients must be monitored closely for autonomic dysreflexia, musculoskeletal injury, and thermal dysregulation.

Various rehabilitation strategies and interventions have been studied for their efficacy in improving prognosis in spinal cord injury (Table 21.3). A systematic review and meta-analysis of over 1000 patients in 31 studies [7] concluded that robotic-assisted gait training significantly improved upper and lower motor function, but did not have a significant effect on walking capacity assessed by timed walking tests. It was suggested that robotic-assisted training improved the therapeutic effectiveness of treadmill training relative to massed practice. Functional electrical stimulation devices, which are commonly used for patients with chronic and subacute spinal cord injury, were found to significantly improve functional upper extremity independence without significantly influencing other motor scores or quality of life. Repetitive transcranial magnetic stimulation (rTMS) devices as

Table 21.3 Functional rehabilitation methods

Functional rehabilitation method	Definition	Citation
Massed practice	Extensive repetition of a rehabilitation exercise with minimal rest between repetitions.	
Treadmill training [23]	Treadmill training with or without body-weight support. Often uses a counterweight-harness system to partially offload the patient's bodyweight. Manual assistance can also be used for postural support.	[23]
Repetitive transcranial magnetic stimulation (rTMS) [24]	Affects the descending corticospinal tract through modulation of motor area cortical excitability.	[24]
Robotic Assisted Training [23]	Computerized, motorized gait orthotic device which is secured to the patient's legs during gait training.	[23]
Functional Electrical Stimulation (FES) [25]	Prolonged peripheral nerve stimulation	[25]
Activity Based Therapy (ABT) [9]	Activity-based intervention including massed practice and treadmill training	[26]

compared to either gait training or sham rTMS, significantly improved walking speed and lower extremity motor scores. Activity-based therapy, including massed practice and treadmill training, did not significantly benefit rehabilitation of spinal cord injury patients compared to controls, which included: no intervention, overground mobility therapy, self-regulated exercises, or conventional rehabilitation programs.

21.2.3 Rehabilitation Psychology

The patient's mental health and perspective of rehabilitation, as well as feelings of safety, support, and control over their lives, are just as important an aspect to their recovery as their physical wellbeing [8]. After spinal cord injury, patients experience various life changes including new bodily limitations, varying levels of pain, and issues with continence, sexuality, fertility, and mental health [9]. This contributes to a sense of losing control over one's body. Functional impairment and pain have a substantial impact on patient quality of life [10]. Comprehensive rehabilitation after spinal cord injury includes an assessment of cognitive, emotional, personality, and social factors that may contribute to the patient's functional capacity and rehabilitation progress [11]. Direct interventions include therapy with the patient that may be one-on-one, group, or family-based. Psychological coping skills are associated with improved psychological distress after SCI [12]. Some studies have suggested that spirituality in patients and their families can play a positive role in post-SCI lifestyle adjustments, life satisfaction, quality of life, and perceived health status, and can contribute to individual and familial resilience [9].

21.2.4 Nutrition

Following SCI, physical changes result in comorbidities that contribute to morbidity and early mortality [13]. Resting metabolism is approximately 15% to 25% lower in SCI patients with functional deficits than in non-disabled counterparts. SCI patients are at increased risk of cardiovascular disease, central obesity, dyslipidemia, hypertension, and insulin resistance. Interrupted bidirectional communication between the central nervous system and sensorimotor targets may have a role in the autonomic and endocrine dysfunction that can affect SCI patients. Changes to the enteric nervous system following SCI may alter physiologic feedback responses to nutrient intake, luminal chemistry, and mechanical distortion. All of these factors may contribute to malnutrition, muscular atrophy, and changes in body composition contributing to worsening physical deconditioning.

Nutrition is an important element of recovery for patients following SCI. Dietary restriction, creatine, and omega-3 dietary supplementation may be helpful but should be individualized [13]. High fiber diets are not recommended for patients with bowel dysfunction. Daily values for macro- and micronutrients should be individualized based on calculated patient metabolism, personalized supplementation, and the degree of mobility limitation from injury.

21.3 Additional Considerations for Patient and Family Support

21.3.1 Peer Mentorship and Support Groups

Peer mentorship programs for patients with SCI allow mentees to discuss topics such as bladder/bowel control, intimacy, and community transition following rehabilitation. Data on the efficacy of these programs are methodologically limited, but qualitative studies suggest benefit [14].

21.3.2 Bowel and Bladder Function

Interview-based studies have, not surprisingly, suggested important challenges to social relationships following SCI due specifically to altered bladder and bowel control [15]. Participants reported feeling like a burden to family, friends, and partners, which they attributed to a lack of independence. The new role that loved ones may have in toileting, changing clothes, or managing incontinence added stress and negatively impacted relationships for SCI patients. Intimacy and disclosing incontinence to new partners is also a concern, attributed to decreased self-confidence. A highly modifiable factor that SCI patients identified as contributory to this lack of confidence was healthcare providers often not discussing specifics of bowel and bladder management post-SCI. Providing the proper counseling, support groups, and contacts for specialists who may provide further insight is beneficial for patient adaptation. Education on the best management for incontinence, as well as improving social environmental factors such as adequate access to public disabled bathrooms, can mitigate social anxiety and isolation for SCI patients.

21.3.3 Employment

Career paths can be drastically changed following SCI. In a systematic quantitative literature review of 102 studies, average employment rate after spinal cord injury was 35% with a range of 15–76% [16]. Average full-time employment was 21%. Post-injury, the average time to return to work was approximately 3.5 years. Employment may improve quality of life by improving mental health and increasing opportunities for social interaction, in addition to reducing financial strain.

21.3.4 Family and Caregiver Support

Spinal cord injury has important implications on family relationships. Long-term care is often necessary following SCI, bringing about major life changes for families and potentially substantial stress on caregivers. As such, there is a need for emotional and social support for families who are caring for a person with SCI.

A systematic review assessing positive and negative impacts of providing care for an adult with SCI on family members included 66 articles and reported three major themes: psychosocial adjustment, the effect of caregiving on marital and family relationships, and caregiver needs and interventions [17]. One-third of the studies reported caregivers with high rates of depression (15–57%) and emotional stress levels, with 38% reporting clinical anxiety. This was highly related to caregiver burden. Caring for an adult family member with SCI is associated with worsened physical and mental health, social functioning, and financial strain [17–19], and is related to the amount and duration of care provided. Interestingly, more depressive symptoms were experienced by couples who had married prior to one partner's injury than among those who had married after injury [17].

These negative effects on families are, however, modifiable. Increased social support for caregivers during times of adjustment has been shown to mitigate levels of depression, anxiety, and perceived burden. Social support was reported to be a source of strength for caregivers, reduced stress levels, and increased well-being [17]. Coping methods were also related to emotional well-being for caregivers, with venting, maladaptive helplessness, and denial all being correlated with poor psychosocial well-being. On the other hand, active coping, acceptance, positive reinterpretation/growth, and social support are protective factors for SCI patient caregivers, associated with lower levels of anxiety and depression [17–19].

Caregivers in an interview-based study reported wanting educational and informational sessions as well as cognitive and behavioral skills for adjusting to a new life with a family member with SCI. Having assistance from professionals allowed the informal caregivers to remain in the role of partner and be able to distance themselves to maintain other roles in life pertaining to work or hobbies [19]. Caregiver training to navigate common problems they may encounter when caring for an SCI patient, as well as peer support, have been shown to improve family function and caregiver adjustment and quality of life [18]. In summary, major negative outcomes associated with caring for SCI patients can be mitigated using interventions focused on the caregiver.

The impact of SCI on parenthood is sometimes overlooked [20]. Parents with disability often have unmet needs regarding adaptive childcare equipment and difficulties receiving housing modifications, transportation, and support. Parental disability may be stigmatized, and assumptions may be made that a disabled parent is unable to be an effective parent. A cohort study of 88 mothers with SCI was compared to 84 without SCI, and found no difference in child adjustment, gender role identity, self-esteem, children's attitude towards each parent, family adjustment, and parental stress and satisfaction. Mothers with SCI were less likely to be employed outside the home, but amongst those who were employed, there was no significant difference in income.

21.4 Summary

The long-term prognosis of SCI depends primarily on the completeness of injury. A significant injury is likely to affect many aspects of a patient's physiology and social relationships. Providing comprehensive rehabilitation and physiologic and social support to patients and their families can have a profound impact on well-being.

References

1. Motiei-Langroudi R, Sadeghian H. Traumatic spinal cord injury: long-term motor, sensory, and urinary outcomes. Asian Spine J. 2017;11(3):412–8. https://doi.org/10.4184/asj.2017.11.3.412.
2. Mahanes D, Muehlschlegel S, Wartenberg KE, Rajajee V, Alexander SA, Busl KM, Creutzfeldt CJ, Fontaine GV, Hocker SE, Hwang DY, Kim KS, Madzar D, Mainali S, Meixensberger J, Varelas PN, Weimar C, Westermaier T, Sakowitz OW. Guidelines for neuroprognostication in adults with traumatic spinal cord injury. Neurocrit Care. 2024;40(2):415–37. https://doi.org/10.1007/s12028-023-01845-8.
3. Badhiwala JH, Wilson JR, Harrop JS, Vaccaro AR, Aarabi B, Geisler FH, Fehlings MG. Early vs late surgical decompression for central cord syndrome. JAMA Surg. 2022;157(11):1024–32. https://doi.org/10.1001/jamasurg.2022.4454.
4. Wang J, Li J, Cai L. Effects of treatment of cervical spinal cord injury without fracture and dislocation in a medium-to long-term follow-up study. World Neurosurg. 2018;113:e515–20. https://doi.org/10.1016/j.wneu.2018.02.071.
5. Sandrow-Feinberg HR, Houlé JD. Exercise after spinal cord injury as an agent for neuroprotection, regeneration and rehabilitation. Brain Res. 2015;1619:12–21. https://doi.org/10.1016/j.brainres.2015.03.052.
6. Jacobs PL, Nash MS. Exercise recommendations for individuals with spinal cord injury. Sports Med (Auckland, N.Z.). 2004;34(11):727–51. https://doi.org/10.2165/00007256-200434110-00003.
7. Duan R, Qu M, Yuan Y, Lin M, Liu T, Huang W, Gao J, Zhang M, Yu X. Clinical benefit of rehabilitation training in spinal cord injury: a systematic review and meta-analysis. Spine. 2021;46(6):E398–410. https://doi.org/10.1097/BRS.0000000000003789.
8. Unger J, Singh H, Mansfield A, Hitzig SL, Lenton E, Musselman KE. The experiences of physical rehabilitation in individuals with spinal cord injuries: a qualitative thematic synthesis. Disabil Rehabil. 2019;41(12):1367–83. https://doi.org/10.1080/09638288.2018.1425745.
9. Jones K, Simpson GK, Briggs L, Dorsett P. Does spirituality facilitate adjustment and resilience among individuals and families after SCI? Disabil Rehabil. 2016;38(10):921–35. https://doi.org/10.3109/09638288.2015.1066884.
10. Erosa NA, Berry JW, Elliott TR, Underhill AT, Fine PR. Predicting quality of life 5 years after medical discharge for traumatic spinal cord injury. Br J Health Psychol. 2014;19(4):688–700. https://doi.org/10.1111/bjhp.12063.

11. Wegener ST, Adams LL, Rohe D. Promoting optimal functioning in spinal cord injury: the role of rehabilitation psychology. Handb Clin Neurol. 2012;109:297–314. https://doi.org/10.1016/B978-0-444-52137-8.00019-X.
12. Scholten EWM, Ketelaar M, Visser-Meily JMA, Roels EH, Kouwenhoven M, POWER Group, Post MWM. Prediction of psychological distress among persons with spinal cord injury or acquired brain injury and their significant others. Arch Phys Med Rehabil. 2020;101(12):2093–102. https://doi.org/10.1016/j.apmr.2020.05.023.
13. Bigford G, Nash MS. Nutritional health considerations for persons with spinal cord injury. Top Spinal Cord Inj Rehabil. 2017;23(3):188–206. https://doi.org/10.1310/sci2303-188.
14. Sweet SN, Hennig L, Pastore OL, Hawley S, Clarke TY, Flaro H, Schaefer L, Gainforth HL. Understanding peer mentorship programs delivered by Canadian SCI community-based organizations: perspectives on mentors and organizational considerations. Spinal Cord. 2021;59(12):1285–93. https://doi.org/10.1038/s41393-021-00721-6.
15. Braaf S, Lennox A, Nunn A, Gabbe B. Social activity and relationship changes experienced by people with bowel and bladder dysfunction following spinal cord injury. Spinal Cord. 2017;55(7):679–86. https://doi.org/10.1038/sc.2017.19.
16. Bloom J, Dorsett P, McLennan V. Investigating employment following spinal cord injury: outcomes, methods, and population demographics. Disabil Rehabil. 2019;41(20):2359–68. https://doi.org/10.1080/09638288.2018.1467968.
17. Wilson CS, DeDios-Stern S, Bocage C, Gray AA, Crudup BM, Russell HF. A systematic review of how spinal cord injury impacts families. Rehabil Psychol. 2022;67(3):273–303. https://doi.org/10.1037/rep0000431.
18. Baker A, Barker S, Sampson A, Martin C. Caregiver outcomes and interventions: a systematic scoping review of the traumatic brain injury and spinal cord injury literature. Clin Rehabil. 2017;31(1):45–60. https://doi.org/10.1177/0269215516639357.
19. Zanini C, Fiordelli M, Amann J, Brach M, Gemperli A, Rubinelli S. Coping strategies of family caregivers in spinal cord injury: a qualitative study. Disabil Rehabil. 2022;44(2):243–52. https://doi.org/10.1080/09638288.2020.1764638.
20. Alexander CJ, Hwang K, Sipski ML. Mothers with spinal cord injuries: impact on marital, family, and children's adjustment. Arch Phys Med Rehabil. 2002;83(1):24–30. https://doi.org/10.1053/apmr.2002.27381.
21. Rupp R, Biering-Sørensen F, Burns SP, Graves DE, Guest J, Jones L, Read MS, Rodriguez GM, Schuld C, Tansey-Md KE, Walden K, Kirshblum S. International standards for neurological classification of spinal cord injury: revised 2019. Top Spinal Cord Inj Rehabil. 2021;27(2):1–22. https://doi.org/10.46292/sci2702-1. PMC8152171.
22. Cohen JT, Marino RJ, Sacco P, Terrin N. Association between the functional independence measure following spinal cord injury and long-term outcomes. Spinal Cord. 2012;50(10):728–33. https://doi.org/10.1038/sc.2012.50.
23. Hornby TG, Zemon DH, Campbell D. Robotic-assisted, body-weight-supported treadmill training in individuals following motor incomplete spinal cord injury. Phys Ther. 2005;85(1):52–66.
24. Kumru H, Benito-Penalva J, Valls-Sole J, Murillo N, Tormos JM, Flores C, Vidal J. Placebo-controlled study of rTMS combined with Lokomat(®) gait training for treatment in subjects with motor incomplete spinal cord injury. Exp Brain Res. 2016;234(12):3447–55. https://doi.org/10.1007/s00221-016-4739-9.
25. Nasser MR, Awad M, Amin I, Samah Assem S. Effect of massed practice and somatosensory stimulation on the upper extremity function in patients with incomplete cervical spinal cord injury. Alex J Med. 2014;50(2):189–96.
26. Jones ML, Evans N, Tefertiller C, Backus D, Sweatman M, Tansey K, Morrison S. Activity-based therapy for recovery of walking in individuals with chronic spinal cord injury: results from a randomized clinical trial. Arch Phys Med Rehabil. 2014;95(12):2239–46.e2. https://doi.org/10.1016/j.apmr.2014.07.400.

The Complexity of Traumatic Spinal Cord Injury Management: Understanding Psychosocial Challenges, Adjustment Dynamics, and Person-Centred Care

22

Ashley Craig, Ilaria Pozzato, Mohit Arora, and James Middleton

22.1 Introduction

Traumatic spinal cord injury (SCI) is a severe neurological condition with devastating physical and psychosocial impacts, leading to reduced life expectancy, diminished quality of life (QoL), and limited social participation [1, 2]. Physical consequences include loss of motor, sensory, and autonomic control at or below the level of the lesion in the cord [3, 4]. Tetraplegia involves damage to the cervical segments, while paraplegia involves damage to the thoracic, lumbar, or sacral segments of the cord. Higher level lesions (e.g., tetraplegia) and complete lesions (with no sensorimotor sparing below level) are usually associated with more severe impairment [4]. Depending on severity, the injury will adversely impact functioning of multiple body systems and functions, requiring specialized acute care and comprehensive, multidisciplinary rehabilitation as soon as possible after the injury, as well as support for community reintegration with access to ongoing medical and

A. Craig (✉)
Faculty of Medicine and Health, The University of Sydney, The Kolling Institute, Northern Sydney Local Health District, Sydney, NSW, Australia

Fellow, College of Clinical Psychology, Sydney, NSW, Australia
e-mail: a.craig@sydney.edu.au

I. Pozzato · M. Arora
Faculty of Medicine and Health, The University of Sydney, The Kolling Institute, Northern Sydney Local Health District, Sydney, NSW, Australia

Senior Research Fellow, Faculty of Medicine and Health, The University of Sydney, The Kolling Institute, Northern Sydney Local Health District, Sydney, NSW, Australia
e-mail: Ilaria.pozzato@sydney.edu.au; mohit.arora@sydney.edu.au

J. Middleton
Faculty of Medicine and Health, The University of Sydney, The Kolling Institute, Northern Sydney Local Health District, Sydney, NSW, Australia
e-mail: james.middleton@sydney.edu.au

E. Brogi et al. (eds.), *Traumatic Spinal Cord Injury*, Hot Topics in Acute Care Surgery and Trauma, https://doi.org/10.1007/978-3-031-99890-4_22

multidisciplinary review and secondary treatment. Furthermore, adults with SCI will need to employ self-management strategies to manage their health and social issues for the remainder of their life [5, 6].

It has been estimated that the majority of adults with SCI cope and adjust well over time after their injury and its associated impairment [7]. However, SCI is highly associated with adverse secondary physical and mental health conditions, presenting continuous lifelong challenges for people with SCI and their families. These include debilitating conditions, such as respiratory infection, bowel and bladder infection, chronic pain, pressure injuries, sexual dysfunction, elevated fatigue, sleep disorder, cognitive impairment, and cardiovascular dysfunction such as autonomic dysreflexia [5]. Furthermore, a large proportion, perhaps as high as 40% of adults with SCI, will experience sub-clinical levels of psychological distress and worryingly, up to 30% will present with a diagnosed mental disorder such as major depressive disorder, anxiety disorder, or alcohol and drug abuse disorder [8, 9]. Due to its catastrophic nature, a SCI will influence every aspect of a person's life, including key interpersonal relationships, where partners or family members of an adult with SCI are vulnerable to relationship conflicts and breakdown in the first 2-years post-injury [10], with many partners or family members experiencing elevated anxiety and depressive mood [11]. This chapter focuses on a deeper understanding of the psychosocial challenges and adjustment dynamics faced by the injured people and their families following a SCI. If left unaddressed, these challenges can significantly complicate SCI management and rehabilitation, ultimately leading to decreased QoL, creating barriers to social reintegration.

22.2 Psychosocial and Psychophysiological Impacts

22.2.1 Quality of Life

Life satisfaction and QoL will be diminished after a SCI [1, 2, 12–14]. Unsurprisingly, domains where most impacts on QoL occur are in the physical functioning domains [1], though psychosocial domains can also be affected, with vitality, social, emotional, and mental health function shown to be significantly below community norms [1, 13–15]. Health-related QoL will be substantially reduced by secondary conditions like fatigue, chronic pain, obesity, and pressure injuries [14, 16–18]. Expectations such as self-efficacy will also influence QoL [1]. Self-efficacy is a measure of a person's expectations and beliefs about their ability to self-manage [5]. Research has shown that for those with normal or robust self-efficacy, no differences in psychosocial QoL domains were found compared to community norms [1]. Whereas, for those with low self-efficacy, QoL was significantly reduced across physical and psychosocial domains [1]. Analysis of a large community survey with adults with SCI [19] found the strongest explanatory factors influencing QoL to be social integration (+0.36 standard deviation or SDs), subjective social position (+0.29), secondary health condition burden (−0.28), activity & participation problem burden (−0.26), day-to-day assistance (−0.26), mental health (+0.18), pain

(−0.16), self-efficacy (+0.15), and vitality (+0.14). It is worth noting that completeness of lesion, sex, age at injury, and time since injury, have not been found to be consistently associated with QoL [1, 5]. However, a higher level of injury does have a diminishing effect on QoL [1]. The following sections illustrate the many challenges to QoL for a person with SCI.

22.2.2 Psychological Distress

Sustaining a SCI will challenge a person's psychosocial resources [20]. Nevertheless, the majority of adults who sustain a SCI, perhaps as high as 70% [7], will cope and adjust well despite the regular challenges experienced in daily living associated with this severe impairment [20]. A prime example involves experiencing grief and sadness related to the injury, which, while potentially distressing, is considered an adaptive reaction to SCI [21]. A clinical challenge, therefore, will be for the health team to distinguish between grief and depression, as a misdiagnosis of depression (when a person is grieving only) or a misdiagnosis of grief (when they are depressed), could interfere with the adjustment and rehabilitation process [5, 21]. Other common life challenges that impact psychological wellbeing and which may cause additional distress include financial and relationship stressors, sleep problems, limited mobility in the community and restricted social access, and difficulties in maintaining and/or obtaining employment.

Nonetheless, this means that around 30% are likely to experience difficulties with mental health problems [5, 20, 22]. Clinically elevated levels of psychological distress are prevalent in comparison to community norms after a SCI [9, 22–26]. Results from a meta-analysis confirmed that psychological distress is clinically elevated after a SCI [27], with data from this meta-analysis indicating that psychological distress had begun to reduce by around 10 years post-SCI [27]. Another meta-analysis indicated that rates of depression following a SCI are high, with as much as 26% of adults with SCI being diagnosed with a probable depression, depending on the time post-injury [9]. Occurrence of post-traumatic stress disorder (PTSD) is thought to lie between 14–40% [28–30], though the higher estimates of PTSD found in some studies will likely be inflated if participants were war veterans with a SCI [30].

As the above illustrates, SCI is associated with substantially elevated occurrence of mental health disorders [22]. This is supported by comparisons to community estimates of mental disorders in Australia. The one-month occurrence of any psychological disorder in the Australian community is estimated to be 13.2%, 3.2% for depressive disorder, 3.4% for any substance use disorder, and almost 1% for PTSD [31]. Further, the 2007 Australian National Survey of Mental Health and Wellbeing study found comparable estimates, with 10% suffering any mental disorder, 2.4% for any depressive disorders, and 1.8% for any substance use disorders [32]. See Table 22.1 for comparison details.

Not only are rates of mental disorders much higher after SCI, rates of mental disorder co-morbidity are also high, indicated by research that employed gold

Table 22.1 Three comparisons of the occurrence of mental disorders (% in the past 2–4 weeks), the first in a SCI sample, and the second and third in Australian community samples

Psychological disorders	Australian sample one year post SCI[a]	Australian community sample[b]	Australian community sample[c]
	% (95% CI)	% (SE)	% (95% CI)
Any psychological disorder	25.3 (20.1–30.5)	13.2 (0.4)	10.0 (9.3–10.8)
Major depressive disorder	14.1 (6.1–22.1)	3.2 (0.2)	2.4 (1.9–2.8)
Substance-induced disorder: Alcohol dependence	8.6 (2.1–15.1)	1.7 (0.1)	–
Substance-induced disorder: Drug dependence	7.0 (1.1–12.9)	0.9 (0.2)	0.6 (0.4–0.9)
Post-traumatic stress disorder	1.4 (0–4.1)	1.3 (0.1)	–
Generalized anxiety disorder	4.2 (0–8.9)	2.0 (0.2)	2.7 (2.2–3.3)
Bipolar disorder	4.2 (0–8.9)	–	1.8 (1.4–2.2)

[a]Craig et al., 2015 [22]
[b]Andrews et al., 2001 [31]
[c]Slade et al., 2009 [32]

standard psychiatric interview techniques to arrive at a diagnosis [22]. Almost 10% of adults were found to meet psychiatric criteria for two mental disorders and 3% met criteria for three mental disorders [22]. Major depressive disorder/episode with a substance use disorder was the most common co-morbidity, followed by major depressive disorder and suicidality. About 4% had a co-morbid PTSD and /or generalized anxiety disorder with depression [22].

22.2.3 Suicide and Self-Neglect

Suicidality is a concern after a severe injury like SCI [26, 33, 34]. A study involving a sample of 9000 people with SCI in the USA found over 6% had committed suicide, and that people with SCI were 4.9 times more likely to commit suicide than the able-bodied community [26]. Research suggests the death rate for suicide has risen, even though deaths from septicaemia, pneumonia, and diseases of the urinary system have decreased [35]. Predictive factors associated with suicide include older age, SCI resulting from a fall, complete neurological lesions, low family or social support, alcohol abuse, and social isolation [36, 37]. Self-neglect involves "indirect self-destructive behavior" [38], which is a concern after SCI. Self-neglect can result in an increased risk of fatality [39], thus, the importance of teaching self-management skills during rehabilitation. A lack of self-management increases risk of conditions like infections and pressure injuries [5]. Finally, attempted suicide can result in severe injuries like SCI, with a study showing survivors were able to return home or to group homes/hostels. However, the authors concluded there was a need for mental health management in the majority, and subsequent suicide rate was found to be high [40].

22.2.4 Mild Cognitive Impairment

Mild cognitive impairment is a prevalent secondary health condition after SCI. It has been estimated that 12 months after the injury, the relative risk of an adult with SCI having mild cognitive impairment was around 13 times that of someone without a SCI, while the odds of an adult with SCI having cognitive impairment were estimated to be almost 18 times greater than that for someone without SCI [41]. Our prospective research found that all five cognitive domains were significantly reduced compared to an able-bodied control group, that is, the executive, attention, perceptual (visuospatial), memory (learning), and language domains [41]. However, a recent network meta-analysis determined that deficits in cognitive function after SCI mostly occurred in the attention and executive function domains, while language and perceptual domains were least affected [42].

A susceptibility to developing mild cognitive impairment after SCI has consequences. For example, we found that those with cognitive impairment were significantly more likely to develop depressive mood and elevated anxiety after they were discharged from SCI rehabilitation, and were transitioning into the community, a time when personal resources will be challenged [41]. Figure 22.1 shows

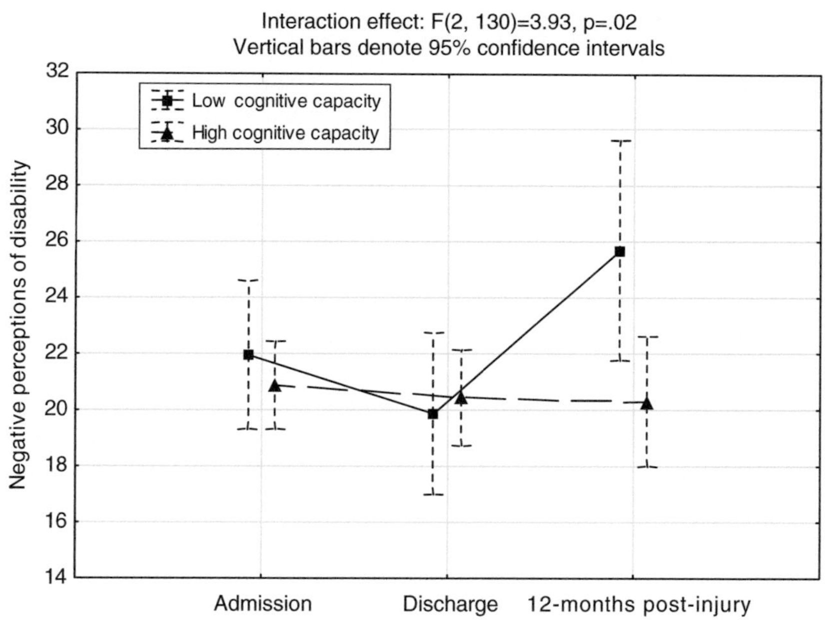

Fig. 22.1 Negative perceptions of disability measured by The Appraisals of DisAbility: Primary and Secondary Scale for adults with SCI who also have mild cognitive impairment (low cognitive capacity) versus those without mild cognitive impairment (high cognitive capacity). The cognitively impaired group was significantly more likely to perceive their injury as unmanageable and in terms of loss and threat. (Note: General linear model multivariate repeated measures analysis with covariates sex, age, and years of education was used)

that a deficit in cognitive capacity also negatively affects other important outcomes, such as how they perceive their disability as assessed by The Appraisals of DisAbility: Primary and Secondary Scale. Without the multidisciplinary support provided during inpatient SCI rehabilitation, after discharge from hospital, adults with low cognitive capacity were more likely to believe their impairment was beyond their control and think negatively about their disability. Furthermore, adults with low cognitive capacity have been shown to be vulnerable to developing conditions such as depression, clinical anxiety, and increased severity of secondary health conditions [5, 41]. In contrast, those with high cognitive capacity did not change their perceptions of disability from rehabilitation through to 12 months post-injury.

Research has concluded that many factors can contribute to the development of mild cognitive impairment after SCI [41, 43, 44]. A traumatic brain injury (TBI), if comorbid with the SCI, can be associated with cognitive impairment [41, 45]. Based on post-traumatic amnesia assessment and cerebral neuroimaging, it was estimated that up to 60% of people with SCI could have a mild TBI [46]. Determining whether a person with SCI has a dual diagnosis of SCI and TBI is often difficult early after the injury, especially when the TBI is of mild severity. In emergency or acute care, an emphasis is placed on medical and surgical stabilization of the SCI and associated injuries, with factors such as hypoxia, use of analgesic medications, surgery, and anaesthesia further complicating diagnostic matters. It is recommended that early cognitive screening (e.g., in emergency and/ or intensive care) for mild TBI be conducted, if possible, as a mild TBI misdiagnosis could lead to medical complications and poorer outcomes from rehabilitation regarding uptake of functional independent living and self-management skills [47].

Additional factors other than TBI are believed to contribute to mild cognitive impairment after a SCI [41, 44]. For example, people with non-traumatic causes of SCI are known to suffer mild cognitive impairment in the absence of a TBI [41]. Pre-morbid learning difficulties and head trauma, fatigue, sleep disorder such as obstructive sleep apnoea, chronic pain, clinically elevated anxiety and depressive mood, polypharmacy, substance abuse, and older age are all suspected to be contributors to cognitive impairment [41]. Post-traumatic inflammation resulting from the repair process after a traumatic SCI may also lead to mild cognitive impairment [48, 49]. For obvious clinical reasons, it is recommended that screening for potential factors contributing to mild cognitive impairment be implemented while participating in SCI rehabilitation [50] and that regular neurocognitive assessment occur in this period [42]. However, a persistent challenge remains the lack of a validated cognitive screening and assessment tool developed specifically to assess people with SCI, taking into consideration their unique impairment profile and the necessity for hands-free testing [51]. A challenge for further research is developing treatments for cognitive impairment after SCI, as there are few interventions, if any, that have been established as effective [43].

22.2.5 Chronic Pain and Pain Catastrophizing

Chronic pain has been defined as persistent pain experienced for at least three months [52]. This definition takes account of expected time for an injury to heal, but also allows for cases where an injury is permanent, as in SCI [53]. Chronic pain is a prevalent condition after SCI, with estimates suggesting up to 80% of people with SCI may experience clinical levels of pain (clinical pain can be defined as ≥4 cut-off out of 10, where 10 is very severe pain or worst pain ever) in both musculoskeletal and neuropathic types of pain [54, 55]. Research in adults with SCI indicates that chronic pain is commonly associated with other comorbid conditions like fatigue and depression, functional limitations, and a greater dependence on pain medications [56] and self-efficacy in people with spinal cord injury [57, 58].

Chronic pain after SCI will lower QoL and be positively associated with cognitive biases like pain catastrophizing [1, 14, 15, 57] and self-efficacy in people with spinal cord injury [1, 59]. Pain catastrophizing involves a negative cognitive appraisal in which someone feels helpless and overwhelmed about their pain. It will also involve intrusive and repetitive thinking with rumination, that is, frequently dwelling on negative feelings and their consequences, and thinking how horrible and disastrous the pain is in their life. The person may also magnify the effects of pain and come to fear pain and any daily activity that may increase their pain [57, 60, 61]. Evidence indicates that pain catastrophizing increases chronic pain by weakening central nervous system analgesic processes, specifically, by adversely influencing centrally mediated diffuse noxious inhibitory control, a mechanism in the pain modulatory process involving bottom-up (spinal) and top-down central nervous system cortical influences [60]. Clearly, pain catastrophizing can be a serious barrier after SCI [57]. It is therefore imperative that SCI rehabilitation begin to address this barrier to the adjustment process through developing effective pain management strategies, psychoeducation, and strengthening appraisals, coping, and beliefs, such as pain self-efficacy [5, 62].

22.2.6 Sleep Disorder and Fatigue

Sleep disturbance associated with disorders such as obstructive sleep apnoea is a common secondary adverse condition after SCI [63–65]. Between 30–60% of adults with SCI will develop obstructive sleep apnoea [64], which may contribute to increased pain and spasticity [63, 64]. Further, poor sleep quality has been strongly associated with negative emotional wellbeing and vitality, higher rates of unemployment, and greater problems with participation in people with SCI [65]. Another related problem is excessive daytime sleepiness, described as a susceptibility to falling asleep during the day [66]. Sleep disorder and excessive daytime sleepiness will diminish QoL and social participation, especially in those with cervical and thoracic lesions and sensorimotor complete injuries [63]. Chronic pain can significantly disrupt sleep quality, and conversely, poor sleep can exacerbate levels of pain [16]. It has been argued that inadequate sleep and associated sleepiness can reduce top-down cortical resources (e.g., attention), leading to decreased ability to perceive and manage pain [67].

Chronic fatigue is another debilitating problem after SCI [68–70]. It is a multifactorial condition that can be defined as excessive chronic tiredness involving feelings of physical and mental exhaustion and negative emotions, such as anxiety and poor mood [69, 71]. Major problems associated with fatigue can include increased chances of errors when performing tasks, reduced motivation, circadian rhythm disruption, and increased risk of anxiety and confusion [14, 69].

22.2.7 Autonomic Nervous System Dysfunction

Dysfunction of the autonomic nervous system (ANS) is a significant problem in adults with SCI and has been linked with poorer cardiovascular health and serious complications, as well as psychological, sleep, cognitive, and fatigue disorders after SCI [3, 66]. ANS dysfunction is more severe in cervical, higher thoracic, and complete lesions [3]. In cervical and thoracic lesions (say at T6 and above), disruption of sympathetic nervous system pathways occurs, resulting in an imbalance of sympathetic and parasympathetic activity, and this can lead to serious cardiovascular problems such as persistent orthostatic hypotension and episodes of uncontrolled hypertension, referred to as autonomic dysreflexia [3]. Autonomic dysreflexia is a life-threatening problem involving unregulated blood pressure control, and even people with lower thoracic lesions can have increased likelihood of uncontrolled hypertension and tachycardia [3]. ANS dysfunction also plays a role in respiratory control, thermoregulation, bowel, bladder, and sexual dysfunction [3], as well as in maintaining emotional and cognitive regulation [72].

Self-regulation of ANS activity, targeting improvement in heart rate variability (HRV) as the main ANS marker, has shown promise as a treatment for cardiovascular health but also depression and trauma-related distress and pain in non-SCI populations [73]. Preliminary evidence has recently been collected for its efficacy with SCI populations [74, 75]. Self-regulation training involves participants learning to regulate their autonomic neuro-cardiac and respiratory activity via computer/mobile app-based feedback of HRV and paced breathing. The benefits of HRV feedback and paced breathing are thought to be due to a combination of strengthening baroreflex homeostasis and vagal afferent pathways, as well as optimizing phase relationships between blood pressure, heart-rate, and brain connectivity [76].

22.2.8 Sexual Problems

The degree of sexual dysfunction (e.g., arousal response, orgasm, and ejaculation) after SCI is influenced by the level and extent of the neurologic lesion, the occurrence of bladder or bowel incontinence, pain, spasticity, fatigue, effect of medications, and by dynamics in interpersonal and social relationships [77]. In a recent large survey of people with SCI in Australia [55], sexual dysfunction was reported as a very common health problem (in 79% of participants), with a notably high proportion (60%) rating it as a severe to extreme condition, and which mostly did not receive adequate treatment (86%). Factors found to enhance sexual adjustment after SCI included frequent sexual activity, experimentation with alternative sexual activities, and a younger age after sustaining a SCI [78]. If the person with an SCI is able to manage and accept the physical restrictions and any negative mental attitude associated with the SCI, they will be more likely to regain an active sexual life with a partner. However, it is recommended that sexual education and counselling be available both during SCI rehabilitation and after discharge when returning home [79]. It should be positive, affirming, and non-judgmental, creating a safe space, and use an organized approach, such as the Ex-PLISSIT (extended permission giving, limited information, specific suggestions, and intensive therapy) model [80].

22.2.9 Social Participation

For optimum health, it is important that an adult with SCI has a degree of personal autonomy that allows them to participate in activities of their own choice in their community [81]. Unfortunately, after discharge from intensive SCI rehabilitation, many will be at risk of diminished personal autonomy and choices while simultaneously experiencing reduced social participation. The majority of people with SCI will engage and participate in their communities [82], however, many will still experience difficulties with social participation that will negatively impact their social network, social and family relationships, and their mental health [37, 81]. While the majority of those with SCI report they are satisfied with their life, many continue to experience limitations in social participation [2, 81]. While adults with a SCI living in the community were found to believe their mobility and social participation were sufficient to conduct daily activities, almost 50% reported their social participation was restricted, including reduced outdoor mobility, and restricted access to employment and educational facilities [83].

22.2.10 Vocation and SCI

The majority of people who sustain a SCI are of working age and employed at the time of their injury, so re-engagement in employment is a necessary goal of SCI rehabilitation and functional recovery. Employment is associated with improved functioning, adjustment, self-esteem, wellbeing, financial independence, and social integration, leading to higher QoL [81, 84–86]. However, rates of employment (around 35%) after SCI are very much lower than before the injury and in the general community [13, 58]. Those individuals with SCI returning to previous jobs do so much earlier than those who are seeking new employment [87].

Factors associated with return to employment after SCI include level of education, type of employment, level and severity of impairment, age at injury, time since injury, sex, being in a relationship, level of social support, vocational counselling, self-efficacy, motivation, discrimination, positive expectations, life satisfaction, extent of secondary conditions, functional capability, and employer role [13, 88, 89]. It is crucial that while participating in intensive SCI rehabilitation, people are introduced to evidence-based vocational rehabilitation services as a continuum of person-centred care, addressing complex interactions between the person with SCI, job and environmental factors [86, 90].

22.3 SCI Rehabilitation

The World Health Organization (WHO) considers SCI rehabilitation a goal-oriented process intended to optimize the healing of remaining function, and which results in the maximum possible physical, psychological, social, and economic independence [91]. This involves coordinated teamwork of medical, nursing, and allied health professionals in conjunction with social, educational, and vocational services. SCI rehabilitation is a process that involves not only physical/medical recovery, but crucially, it also requires psychological and cognitive recovery and social reintegration of the person into the community, including return to employment if possible [91].

The WHO Rehabilitation 2030 initiative draws attention to the profound unmet need for rehabilitation worldwide and highlights the importance of strengthening health systems to provide rehabilitation [92]. In addition, the WHO's Comprehensive Mental Health Action Plan (2013–2030) has added new targets to ensure that emergency plans include mental health and psychosocial support, mental health to be integrated into primary health care, and a focus on research for mental health is expanded [93].

People sustaining an acute SCI are usually transferred from emergency and intensive medical care to specialist SCI rehabilitation centres where they commence SCI specialist rehabilitation, involving comprehensive, multidisciplinary management (e.g., medical and nursing management, physiotherapy, occupational therapy, psychological therapy and dietary management). Primarily, it is designed to assist reintegration back into the community by treating secondary medical conditions, functional retraining (e.g., skills to transfer, wheelchair mobility), establishing self-management skills, and reinforcing resilience and adjustment in response to functional impairment, ongoing disability, and changed life circumstances. Restoration of pre-injury relationships, daily life activities and roles, and social opportunities are priorities for successful rehabilitation [4]. To achieve this, length of stay in SCI rehabilitation is generally between 2 and 6 months, however, length of stay varies between countries depending on the health and medical insurance schemes, injury severity, and personal circumstances. Factors determining optimal length of stay for SCI rehabilitation are unidentified, so this area requires substantial investigation.

There is evidence that life expectancy is improving for people participating in SCI rehabilitation [94, 95]. This is believed to be due, at least in part, to early diagnosis, more efficient roadside resuscitation and management, rapid transfer to a specialized major trauma service, improved management of secondary conditions, and the establishment of committed long-term medical follow-up processes by SCI specialists [4]. However, life expectancy is still well below that in the able-bodied community [34, 96]. On a positive note, advances in SCI rehabilitation are ongoing [97] and supported by innovative research and development, ranging from investigating improvements in valid strategies for determining cognitive capacity and treatment specific to SCI [43] to exploring stimulation techniques to recover function [98].

Given medical care has evolved and become more effective, survival rates have improved, and it has been argued that emphasis should now be on establishing acceptable QoL for paediatric and adult patients with SCI [1, 13, 14]. For example, addressing the abovementioned psychosocial challenges in those participating in SCI rehabilitation and when living in the community after discharge, will strengthen QoL [1]. Establishing patient or person-centred care (PCC) in SCI rehabilitation, and possibly earlier in acute care settings, is also a necessary goal that the authors believe will improve adjustment and resilience outcomes in people with SCI [7, 99]. PCC is an inclusive approach distinguished by individualized care, based on the needs of each person, and that encourages patients to be autonomous by participating in their care [99]. Please refer to Table 22.2 for the core elements of PCC.

It is important to comment on the role of peer and family support in the SCI rehabilitation process. A peer support person in this area is generally someone with the experience of living with a SCI. As such, they are able to provide non-clinical and practical advice about living with a SCI. The aim of peer support is to assist the person with a SCI, either during rehabilitation or after discharge when living in the community, to regain best possible independence, to strengthen connections within the community, and to offer tips and advice about self-management skills that are

Table 22.2 The core elements of person-centred care that should be employed during SCI rehabilitation [102, 103]

➢	The person with SCI is unique and has their own set of needs, preferences, values, emotions, beliefs, worries and expectations.
➢	The person with SCI is involved with the health professional in decision making and treatment planning.
➢	A genuine reciprocal and caring relationship is developed between the person with SCI and the healthcare professional in the SCI multidisciplinary treatment team.
➢	An open communication is nurtured between the person with SCI and the health professional, involving appropriate socially skilled verbal and non-verbal behaviours, open-ended questions, reviewing and simplifying information, making eye contact, and so on.
➢	The health professional is professionally experienced and expert in SCI rehabilitation, has a commitment to evidence-based practice, has a basic understanding of psychological skills, and a tolerant, respectful, compassionate commitment to the person with SCI.
➢	Teamwork and teambuilding within and between disciplines/ healthcare providers, as well as up-skilling teams through training and educational programs.

necessary for everyday living (Spinal Cord Injuries Australia; https://scia.org.au/peer-support/). It is usually assumed that peer support is beneficial for individuals with a new SCI; however, recent research showed that those who reported more help from peers were no better adjusted than those who reported less interaction with a peer [100]. Further, those who were more satisfied with peer support reported greater adjustment, and peer support was more effective for those who had little family or friends support [100]. Also, individuals who received intensive peer mentoring during and after discharge from rehabilitation showed greater gains in self-efficacy and had fewer days of unplanned rehospitalization in the first 180 days after discharge [101].

22.4 A Unified SCI Rehabilitation Management Framework

Employing the biopsychosocial model of care for SCI rehabilitation as a unified rehabilitation management framework is key to the delivery of SCI rehabilitation in a PCC approach [7, 104, 105]. This model views a person's health and well-being as the outcome of interconnected physical, psychological, and social factors. Therefore, it advocates for rehabilitation as a comprehensive and interdisciplinary intervention that encompasses physiological, psychological, and social domains. Each of these domains is equally important and necessary and plays a significant role in influencing the capacity of a person with SCI to adjust and thrive [7, 106]. It is the authors' belief that conducting SCI rehabilitation within the scope and framework of the biopsychosocial model will optimize PCC for these individuals and enhance adjustment and resilience. Healthcare professionals in the SCI multidisciplinary team are in a unique situation to provide the best physical health care, but also optimal psychosocial health care to inpatients with a SCI during rehabilitation soon after the injury.

Recently, a theory has been proposed to explain how rehabilitation may assist patients, improve understanding of rehabilitation dynamics, and improve health services in cases of permanent injury and impairment such as SCI [107]. The theory asserts that people continuously adapt to change throughout their lives, and when faced with impairment or illness, they must adapt and adjust to maintain equilibrium across the various biopsychosocial domains that characterize a person's life. The theory also suggests that behaviour change and adjustment are governed by a central homeostatic mechanism [107]. Rehabilitation plays a key role in helping the person to adjust to the changes brought about by the SCI. This involves factors like accurate diagnosis and formulation, optimizing the environment, and supporting self-management and recovery of remaining function [107]. According to this theory, the person with SCI should be the central active agent within the rehabilitation setting, facilitating adjustment as advocated by the biopsychosocial model and PCC [107].

22.5 Adjustment Dynamics After SCI

When attempting to explain the dynamics involved in adjustment after SCI, it is necessary to refer to psychosocial theories that contribute to an understanding of the process [5]. Such theories include the Response Shift Theory, which emphasizes the need to adapt when challenged by distressing events like injury and impairment [108]. Another influential model is the transactional model of stress and coping [109], which asserted that a person's capacity to adjust to life challenges is a result of transactions that occur between the person and their environment, including appraisal-reappraisal processes, and this theory has been applied to adjustment after SCI [110]. Last, the health belief model [111], contended that health status is a product of expectations and perceptions, including perceived barriers and perceived susceptibility [112].

22.5.1 The SCI Adjustment Model

The SCI adjustment model (SCIAM), presented in a simplified form in Fig. 22.2, was developed with reference to the above theories/models, as well as the Biopsychosocial Model [62, 104]. SCIAM explains the dynamic processes believed to occur in the process of adjustment after SCI. While it is accepted that SCIAM simplifies such a complex process, it assumes adjustment is a complex non-linear process over time and that life events and challenges will influence adjustment [5]. Importantly, SCIAM stresses the central role that appraisal and re-appraisal play in the adjustment process, such as perceptions like self-efficacy or catastrophizing thinking styles. SCIAM also contends that multiple moderators will influence adjustment outcomes. Moderators (shown in the brown boxes in Table 22.2) include pre-injury health, cultural factors, medications, personality, age, cognitive capacity, pain intensity and interference, level of psychological distress, biological factors, and religious and political factors [62, 113]. Furthermore, these moderators are suggested to contribute in an interactive, non-linear, and reciprocal manner [62]. Moderators will also act on mediators (e.g., appraisal and re-appraisal dynamics) as well as expectations following a coping strategy in response to the appraisal re-appraisal process. It is hoped that SCIAM will facilitate the understanding of the adjustment processes in the SCI multidisciplinary team, and thus improve SCI rehabilitation outcomes.

The mediators, depicted as the "Appraisal-reappraisal" yellow box in Fig. 22.2, have been labelled the "engine room" of adjustment, given that this mediator process is where the person makes decisions about what is important and relevant (appraisal-reappraisal), leading to a decision about a course of action (coping strategy). As shown in Fig. 22.2, these mediators can include factors like self-efficacy, cognitive distortions such as catastrophizing thinking, perceived barriers to change, and self-esteem [62, 114]. The results of this "engine room" dynamic result in a person employing a coping strategy, with the success or failure of the coping strategy providing feedback to the person's "engine room", resulting in secondary

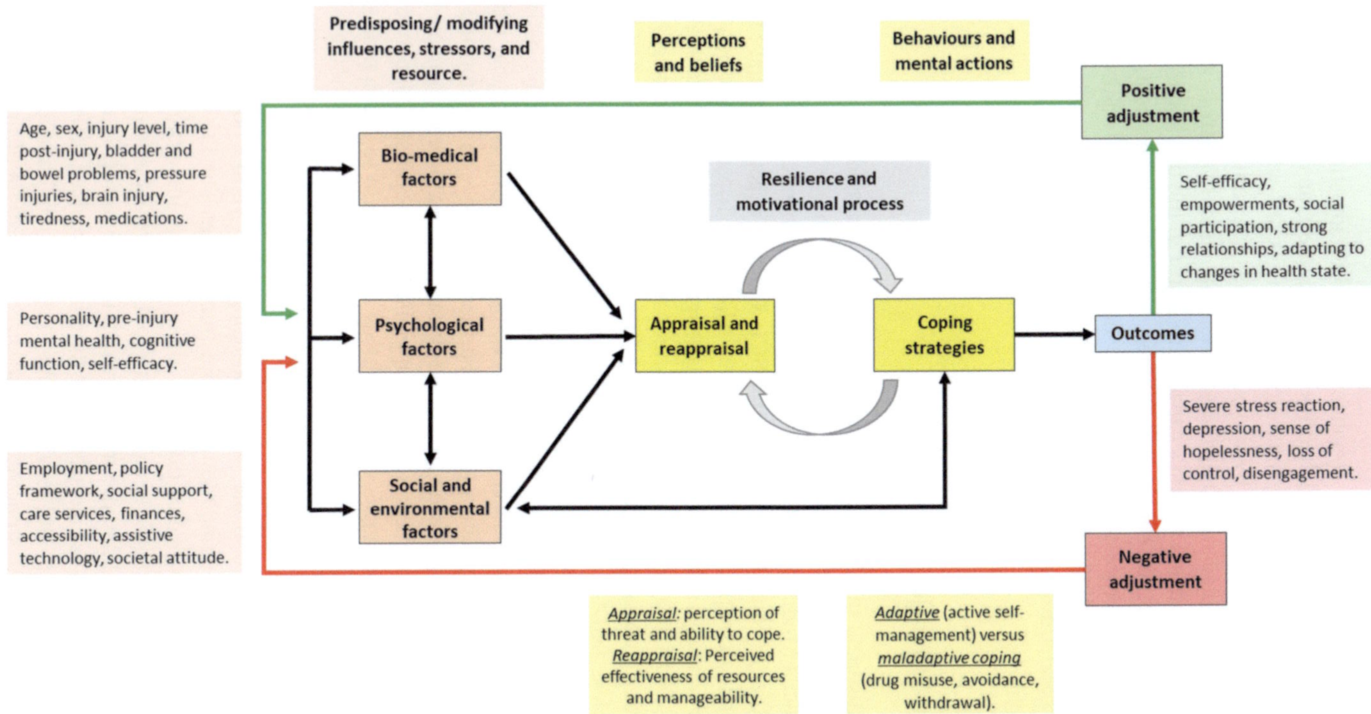

Fig. 22.2 Shows the SCI adjustment model, the relationship among moderators, mediators, and medium to long-term outcomes, and how people with SCI adapt and adjust over time to their injury. (Adapted from [62])

appraisal processing that leads to either persistence with a coping strategy or, if problematic, an adoption of alternative coping strategies. Of course, the model shows that this "engine room" dynamic is influenced by moderators at any particular point in time. SCIAM predicts that a person will positively (green box in Fig. 22.2) or negatively adjust (red box). Substantial support from controlled research is accumulating for SCIAM [5, 22, 62, 67, 114–116].

22.6 The Need for Psychosocial Guidelines in SCI Rehabilitation

Healthcare professionals working within SCI rehabilitation are in an ideal position to provide not only physical health care, but also psychosocial health care to inpatients adjusting to a new SCI. The value of integrating psychosocial care guidelines and employing PCC goals into the SCI rehabilitation setting will, arguably, constructively influence how these patients recover and adjust to their injury [7]. However, healthcare professionals working in SCI rehabilitation settings may not have the necessary training to apply psychosocial care as part of standard practice [7]. To establish and enhance PCC within SCI rehabilitation, the authors believed it was necessary to develop and integrate psychosocial guidelines into SCI rehabilitation, which were designed for use by the multiple health professional disciplines working in SCI rehabilitation [117]. Psychosocial guidelines were initially developed in 2008 to address this issue, with the most recent version of the guidelines upgraded in 2023 [50]. These guidelines are now available online: https://aci.health.nsw.gov.au/networks/spinal-cord-injury/resources/psychosocial-care, and are composed of three separate sections: Recommendations, Models of Care, and Background and Methodology.

Arguably, psychosocial factors influence every aspect of SCI rehabilitation. Therefore, these guidelines were designed to address the multiple psychosocial domains believed to influence adjustment and resilience outcomes following SCI [105]. For example, healthcare professionals working in the acute and rehabilitation phases need to have the confidence to screen for symptoms of mild cognitive impairment and mental health comorbidities in their patients, and in response, have the confidence to integrate and adopt psychosocial care strategies that assist in referral processes, as well as promote an environment in which the patient can cope and adjust. Additionally, the psychosocial guidelines have been designed to support strategies for effective communication between staff in the multidisciplinary team and patients, the eventual aim being to have a unified team approach that will support and motivate patients with SCI during their rehabilitation phase. To gain a detailed grasp of the psychosocial guidelines, the reader is advised to consult the three psychosocial guideline documents mentioned above. However, a summary of some general principles discussed in the 2023 psychosocial guidelines is provided below:

(i) Rehabilitation services for people with a new SCI should be designed around PCC so as to promote a safe environment and appropriate health care that will assist the person with SCI to adjust and develop resilience.
(ii) Provision of PCC and psychosocial care is dependent on the skills of health care staff working in SCI rehabilitation to detect signs and symptoms of distress. This includes the need for an awareness of what an appropriate response is to a range of matters that may occur (e.g., such as suicidal ideation).
(iii) Given the shock and distress associated with the early stages of the SCI, health professional staff in the multidisciplinary rehabilitation team should provide generous emotional and social support, thereby strengthening the relationship between the person with SCI and members of the rehabilitation team.
(iv) Health professionals working in the SCI rehabilitation team should be trained to use effective communication skills, and importantly, communication should be adapted to the person's level of understanding and health literacy. Effective communication skills also need to be used in interactions with the family of a person with SCI. The guidelines stress that effective communication is based upon empathy and active listening.
(v) Patients in SCI rehabilitation should be provided with timely and targeted information appropriate to their cognitive capacity. Patients with a new SCI require accurate information to assist their active engagement about treatment options. Factors that may act as barriers to decision-making include age, gender, culture, attitudes, opinions, level of education, past experiences, emotional readiness, degree of trust and confidence in the health care system or clinician, and the communication skills of both parties.
(vi) The need for goal-planning to occur for each person with SCI [112]. Goal planning can positively influence adjustment outcomes, and all the multidisciplinary staff in the team should be trained to develop goal planning skills [112]. Effective goal planning has four main purposes: improving rehabilitation outcomes, assessing outcomes, enhancing the autonomy of the person with SCI, and meeting contractual, legislative or professional requirements [118].
(vii) The needs of each patient should be carefully assessed. The Stoke Mandeville Spinal Needs Assessment Checklist (SMS-NAC; [119]) is a validated and reliable tool used to guide goal planning [120]. The SMS-NAC provides evidence-based outcomes so that the needs of patients with SCI are better understood, hopefully leading to improved adjustment [121].
(viii) The psychosocial guidelines also stress the importance of the following in SCI inpatient rehabilitation: each SCI patient should be allocated a keyworker from the rehabilitation team who has primary responsibility for coordinating the care for the patient; valid assessment of care at admission and discharge directly related to goal planning should be conducted, including regular goal planning meetings, and collaborative goal setting also conducted with the patient, their family and the treating team.

(ix) The provision of evidence-based treatments for conditions like substance abuse, mental health disorders, neuropathic pain, and suicidality, either within SCI rehabilitation by a clinical psychologist or liaison psychiatrist or referred externally to the SCI Unit to a specialist centre.

It must be clear that the psychosocial guide is not a substitute for the knowledge and skill of individual practitioners, nor does it attempt to impose clinical guidelines on medical and physical treatments. It was designed to be used in conjunction with the clinician's judgment and experience within the context of the client-practitioner relationship. The overall purpose of the guide is to enhance the psychosocial care of people with SCI when in SCI rehabilitation, as well as to strengthen the knowledge, skills, and confidence in identifying and dealing with psychosocial challenges of health professionals, who are not skilled in mental health or psychological practices [50]. An additional associated innovation based on these guidelines has involved the development of a SCI psychosocial screen and training package based on the SCIAM model [122]. This toolkit provides strategies for the whole rehabilitation team, so they are better equipped to distinguish between grief and depression and receive information on the appropriate use of brief standardized screens for assessing mental health issues such as mood, anxiety, pain, trauma, substance use, and psychoses.

22.7 Conclusions

This chapter has provided a detailed description of evidence on the psychosocial impacts associated with SCI, hopefully increasing the understanding of health professionals working in acute care settings and SCI rehabilitation. As SCI is a very complex injury with permanent disability and lifelong impacts, it is crucial that health professionals understand the profound influence that psychosocial factors will have on the ability of persons to recover and adjust to the injury, and to achieve optimal levels of quality of life and wellbeing. Furthermore, it is essential that SCI rehabilitation be person-centred, with the inclusion of formal psychosocial guidelines being an important consideration for achieving PCC. Therefore, a further aim of this chapter was to provide an overview of the challenges that a person with SCI will likely encounter in their daily life, especially during their stay in the intensive inpatient phase of SCI rehabilitation, with particular focus on social and psychological aspects. These challenges were discussed in the light of an overarching unifying framework called the Biopsychosocial Model. Employing this framework, a model that explains the complex non-linear processes involved in adjustment after SCI was presented, called SCIAM. This model was designed to clarify how numerous factors, namely moderators and mediators, can influence the complex process of adjustment over time. Importantly, the relationship of this adjustment model to the processes involved in SCI rehabilitation were also discussed, with an aim of improving rehabilitation strategies and outcomes.

No detail is presented in this chapter about the specific psychosocial factors associated with managing younger people with a SCI, that is, from the very young up to the mid-teen years, because of the lack of controlled research in this age range. This is a challenge for future research. In terms of future professional practice in SCI rehabilitation, it is essential that research be translated and implemented at the coal-face, that is, applied and tested in clinical practice contexts within SCI Units. We believe strongly that translation of research findings can be applied in SCI rehabilitation within a PCC approach, and that such a union will make unique and valuable contributions to the multi-disciplinary health professional team involved in SCI rehabilitation. We hope this chapter stimulates researchers and clinicians to become involved in future research in this very severe injury.

Acknowledgement We acknowledge financial support from NSW Ministry of Health SCI Grant 2020 and a NSW icare SCI Cognitive Grant 2023–25.

References

1. Middleton J, Tran Y, Craig A. Relationship between quality of life and self-efficacy in persons with spinal cord injuries. Arch Phys Med Rehabil. 2007;88(12):1643–8.
2. Tasiemski T, Kujawa J, Tederko P, Rubinelli S, Middleton JW, Craig A, et al. Comparison of life satisfaction in persons with spinal cord injury living in 22 countries with different economic status. Arch Phys Med Rehabil. 2022;103(7):1285–93.
3. Krassioukov A. Autonomic function following cervical spinal cord injury. Resp Physiol Neurobiol. 2009;169(2):157–64.
4. Middleton JW, Cameron ID. Introduction to physical injuries, recovery and adversity following motor vehicle crashes. In: Craig A, Guest R, editors. Adversity after the crash: the physical, psychological and social burden of motor vehicle crashes. New York: Nova Science; 2019. p. 3–35.
5. Craig A, Tran Y, Arora M, Pozzato I, Middleton JW. Investigating dynamics of the spinal cord injury adjustment model: mediation model analysis. J Clin Med. 2022;11(15):4557.
6. Middleton JW, Arora M, Jerram KAS, Bourke J, McCormick M, O'Leary D, et al. Co-design of the spinal cord injury health maintenance tool to support self-management: a mixed-methods approach. Top Spinal Cord Inj Rehabil. 2024;30(1):59–73.
7. Sandalic D, Arora M, Pozzato I, Simpson G, Middleton J, Craig A. A narrative review of research on adjustment to spinal cord injury and mental health: gaps, future directions, and practice recommendations. Psychol Res Behav Manage. 2022;15:1997–2010.
8. Craig A, Tran Y, Middleton J. Psychological morbidity and spinal cord injury: a systematic review. Spinal Cord. 2009;47(2):108–14.
9. Williams R, Murray A. Prevalence of depression after spinal cord injury: a meta-analysis. Arch Phys Med Rehabil. 2015;96(1):133–40.
10. Kreuter M. Spinal cord injury and partner relationships. Spinal Cord. 2000;38(1):2–6.
11. Melanie C, Paul K, Navtej S. The association between threat appraisals and psychological adjustment in partners of people with spinal cord injuries. Rehabil Psychol. 2007;52(4):470–7.
12. Geyh S, Nick E, Stirnimann D, Ehrat S, Müller R, Michel F. Biopsychosocial outcomes in individuals with and without spinal cord injury: a swiss comparative study. Spinal Cord. 2012;50(8):614–22.
13. Ottomanelli L, Lind L. Review of critical factors related to employment after spinal cord injury: implications for research and vocational services. J Spinal Cord Med. 2009;32(5):503–31.

14. Wijesuriya N, Tran Y, Middleton J, Craig A. Impact of fatigue on the health-related quality of life in persons with spinal cord injury. Arch Phys Med Rehabil. 2012;93(2):319–24.
15. Kennedy P, Lude P, Taylor N. Quality of life, social participation, appraisals and coping post spinal cord injury: a review of four community samples. Spinal Cord. 2006;44(2):95–105.
16. Jensen MP, Gould EM, Victor TW, Gammaitoni AR, White RE, Galer BS. The relationship of changes in pain quality to pain interference and sleep quality. J Pain. 2010;11(8):782–8.
17. Shojaei MH, Alavinia SM, Craven BC. Management of obesity after spinal cord injury: a systematic review. J Spinal Cord Med. 2017;40(6):783–94.
18. Atkinson RA, Cullum NA. Interventions for pressure ulcers: a summary of evidence for prevention and treatment. Spinal Cord. 2018;56(3):186–98.
19. Kifley A, Arora M, Nunn A, Marshall R, Geraghty T, Weber G, et al. Australian arm of the international spinal cord injury (aus-insci) community survey: 3. Drivers of quality of life in people with spinal cord injury. Spinal Cord. 2023;61(3):185–93.
20. Guest R, Craig A, Nicholson Perry K, Tran Y, Ephraums C, Hales A, et al. Resilience following spinal cord injury: a prospective controlled study investigating the influence of the provision of group cognitive behavior therapy during inpatient rehabilitation. Rehabil Psychol. 2015;60(4):311–21.
21. Klyce DW, Bombardier CH, Davis TJ, Hartoonian N, Hoffman JM, Fann JR, et al. Distinguishing grief from depression during acute recovery from spinal cord injury. Arch Phys Med Rehabil. 2015;96(8):1419–25.
22. Craig A, Nicholson Perry K, Guest R, Tran Y, Dezarnaulds A, Hales A, et al. Prospective study of the occurrence of psychological disorders and comorbidities after spinal cord injury. Arch Phys Med Rehabil. 2015;96(8):1426–34.
23. Hancock K, Craig A, Tennant C, Chang E. The influence of spinal cord injury on coping styles and self-perceptions: a controlled study. ANZ J Psychiatry. 1993;27(3):450–6.
24. Craig AR, Hancock K, Chang E. The influence of spinal cord injury on coping styles and self-perceptions two years after the injury. ANZ J Psychiatry. 1994;28(2):307–12.
25. Hoffman JM, Bombardier CH, Graves DE, Kalpakjian CZ, Krause JS. A longitudinal study of depression from 1 to 5 years after spinal cord injury. Arch Phys Med Rehabil. 2011;92(3):411–8.
26. Bombardier CH, Azuero CB, Fann JR, Kautz DD, Richards JS, Sabharwal S. Management of mental health disorders, substance use disorders, and suicide in adults with spinal cord injury: clinical practice guideline for healthcare providers. Top Spinal Cord Inj Rehabil. 2021;27(2):152–224.
27. Craig A, Tran Y, Guest R, Gopinath B, Jagnoor J, Bryant RA, et al. Psychological impact of injuries sustained in motor vehicle crashes: systematic review and meta-analysis. BMJ Open. 2016;6(9):e011993.
28. Chung MC, Preveza E, Papandreou K, Prevezas N. The relationship between posttraumatic stress disorder following spinal cord injury and locus of control. J Affect Disord. 2006;93(1–3):229–32.
29. Kennedy P, Evans MJ. Evaluation of post traumatic distress in the first 6 months following sci. Spinal Cord. 2001;39(7):381–6.
30. Ullrich PM, Smith BM, Poggensee L, Evans CT, Stroupe KT, Weaver FM, et al. Pain and post-traumatic stress disorder symptoms during inpatient rehabilitation among operation enduring freedom/operation iraqi freedom veterans with spinal cord injury. Arch Phys Med Rehabil. 2013;94(1):80–5.
31. Andrews G, Henderson S, Hall W. Prevalence, comorbidity, disability and service utilisation: overview of the australian national mental health survey. Br J Psychiatry. 2001;178(2):145–53.
32. Slade T, Johnston A, Oakley Browne MA, Andrews G, Whiteford H. 2007 national survey of mental health and wellbeing: methods and key findings. ANZ J Psychiatry. 2009;43(7):594–605.

33. Kennedy P, Garmon-Jones L. Self-harm and suicide before and after spinal cord injury: a systematic review. Spinal Cord. 2017;55(1):2–7.
34. Savic G, DeVivo MJ, Frankel HL, Jamous MA, Soni BM, Charlifue S. Long-term survival after traumatic spinal cord injury: a 70-year british study. Spinal Cord. 2017;55(7):651–8.
35. Soden RJ, Walsh J, Middleton JW, Craven ML, Rutkowski SB, Yeo JD. Causes of death after spinal cord injury. Spinal Cord. 2000;38(10):604–10.
36. Kishi Y, Robinson RG. Suicidal plans following spinal cord injury: a six month study. J Neuropsychiatry Clin Neurosci. 1996;8(4):442–5.
37. Charlifue S, Gerhart K. Community integration in spinal cord injury of long duration. Neuro Rehabil. 2004;19(2):91–101.
38. Nehemkis A, Groot H. Indirect self-destructive behavior in spinal cord injury. In: Faberon N, editor. The many faces of suicide. New york: Mcgraw-Hill; 1980. p. 99–115.
39. Wilcox NE, Stauffer ES. Follow-up of 423 consecutive patients admitted to the spinal cord centre, Rancho Los Amigos Hospital, 1 January to 31 December 1967. Spinal Cord. 1972;10(2):115–22.
40. Stanford RE, Soden R, Bartrop R, Mikk M, Taylor TK. Spinal cord and related injuries after attempted suicide: psychiatric diagnosis and long-term follow-up. Spinal Cord. 2007;45(6):437–43.
41. Craig A, Guest R, Tran Y, Middleton J. Cognitive impairment and mood states after spinal cord injury. J Neurotrauma. 2017;34(6):1156–63.
42. Sandalic D, Craig A, Tran Y, Arora M, Pozzato I, McBain C, et al. Cognitive impairment in individuals with spinal cord injury: findings of a systematic review with robust variance and network meta-analyses. Neurology. 2022;99:e1779–e90.
43. Li Y, Hu Y, Pozzato I, Arora M, Schoffl J, McBain C, et al. Efficacy of interventions to improve cognitive function in adults with spinal cord injury: a systematic review. J Neurotrauma. 2024. https://doi.org/10.1089/neu.2024.0032.
44. Alcántar-Garibay O, Incontri-Abraham D, Ibarra A. Spinal cord injury-induced cognitive impairment: a narrative review. Neural Reg Res. 2022;17(12):2649.
45. Bradbury CL, Wodchis WP, Mikulis DJ, Pano EG, Hitzig SL, McGillivray CF, et al. Traumatic brain injury in patients with traumatic spinal cord injury: clinical and economic consequences. Arch Phys Med Rehabil. 2008;89(12 Suppl):S77–84.
46. Macciocchi S, Seel RT, Thompson N, Byams R, Bowman B. Spinal cord injury and co-occurring traumatic brain injury: assessment and incidence. Arch Phys Med Rehabil. 2008;89(7):1350–7.
47. Sandalic D, Craig A, Arora M, Pozzato I, Simpson G, Gopinath B, et al. A prospective cohort study investigating contributors to mild cognitive impairment in adults with spinal cord injury: study protocol. BMC Neurol. 2020;20(1):341.
48. Ankeny DP, Popovich PG. Mechanisms and implications of adaptive immune responses after traumatic spinal cord injury. Neuroscience. 2009;158(3):1112–21.
49. Wu J, Zhao Z, Kumar A, Lipinski MM, Loane DJ, Stoica BA, et al. Endoplasmic reticulum stress and disrupted neurogenesis in the brain are associated with cognitive impairment and depressive-like behavior after spinal cord injury. J Neurotrauma. 2016;33(21):1919–35.
50. Craig A, Arora M, Middleton JW, SCI Cog Study Group. Psychosocial care of adults with spinal cord injuries guide. St Leonards: NSW Agency for Clinical Innovation; 2023.
51. Sandalic D, Tran Y, Craig A, Arora M, Pozzato I, Simpson G, et al. The need for a specialized neurocognitive screen and consistent cognitive impairment criteria in spinal cord injury: analysis of the suitability of the neuropsychiatry unit cognitive assessment tool. J Clin Med. 2022;11(12):3344.
52. Apkarian AV, Baliki MN, Geha PY. Towards a theory of chronic pain. Prog Neurobiol. 2009;87(2):81–97.
53. Siddall PJ, Cousins MJ. Persistent pain as a disease entity: implications for clinical management. Anesth Analg. 2004;99(2):510–20.

54. Siddall PJ, McClelland JM, Rutkowski SB, Cousins MJ. A longitudinal study of the prevalence and characteristics of pain in the first 5 years following spinal cord injury. Pain. 2003;103(3):249–57.
55. Middleton JW, Arora M, Kifley A, Clark J, Borg SJ, Tran Y, et al. Australian arm of the international spinal cord injury (aus-insci) community survey: 2. Understanding the lived experience in people with spinal cord injury. Spinal Cord. 2022;60(12):1069–79.
56. Craig A, Tran Y, Siddall P, Wijesuriya N, Lovas J, Bartrop R, et al. Developing a model of associations between chronic pain, depressive mood, chronic fatigue, and self-efficacy in people with spinal cord injury. J Pain. 2013;14(9):911–20.
57. Craig A, Guest R, Tran Y, Nicholson Perry K, Middleton J. Pain catastrophizing and negative mood states after spinal cord injury: transitioning from inpatient rehabilitation into the community. J Pain. 2017;18(7):800–10.
58. Kennedy P, Hasson L. The relationship between pain and mood following spinal cord injury. J Spinal Cord Med. 2017;40(3):275–9.
59. Budh CN, Osteråker AL. Life satisfaction in individuals with a spinal cord injury and pain. Clin Rehabil. 2007;21(1):89–96.
60. Quartana PJ, Campbell CM, Edwards RR. Pain catastrophizing: a critical review. Exp Rev Neurother. 2009;9(5):745–58.
61. Velly AM, Look JO, Carlson C, Lenton PA, Kang W, Holcroft CA, et al. The effect of catastrophizing and depression on chronic pain—a prospective cohort study of temporomandibular muscle and joint pain disorders. Pain. 2011;152(10):2377–83.
62. Craig A, Tran Y, Middleton J. Theory of adjustment following severe neurological injury: evidence supporting the spinal cord injury adjustment model. In: Costa A, Villalba E, editors. Horizons Neuroscience Research, vol. 29. New York: Nova Science Publishers. p. 117–139.
63. Leduc BE, Dagher JH, Mayer P, Bellemare F, Lepage Y. Estimated prevalence of obstructive sleep apnea–hypopnea syndrome after cervical cord injury. Arch Phys Med Rehabil. 2007;88(3):333–7.
64. Berlowitz DJ, Spong J, Gordon I, Howard ME, Brown DJ. Relationships between objective sleep indices and symptoms in a community sample of people with tetraplegia. Arch Phys Med Rehabil. 2012;93(7):1246–52.
65. Graco M, Arora M, Berlowitz DJ, Craig A, Middleton JW. The impact of sleep quality on health, participation and employment outcomes in people with spinal cord injury: analyses from a large cross-sectional survey. Ann Phys Rehabil Med. 2023;66(5):101738.
66. Craig A, Rodrigues D, Tran Y, Guest R, Middleton J. Daytime sleepiness and its relationships to fatigue and autonomic dysfunction in adults with spinal cord injury. J Psychosom Res. 2018;112:90–8.
67. Craig A, Tran Y, Guest R, Middleton J. Excessive daytime sleepiness in adults with spinal cord injury and associations with pain catastrophizing and pain intensity. Spinal Cord. 2020;58(7):831–9.
68. Fawkes-Kirby TM, Wheeler MA, Anton HA, Miller WC, Townson AF, Weeks CAO. Clinical correlates of fatigue in spinal cord injury. Spinal Cord. 2008;46(1):21–5.
69. Craig A, Tran Y, Wijesuriya N, Middleton J. Fatigue and tiredness in people with spinal cord injury. J Psychosom Res. 2012;73(3):205–10.
70. van Diemen T, Lankveld W, Leeuwen C, Post M, Nes I. Multidimensional fatigue during rehabilitation in persons with recently acquired spinal cord injury. J Rehabil Med. 2016;48(1):27–32.
71. Craig A, Tran Y, Wijesuriya N, Boord P. A controlled investigation into the psychological determinants of fatigue. Biol Psychol. 2006;72(1):78–87.
72. Quadt L, Critchley H, Nagai Y. Cognition, emotion, and the central autonomic network. Autonom Neurosci. 2022;238:102948.
73. Burlacu A, Brinza C, Popa IV, Covic A, Floria M. Influencing cardiovascular outcomes through heart rate variability modulation: a systematic review. Diagnostics. 2021;11(12):2198.

74. Craig A, Pozzato I, Arora M, Middleton J, Rodrigues D, McBain C, et al. A neuro-cardiac self-regulation therapy to improve autonomic and neural function after sci: a randomized controlled trial protocol. BMC Neurol. 2021;21(1):329.
75. Schoffl J, Arora M, Pozzato I, McBain C, Rodrigues D, Vafa E, et al. Heart rate variability biofeedback in adults with a spinal cord injury: a laboratory framework and case series. J Clin Med. 2023;12(24):7664.
76. Lehrer PM, Gevirtz R. Heart rate variability biofeedback: how and why does it work? Front Psychol. 2014;5:756.
77. Sramkova T, Skrivanova K, Dolan I, Zamecnik L, Sramkova K, Kriz J, et al. Women's sex life after spinal cord injury. Sex Med. 2017;5(4):e255–e9.
78. Siösteen A, Lundqvist C, Blomstrand C, Sullivan L, Sullivan M. Sexual ability, activity, attitudes and satisfaction as part of adjustment in spinal cord-injured subjects. Spinal Cord. 1990;28(5):285–95.
79. Krueger H, Noonan VK, Williams D, Trenaman LM, Rivers CS. The influence of depression on physical complications in spinal cord injury: behavioral mechanisms and health-care implications. Spinal Cord. 2013;51(4):260–6.
80. Mohammadi Z, Maasoumi R, Vosoughi N, Eftekhar T, Soleimani M, Montazeri A. The effect of the ex-plissit model-based psychosexual counseling on improving sexual function and sexual quality of life in gynecologic cancer survivors: a randomized controlled clinical trial. Support Care Cancer. 2022;30(11):9117–26.
81. Craig A, Nicholson Perry K, Guest R, Tran Y, Middleton J. Adjustment following chronic spinal cord injury: determining factors that contribute to social participation. Br J Health Psychol. 2015;20(4):807–23.
82. Pollard C, Kennedy P. A longitudinal analysis of emotional impact, coping strategies and post-traumatic psychological growth following spinal cord injury: a 10-year review. Br J Health Psychol. 2007;12:347–62.
83. Larsson Lund M, Nordlund A, Nygård L, Lexell J, Bernspång B. Perceptions of participation and predictors of perceived problems with participation in persons with spinal cord injury. J Rehabil Med. 2005;37(1):3–8.
84. Krause JS, Saunders LL, Acuna J. Gainful employment and risk of mortality after spinal cord injury: effects beyond that of demographic, injury and socioeconomic factors. Spinal Cord. 2012;50(10):784–8.
85. Hay-Smith EJC, Dickson B, Nunnerley J, Anne Sinnott K. "The final piece of the puzzle to fit in" : an interpretative phenomenological analysis of the return to employment in New Zealand after spinal cord injury. Disabil Rehabil. 2013;35(17):1436–46.
86. Hilton G, Unsworth CA, Murphy GC, Browne M, Olver J. Longitudinal employment outcomes of an early intervention vocational rehabilitation service for people admitted to rehabilitation with a traumatic spinal cord injury. Spinal Cord. 2017;55(8):743–52.
87. Krause JS, Terza JV, Saunders LL, Dismuke CE. Delayed entry into employment after spinal cord injury: factors related to time to first job. Spinal Cord. 2010;48(6):487–91.
88. Hilton G, Unsworth C, Murphy G. The experience of attempting to return to work following spinal cord injury: a systematic review of the qualitative literature. Disabil Rehabil. 2018;40(15):1745–53.
89. Trenaman L, Miller WC, Querée M, Escorpizo R. Modifiable and non-modifiable factors associated with employment outcomes following spinal cord injury: a systematic review. J Spinal Cord Med. 2015;38(4):422–31.
90. Middleton JW, Johnston D, Murphy G, Ramakrishnan K, Savage N, Harper R, et al. Early access to vocational rehabilitation for spinal cord injury inpatients. J Rehabil Med. 2015;47(7):626–31.
91. World Health Organisation. A glossary of terms for community health care and services for older persons. Kobe: WHO Centre for Health Development; 2004.
92. Gimigliano F, Negrini S. The world health organization "rehabilitation 2030: a call for action". Eur J Phys Rehabil Med. 2017;53(2):155–68.

93. World Health Organization. Comprehensive mental health action plan 2013–2030. Geneva: WHO; 2021. Available from: https://www.who.int/publications/i/item/9789240031029.
94. DeVivo MJ, Stover SL. Long-term survival and causes of death. In: Stover SL, DeLisa JA, Whiteneck GG. (Eds) Spinal cord injury: Clinical outcomes from the model systems. Baltimore: Aspen, p. 289–315.
95. Middleton JW, Dayton A, Walsh J, Rutkowski SB, Leong G, Duong S. Life expectancy after spinal cord injury: a 50-year study. Spinal Cord. 2012;50(11):803–11.
96. Shavelle RM, DeVivo MJ, Brooks JC, Strauss DJ, Paculdo DR. Improvements in long-term survival after spinal cord injury? Arch Phys Med Rehabil. 2015;96(4):645–51.
97. Arora M, Craig AR. Spinal cord injuries: advances in rehabilitation. J Clin Med. 2024;13:1782.
98. Samejima S, Shackleton C, Malik RN, Cao K, Bohorquez A, Nightingale TE, et al. Spinal cord stimulation prevents autonomic dysreflexia in individuals with spinal cord injury: a case series. J Clin Med. 2023;12(8):2897.
99. Lindberg J, Kreuter M, Taft C, Person LO. Patient participation in care and rehabilitation from the perspective of patients with spinal cord injury. Spinal Cord. 2013;51(11):834–7.
100. McLeod J, Davis CG. Community peer support among individuals living with spinal cord injury. J Health Psychol. 2023;28(10):943–55.
101. Gassaway J, Jones ML, Sweatman WM, Hong M, Anziano P, DeVault K. Effects of peer mentoring on self-efficacy and hospital readmission after inpatient rehabilitation of individuals with spinal cord injury: a randomized controlled trial. Arch Phys Med Rehabil. 2017;98(8):1526–34.
102. Kitson A, Marshall A, Bassett K, Zeitz K. What are the core elements of patient-centred care? A narrative review and synthesis of the literature from health policy, medicine and nursing. J Adv Nurs. 2013;69(1):4–15.
103. Scholl I, Zill JM, Härter M, Dirmaier J. An integrative model of patient-centeredness–a systematic review and concept analysis. PLoS One. 2014;9(9):e107828.
104. Engel GL. The need for a new medical model: a challenge for biomedicine. Science. 1977;196(4286):129–36.
105. McBain C, Sarandrea AM, Pozzato I, Myles D, Bourke J. (submitted) Implementing psychosocial guidelines into specialized spinal cord injury rehabilitation units to strengthen person-centred health care: protocol for a mixed-methods study. BMC Health Services. 2024.
106. Budd MA, Gater DR Jr, Channell I. Psychosocial consequences of spinal cord injury: a narrative review. J Personal Med. 2022;12(7):1178.
107. Wade DT. A general theory of rehabilitation: rehabilitation catalyses and assists adaptation to illness. Clin Rehabil. 2024;38(4):429–42.
108. Sprangers MAG, Schwartz CE. Integrating response shift into health-related quality of life research: a theoretical model. Soc Sci Med. 1999;48(11):1507–15.
109. Folkman S. Stress: appraisal and coping. In: Gellman MD, editor. Encyclopedia of behavioral medicine. Springer International Publishing; 2020. p. 2177–9.
110. Boekamp JR, Overholser JC, Schubert DSP. Depression following a spinal cord injury. Int J Psychiatry Med. 1996;26(3):329–49.
111. Janz NK, Becker MH. The health belief model: a decade later. Health Educ Q. 1984;11(1):1–47.
112. Duff J, Kennedy P. Spinal cord injury (chapter 14). In: Llewelyn S, Kennedy P, editors. Handbook of clinical health psychology. Chichester: John Wiley and Son Ltd; 2003. p. 251–78.
113. Craig A, Duff J, Middleton J. 8.17 - Spinal cord injuries. In: Asmundson GJG, Crombez G, editors. Comprehensive clinical psychology. Vol 8: Health Psychology. 2nd ed. Oxford: Elsevier; 2022. p. 301–28.
114. van Diemen T, Crul T, van Nes I, Geertzen JH, Post MW. Associations between self-efficacy and secondary health conditions in people living with spinal cord injury: a systematic review and meta-analysis. Arch Phys Med Rehabil. 2017;98(12):2566–77.

115. Craig A, Wijesuriya N, Tran Y. The influence of self-efficacy on mood states in people with spinal cord injury. ISRN Rehabil. 2013;1:232978.
116. Peter C, Müller R, Post MW, van Leeuwen CM, Werner CS, Geyh S. Psychological resources, appraisals, and coping and their relationship to participation in spinal cord injury: a path analysis. Arch Phys Med Rehabil. 2014;95(9):1662–71.
117. Middleton J, Nicholson Perry K, Craig A. Development of a guide for the psychosocial care of people with spinal cord injury: introduction and practice implications. Int J Phys Med Rehabil. 2014;2:226–31.
118. Levack WMM, Weatherall M, Hay-Smith EJC, Dean SG, McPherson K, Siegert RJ. Goal setting and strategies to enhance goal pursuit for adults with acquired disability participating in rehabilitation. Cochrane Database Syst Rev. 2015;20(7):CD009727.
119. Kennedy P, Hamilton LR. The needs assessment checklist: a clinical approach to measuring outcome. Spinal Cord. 1999;37(2):136–9.
120. Berry C, Kennedy P. A psychometric analysis of the needs assessment checklist (NAC). Spinal Cord. 2003;41(9):490–501.
121. Duff J, Jones K, Eaton R. A clinical perspective on rehabilitation outcome measures following an acute spinal cord injury. In: 57th International Spinal Cord Injury (ISCoS) Conference, Sydney (poster); 2018.
122. Emotional Wellbeing Toolkit: A Clinicians Guide to working with SCI. NSW State Spinal Cord Injury Service Strategy for the Psychosocial Care of People with Spinal Cord Injury. 2016. https://aci.health.nsw.gov.au/networks/spinal-cord-injury/resources/emotional-wellbeing

MIX
Papier aus verantwortungsvollen Quellen
Paper from responsible sources
FSC® C105338

If you have any concerns about our products,
you can contact us on
ProductSafety@springernature.com

In case Publisher is established outside the EU,
the EU authorized representative is:
Springer Nature Customer Service Center GmbH
Europaplatz 3, 69115 Heidelberg, Germany

Printed by Libri Plureos GmbH
in Hamburg, Germany